Aging, Natural Bioactive Compounds and Non-communicable Chronic-Degenerative Diseases

Aging, Natural Bioactive Compounds and Non-communicable Chronic-Degenerative Diseases

Guest Editors

Nicola Di Daniele
Annalisa Noce

MDPI

Basel • Beijing • Wuhan • Barcelona • Belgrade • Novi Sad • Cluj • Manchester

Guest Editors
Nicola Di Daniele
Department of Systems Medicine
University of Rome Tor Vergata
Rome
Italy

Annalisa Noce
Department of Systems Medicine
University of Rome Tor Vergata
Rome
Italy

Editorial Office
MDPI AG
Grosspeteranlage 5
4052 Basel, Switzerland

This is a reprint of the Special Issue, published open access by the journal *Nutrients* (ISSN 2072-6643), freely accessible at: https://www.mdpi.com/journal/nutrients/special_issues/Bioactive_Aging.

For citation purposes, cite each article independently as indicated on the article page online and as indicated below:

Lastname, A.A.; Lastname, B.B. Article Title. *Journal Name* **Year**, *Volume Number*, Page Range.

ISBN 978-3-7258-7138-4 (Hbk)
ISBN 978-3-7258-7139-1 (PDF)
https://doi.org/10.3390/books978-3-7258-7139-1

Contents

nutrients

MDPI

Editorial

Aging, Natural Bioactive Compounds and Non-Communicable Chronic Degenerative Diseases

Annalisa Noce [1,2,*] and Nicola Di Daniele [1,3]

1 Department of Systems Medicine, University of Rome Tor Vergata, 00133 Rome, Italy; didaniele@med.uniroma2.it
2 UOSD Nephrology and Dialysis, Policlinico Tor Vergata, 00133 Rome, Italy
3 Fondazione Leonardo per le Scienze Mediche Onlus, Policlinico Abano, 35031 Abano Terme, Italy
* Correspondence: annalisa.noce@uniroma2.it; Tel.: +39-0620902194

In recent decades, the world has witnessed a major demographic change characterized by an aging of the general population. Across the globe, the number of people aged 65 and over is increasing enormously; between 1990 and 2017, the percentage of elderly people increased globally from 6.1% to 8.8%, and it is estimated that their number will reach approximately 1.5 billion (i.e., 16% of the world population) by 2050 [1,2]. The aging of the world's population could have enormous repercussions on Health Systems due to the numerous age-related chronic diseases [3–6]. Although aging is a physiological process, it is closely related to the increased risk of non-communicable chronic degenerative disease (NCCDD) onset, such as diabetes mellitus, arterial hypertension, chronic kidney disease (CKD), neurodegenerative diseases, cancers, chronic respiratory diseases, and cardiovascular diseases [7,8]. There are multiple biological mechanisms underlying the predisposition for these ailments, including increases in oxidative stress and the chronic inflammatory state [9,10].

Numerous recent studies have aimed at investigating new possible strategies to counteract the aging and the onset of NCCDDs. Many have focused on the use of adjuvant treatments, free of side effects, based on natural bioactive compound (NBC) consumption. NBCs are molecules of various nature and origin, mainly contained in plant-based foods, capable of exerting several beneficial effects on human health [11–13]. Specifically, they can perform important anti-aging actions; for example, they are able to delay the aging and reduce the risk of aging-related diseases, prolonging lifespan and promoting the well-being of the individual through the regulation of various physiological processes [14–20].

In our Special Issue, we explore, through reviews and original articles, this interesting field.

Di Lauro et al. (contribution 1) examined the close bidirectional correlation between the gut microbiota alterations and the migraine onset, involving the gut–brain axis, and how this axis can influence the NCCDDs risk. The Authors highlighted the importance of proper nutrition, the consumption of specific NBCs, and lifestyle in order to combat migraines in NCCDDs patients. In the same context, Derkaczew et al. (contribution 2) studied new possible adjuvant treatments for neurodegenerative diseases (such as Alzheimer's disease, Parkinson's disease, and Huntington's disease) based on myo-inositol and its derivatives. The Authors concluded that dietary supplementation with myo-inositol exhibited a promising effect in the treatment of these neurodegenerative disorders and could be a valid support for alleviating the depressive symptoms associated with them. Furthermore, the neuroprotective and anti-neuroinflammatory effect of the metabolites of the plant *Allium hookeri*, a member of the genus Allium, was also demonstrated by the study conducted by Doan et al. (contribution 3). Specifically, the Authors used a non-targeted metabolomics approach to comprehensively profile the chemical composition of metabolites in *A. hookeri*. The Authors emphasized N-trans-feruloyltyramine as the most potent neuroprotective compound of the studied plant, able to mitigate senescence-associated neurological diseases. In addition, Yoon et al. (contribution 4) examined the potential therapeutic properties of fermented ginseng berry extract as adjuvant treatment for Alzheimer's disease. The Authors highlighted how high levels of active ginsenosides in fermented ginseng exert neuroprotective effects and improve cognitive functions through antioxidant properties and acetylcholinesterase inhibitory activities. Moreover, Zhou et al. (contribution 5) evaluated the mechanism of the anti-hypoxic neuroprotective effect of chebulic acid, isolated from Terminalia chebula, both in vitro and in vivo. In vitro results showed that chebulic acid seems to protect against oxygen–glucose deprivation/reoxygenation-induced neurotoxicity in SH-SY5Y cells, through an important indirect antioxidant action; in vivo results showed, instead, that treatment with chebulic acid determines a significant decrease in ischemic infarct volume and an improvement in motor performance in mice at 24 h after stroke. The study, therefore, lays the foundation for a possible new chebulic acid-based drug for the control of ischemic stroke in humans.

With regard to cardiovascular risk, Marrone et al. (contribution 6) investigated the cardioprotective effects of minor polar compounds (such as oleocanthal, oleacin, tyrosol, and hydroxytyrosol) in extra virgin olive oil (EVOO) on CKD patients. Specifically, the Authors revealed, for the first time, important anti-inflammatory effects and significant improvements in lipid and purine metabolism, atherogenic indices, and body composition, exerted by the minor polar compounds of EVOO in nephropathic patients.

Ranogajec et al. (contribution 7) explored the effects of NBCs consumption, contained in plant-based foods, on the improvement of lung function in patients with chronic obstructive pulmonary disease (COPD). In particular, the Authors estimated the dietary phytochemical index (DPI) and revealed the DPI's association with the improvement of lung function, strength, and function of inspiratory muscles and peripheral muscles in COPD patients. The Authors concluded that a higher intake of phytochemicals could be useful as dietary intervention in COPD treatment.

Finally, Wu et al. (contribution 8) focused their study on the role of the Mediterranean diet, which encourages a high consumption of plant-based foods, in promoting healthy aging. In particular, the Authors analyzed dietary data from over 7000 subjects, highlighting how a higher adherence to the Mediterranean diet showed a positive correlation with levels of soluble Klotho, a marker related to aging. A lower odds ratio for aging was, thus, observed in subjects who had a higher adherence to the Mediterranean diet.

In light of the conclusions of all the Authors who brilliantly contributed to our Special Issue, it is possible to affirm that the use of NBCs, mainly contained in plant-based foods, represents an important adjuvant strategy to counteract the onset of age-related NCCDDs and to slow down their progression.

Conflicts of Interest: The authors declare no conflicts of interest.

List of Contributions:

1. Di Lauro, M.; Guerriero, C.; Cornali, K.; Albanese, M.; Costacurta, M.; Mercuri, N.B.; Di Daniele, N.; Noce, A. Linking Migraine to Gut Dysbiosis and Chronic Non-Communicable Diseases. *Nutrients* **2023**, *15*, 4327. https://doi.org/10.3390/nu15204327.

2. Derkaczew, M.; Martyniuk, P.; Osowski, A.; Wojtkiewicz, J. Cyclitols: From Basic Understanding to Their Association with Neurodegeneration. *Nutrients* **2023**, *15*, 2029. https://doi.org/10.3390/nu15092029.
3. Doan, T.P.; Zhang, M.; An, J.P.; Ponce-Zea, J.E.; Mai, V.H.; Ryu, B.; Park, E.J.; Oh, W.K. Metabolite Profiling of Allium hookeri Leaves Using UHPLC-qTOF-MS/MS and the Senomorphic Activity of Phenolamides. *Nutrients* **2023**, *15*, 5109. https://doi.org/10.3390/nu15245109.
4. Yoon, E.J.; Ahn, J.W.; Kim, H.S.; Choi, Y.; Jeong, J.; Joo, S.S.; Park, D. Improvement of Cognitive Function by Fermented Panax ginseng C.A. Meyer Berries Extracts in an AF64A-Induced Memory Deficit Model. *Nutrients* **2023**, *15*, 3389. https://doi.org/10.3390/nu15153389.
5. Zhou, R.; Lin, K.; Leng, C.; Zhou, M.; Zhang, J.; Li, Y.; Liu, Y.; Ye, X.; Xu, X.; Sun, B.; et al. Chebulic Acid Prevents Hypoxia Insult via Nrf2/ARE Pathway in Ischemic Stroke. *Nutrients* **2022**, *14*, 5390. https://doi.org/10.3390/nu14245390.
6. Marrone, G.; Urciuoli, S.; Di Lauro, M.; Ruzzolini, J.; Ieri, F.; Vignolini, P.; Di Daniele, F.; Guerriero, C.; Nediani, C.; Di Daniele, N.; et al. Extra Virgin Olive Oil and Cardiovascular Protection in Chronic Kidney Disease. *Nutrients* **2022**, *14*, 4265. https://doi.org/10.3390/nu14204265.
7. Ranogajec, A.; Ilic, A.; Benko Mestrovic, S.; Rumbak, I. Effect of Phytochemical-Rich Food Intake on Respiratory and Muscle Function in Middle-Aged Patients with COPD: A Cross-Sectional Study. *Nutrients* **2024**, *16*, 3962. https://doi.org/10.3390/nu16223962.
8. Wu, S.E.; Chen, Y.J.; Chen, W.L. Adherence to Mediterranean Diet and Soluble Klotho Level: The Value of Food Synergy in Aging. *Nutrients* **2022**, *14*, 3910. https://doi.org/10.3390/nu14193910.

References

1. Cheng, X.; Yang, Y.; Schwebel, D.C.; Liu, Z.; Li, L.; Cheng, P.; Ning, P.; Hu, G. Population ageing and mortality during 1990–2017: A global decomposition analysis. *PLoS Med.* **2020**, *17*, e1003138. [CrossRef] [PubMed]
2. Lutz, W.; Sanderson, W.; Scherbov, S. The coming acceleration of global population ageing. *Nature* **2008**, *451*, 716–719. [CrossRef] [PubMed]
3. Mitchell, E.; Walker, R. Global ageing: Successes, challenges and opportunities. *Br. J. Hosp. Med.* **2020**, *81*, 1–9. [CrossRef] [PubMed]
4. Ismail, Z.; Ahmad, W.I.W.; Hamjah, S.H.; Astina, I.K. The Impact of Population Ageing: A Review. *Iran J. Public Health* **2021**, *50*, 2451–2460. [CrossRef] [PubMed]
5. Sander, M.; Oxlund, B.; Jespersen, A.; Krasnik, A.; Mortensen, E.L.; Westendorp, R.G.; Rasmussen, L.J. The challenges of human population ageing. *Age Ageing* **2015**, *44*, 185–187. [CrossRef] [PubMed]
6. Atella, V.; Piano Mortari, A.; Kopinska, J.; Belotti, F.; Lapi, F.; Cricelli, C.; Fontana, L. Trends in age-related disease burden and healthcare utilization. *Aging Cell* **2019**, *18*, e12861. [CrossRef] [PubMed]
7. Jaul, E.; Barron, J. Age-Related Diseases and Clinical and Public Health Implications for the 85 Years Old and Over Population. *Front. Public Health* **2017**, *5*, 335. [CrossRef] [PubMed]
8. Kennedy, B.K.; Berger, S.L.; Brunet, A.; Campisi, J.; Cuervo, A.M.; Epel, E.S.; Franceschi, C.; Lithgow, G.J.; Morimoto, R.I.; Pessin, J.E.; et al. Geroscience: Linking aging to chronic disease. *Cell* **2014**, *159*, 709–713. [CrossRef] [PubMed]
9. Li, Z.; Zhang, Z.; Ren, Y.; Wang, Y.; Fang, J.; Yue, H.; Ma, S.; Guan, F. Aging and age-related diseases: From mechanisms to therapeutic strategies. *Biogerontology* **2021**, *22*, 165–187. [CrossRef] [PubMed]
10. Serrano, A.; Ros, G.; Nieto, G. Bioactive Compounds and Extracts from Traditional Herbs and Their Potential Anti-Inflammatory Health Effects. *Medicines* **2018**, *5*, 76. [CrossRef] [PubMed]
11. Noce, A.; Di Lauro, M.; Di Daniele, F.; Pietroboni Zaitseva, A.; Marrone, G.; Borboni, P.; Di Daniele, N. Natural Bioactive Compounds Useful in Clinical Management of Metabolic Syndrome. *Nutrients* **2021**, *13*, 630. [CrossRef] [PubMed]
12. Lianou, A.D.; Lianos, G.D.; Schizas, D.; Machairas, N.; Mitsis, M.; Alexiou, G.A. Natural Compounds and Cancer: Current Evidences. *Maedica* **2024**, *19*, 621–628. [CrossRef] [PubMed]
13. Narayanankutty, A.; Famurewa, A.C.; Oprea, E. Natural Bioactive Compounds and Human Health. *Molecules* **2024**, *29*, 3372. [CrossRef] [PubMed]
14. Song, L.; Zhang, S. Anti-Aging Activity and Modes of Action of Compounds from Natural Food Sources. *Biomolecules* **2023**, *13*, 1600. [CrossRef] [PubMed]
15. Owona, B.A.; Abia, W.A.; Moundipa, P.F. Natural compounds flavonoids as modulators of inflammasomes in chronic diseases. *Int. Immunopharmacol.* **2020**, *84*, 106498. [CrossRef] [PubMed]

16. Du, B.; Xu, B. Natural Bioactive Compounds Exerting Health-Promoting Effects by Ameliorating Oxidative Stress. *Antioxidants* **2025**, *14*, 85. [CrossRef] [PubMed]
17. Balsano, C.; Alisi, A. Antioxidant effects of natural bioactive compounds. *Curr. Pharm. Des.* **2009**, *15*, 3063–3073. [CrossRef] [PubMed]
18. Cuffaro, D.; Digiacomo, M.; Macchia, M. Dietary Bioactive Compounds: Implications for Oxidative Stress and Inflammation. *Nutrients* **2023**, *15*, 4966. [CrossRef] [PubMed]
19. Noce, A.; Marrone, G.; Urciuoli, S.; Di Daniele, F.; Di Lauro, M.; Pietroboni Zaitseva, A.; Di Daniele, N.; Romani, A. Usefulness of Extra Virgin Olive Oil Minor Polar Compounds in the Management of Chronic Kidney Disease Patients. *Nutrients* **2021**, *13*, 581. [CrossRef] [PubMed]
20. Romani, A.; Bernini, R.; Noce, A.; Urciuoli, S.; Di Lauro, M.; Pietroboni Zaitseva, A.; Marrone, G.; Di Daniele, N. Potential Beneficial Effects of Extra Virgin Olive Oils Characterized by High Content in Minor Polar Compounds in Nephropathic Patients: A Pilot Study. *Molecules* **2020**, *25*, 4757. [CrossRef] [PubMed]

nutrients

MDPI

Article

Effect of Phytochemical-Rich Food Intake on Respiratory and Muscle Function in Middle-Aged Patients with COPD: A Cross-Sectional Study

Alda Ranogajec [1,2], Ana Ilić [2,*], Snježana Benko Meštrović [1,3] and Ivana Rumbak [2]

[1] Special Hospital for Pulmonary Diseases, Rockefellerova 3, 10000 Zagreb, Croatia; avilogorac@gmail.com (A.R.); snjezanabenkom@gmail.com (S.B.M.)

[2] Department of Food Quality Control, Faculty of Food Technology and Biotechnology, University of Zagreb, Pierottijeva 6, 10000 Zagreb, Croatia; ivana.rumbak@pbf.unizg.hr

[3] Physiotherapy Department, University of North, Jurja Križanića 31b, 42000 Varaždin, Croatia

* Correspondence: ana.ilic@pbf.unizg.hr; Tel.: +385-1-4605-011

Abstract: Background: It is known that the consumption of single phytochemicals improves respiratory function in chronic obstructive pulmonary disease (COPD) patients. Since phytochemicals have a synergistic effect on health, a more comprehensive analysis is needed. The aim of this study was to estimate the intake of phytochemicals using the dietary phytochemical index (DPI) and assess their association with respiratory function, inspiratory muscle strength and function, and peripheral muscle strength. **Methods**: This study was conducted at the Special Hospital for Pulmonary Diseases in Zagreb (September 2023 to May 2024). The DPI was assessed using three 24 h recalls from 71 COPD patients (66.5 ± 8.4 years; 53.5% men). Anthropometric measurements, respiratory function, inspiratory muscle function and strength, and peripheral muscle strength were assessed during pulmonary rehabilitation following standard protocols. **Results**: Patients were divided into DPI tertiles with mean values of 7.3 ± 3.0, 16.0 ± 3.0, and 32.2 ± 8.8, respectively. After controlling for confounding factors, a significant association was found between DPI tertiles and FEV_1 (p-trend < 0.001), FVC (p-trend = 0.002), FEV_1/FVC (p-trend < 0.001), MIP (p-trend = 0.012), and MSUE (p-trend = 0.002). In addition, an inverse association was found between DPI tertiles and diaphragm thickness during inhalation (p-trend = 0.012) and exhalation (p-trend = 0.013). **Conclusions**: This study suggests that a higher intake of phytochemicals could be beneficial in dietary interventions for COPD therapy. Future prospective studies are needed to confirm these findings.

Keywords: chronic obstructive pulmonary disease; dietary phytochemical index; diaphragm thickness; FEV_1; FVC; MIP; peripheral muscle strength; pulmonary rehabilitation

1. Introduction

By definition, chronic obstructive pulmonary disease (COPD) is a chronic, non-communicable lung disease characterized by airflow limitation and respiratory symptoms such as shortness of breath, cough, expectoration, wheezing, etc. [1]. COPD is a multifactorial systemic disease that can develop from several causes (alpha-1 antitrypsin deficiency, abnormal lung development, severe respiratory infections and childhood asthma, air pollution, occupational exposures, etc.), with the main risk factor being exposure to tobacco (active or passive) [1–3]. It is recognized that some of the comorbidities such as heart disease, cancer, poor mental health, musculoskeletal disorders, gastrointestinal disorders, endocrine and metabolic disorders, sleep disorders, malnutrition, and other diseases associated with poor nutrition are associated with COPD [3]. According to estimates, COPD caused 3.3 million deaths in 2019, making it the third most common cause of death worldwide, and the trend is rising [3–5].

The most important treatment approach for patients with COPD is pulmonary rehabilitation, which combines pharmacotherapy and supplemental oxygen therapy with exercise training, education, and behavior change [6]. Education may include nutritional therapy and dietary behavior modification due to the high prevalence of nutritional depletion in patients with COPD [7]. Nutritional interventions that focus on regulating body mass and reducing the degree of malnutrition as part of pulmonary rehabilitation may improve COPD outcomes [8,9]. In addition, according to the systematic reviews and meta-analyses, unhealthy eating habits are associated with a higher risk of COPD [10–12]. Most studies focus on improving respiratory function and nutritional status by providing certain nutrients such as protein, vitamin E, and vitamin D or taking Oral Nutritional Supplements (ONSs). Since there has been a recent shift to looking at the diet as a whole rather than focusing on a single nutrient, it has been found that patients who followed the Dietary Approaches to Stop Hypertension (DASH) and the Mediterranean diet (MedDiet) had better respiratory function [13–16]. Both DASH and the MedDiet are characterized by a high intake of whole grains, fruits and vegetables, and plant-based proteins and a lower intake of red meat, processed foods, and salt [17,18]. Indeed, a higher intake of fruit and vegetables is associated with lower risk of COPD [11,19–21]. It has been hypothesized that consumption of fruit and vegetables, as a good source of phytochemicals, may reduce the oxidative stress that often occurs in COPD patients [22–25]. The link between phytochemical intake and respiratory function in patients with COPD is still unclear. However, in the literature several studies have highlighted the benefit of intake of individual phytochemicals to reduce the symptoms of COPD and prevent lung cancer. COPD is an inflammatory disease and, in addition, most COPD patients were smokers or continue to smoke after diagnosis, which can further exacerbate oxidative damage and prolong immune responses [26]. Therefore, phytochemicals can act as antioxidants and reduce the expression of genes that promote the immune system and increase mucus secretion [26,27]. Carotenoids, of which lycopene is one of the most interesting, are among the phytochemicals proposed as a therapy for patients with lung disease. Carotenoids are thought to activate the NRF2/HO-1 signaling pathway, which inhibits transcription factors, namely nuclear factor-kappa B (NF-κB) [27–29]. The second type of interesting phytochemicals is flavonoids, whose higher uptake improves FEV_1. One of the suggested underlying mechanisms is that they reduce oxidative stress and increase PaO_2 [30,31]. Moreover, the flavonoid resveratrol from wine appears to inhibit inflammatory cytokines and the activation of NF-κB and AP-1, while stimulating GSH synthesis [32,33]. Curcumin is one of the phytochemicals that have been studied in relation to lung disease. Curcumin is thought to inhibit the synthesis of NF-κB, particularly in smokers, and can enhance the effects of glucocorticoids [34,35].

Phytochemicals are secondary metabolites that are mainly found in plant foods and whose intake has a positive effect on health [36,37]. However, there is no recommendation for their intake as there is lack of information on their quantity in foods and their bioavailability and accessibility after processing and metabolism [36,38–40]. To address this problem, McCarty proposed the dietary phytochemical index (DPI) as a tool to determine the intake of phytochemicals [41]. The DPI is based on the daily energy intake from foods rich in phytochemicals. Therefore, the DPI enables the indirect assessment of the intake of various phytochemicals through the assessment of food intake. Further, the DPI has been used in several epidemiologic studies and linked phytochemical intake to disease outcomes, e.g., migraine [42], gastric ulcer [43], multiple sclerosis [44], various cancers [45–49], mental disorders [50,51], metabolic syndrome [52], skeletal disorders [53,54], cardiovascular diseases [55–58], nutritional status [59,60], non-alcoholic fatty liver disease [61], etc. To our knowledge, this has not yet been observed in patients with COPD.

To better understand the relationship between the intake of phytochemicals and the health status of adult COPD patients, this study aims to estimate the intake of phytochemicals using the DPI and to observe the relationship between the DPI and respiratory function (forced expiratory volume in the first second and forced vital capacity). Since muscle strength is a risk factor for poorer outcomes, this study also aims to observe the association between the DPI and inspiratory muscle strength and function (maximum inspiratory pressure, diaphragm thickness in inhalation and exhalation), and peripheral muscle strength.

2. Materials and Methods

2.1. Settings and Participants

This cross-sectional study was conducted from September 2023 to May 2024 at the Special Hospital for Pulmonary Diseases in Zagreb, Croatia. Participants were recruited via the day clinic during pulmonary rehabilitation. The inclusion criterion was the presence of COPD, which was assessed using the Global Initiative for Chronic Obstructive Lung Diseases (GOLD) scale [62]. During the recruitment phase, patients were recruited who were diagnosed with COPD between 6 and 30 years ago. The exclusion criteria were as follows: use of long-term oxygen therapy; overlapping conditions with asthma; use of systemic corticosteroid therapy in the last six months; implanted pacemaker or other electrical implant; neuromuscular disease, phrenic nerve injury, or a condition following cerebrovascular accident with residual hemiparesis; history of lung surgery; and autoimmune, neurological, or other systemic diseases that could affect respiratory function. During the recruitment period, a total of 102 patients were eligible for the study. However, after applying the exclusion criteria, 73 patients were included in the study (72%). After data collection, two additional patients were excluded for the purposes of the present study because they had not completed the 24 h recalls. Finally, data from 71 (70%) adult patients with COPD (45 to 85 years) were analyzed. An a priori analysis to estimate the sample size was performed using the GPower program (version 3.1.9.2; Heinrich Heine University Dusseldorf, Dusseldorf, Germany). The a priori analysis was performed assuming a power of 80%, a significance level of $\alpha = 0.05$, an expected effect of 0.15, and at least 2 existing predictors (sex and smoking). Respiratory function was used as the primary outcome to assess the expected effect. This analysis indicated that at least 68 patients should be included in the study. General information about the participants was collected through interviews during pulmonary rehabilitation and through the Hospital Information System software (version 212.0.000¸IN2 Ltd., Zagreb, Croatia).

Each patient was informed of the study protocols and gave written consent to participate in the study. Participants were free to withdraw their consent at any time during or after data collection. The study protocols were designed and conducted in accordance with the Declaration of Helsinki. In addition, the protocols were approved by the Ethics Committee of the School of Medicine, University of Zagreb (reference number: 251-59-10106-23-111/203, class: 641-01/23-02/01).

2.2. Dietary Assessment

Data on consumed food and drink were collected using 24 h recalls on three non-consecutive days within the first two weeks of recruitment. Each patient was interviewed individually by trained dietitians from the research team using a 5-step protocol. Portion size was estimated using kitchen utensils (cups, spoons, plates, etc.), packaging/portion sizes of packaged foods, or in grams if participants knew the weight of food and drink consumed. In addition, the brands of packaged foods and food supplements were recorded. The conversion of the collected data into energy and macronutrient intake was carried out using the Prehrana software (version 1.0; Infosistem Plc., Zagreb, Croatia). The software contains national food composition tables [63] and is supplemented by data on packaged foods and food supplements from their nutrition labels. The observed individual means method was used to present daily energy and energy intake from food items that are considered good sources of phytochemicals [64].

2.3. Dietary Phytochemical Index

For each patient, the DPI was calculated according to the proposed method as the ratio between the daily energy intake from foods that are good sources of phytochemicals and the total daily energy intake multiplied by 100 [41]. Food items that are high in phytochemicals include the following: fruit, including natural fruit juices, vegetables (including natural vegetable juices and tomato sauces), plant-based protein food (dry legumes, nuts, and seeds), whole grains (grains, flour/semolina, bread and rolls, cereals, and pasta), and other phytochemical-rich food (herbs, spices, coffee, tea, soy products, cocoa, beer and wine, and olive oil). Due to their low content of phytochemicals, potatoes and picked fruit and vegetables were excluded from the estimation of the DPI [41,46,53,58,59].

2.4. Anthropometric and Body Composition Assessments

An anthropometric assessment was performed during the visit to the pulmonary rehabilitation day clinic. Body height was measured to the nearest 0.1 cm using a stadiometer (SECA 799, Hamburg, Germany). Body weight was measured to the nearest 0.1 kg using a combination digital scale with bioelectrical impedance (TANITA MC-780MA P, Tanita Corp., Tokyo, Japan). Body mass index (BMI; kg/m^2) was calculated for each patient based on body mass and weight measurements. Patients were classified according to the BMI classification proposed by the World Health Organization [65].

The body composition assessment (TANITA MC-780MA P, Tanita Corp., Tokyo, Japan) includes several analyses from which the percentage of body fat and appendicular muscle mass (kg) were extracted for the purposes of this study. The appendicular skeletal muscle index (SMI; km/m^2) was calculated for each patient from the appendicular muscle mass data obtained. The cut-off value for men and women for the SMI was taken from the ESPEN guidelines [66].

2.5. Respiratory Function Assessments

FEV_1 and FVC were measured with a Medisoft HypAir PFT System (Medisoft, Sorrines, Belgium) in seated position. Expiratory flow is measured by having the patient inhale as deeply as possible and exhale forcefully and completely as quickly as possible into a device that records the volume of exhaled air (FVC) as a percentage of the predicted value for age and sex and the volume of air exhaled in the first second (FEV_1) as a percentage of the predicted value for age and sex. It is normally 80% of the FVC. We repeated the measurement at least 3 times with an interval of 90 s between each measurement in COPD patients and recorded the highest value obtained [67].

2.6. Inspiratory Muscle Strength and Function Assessment

The assessment of inspiratory muscle strength and function includes maximum inspiratory pressure (MIP) and diaphragm thickness at the end of inhalation (T min) and exhalation (T max).

MIP was measured using the PowerBreathe device (PowerBreathe International Ltd., Southam, England, UK). The MIP value reflects the strength of the diaphragm and the extra-diaphragmatic inspiratory muscles. The patient should be in a sitting position and have a blocked nose, for which a tick is provided. The patient first inhales and exhales normally through the mouthpiece several times, then exhales slowly and to the end (to the residual volume), and then inhales as forcefully as possible. The breath must last at least 1.5 s and the maneuver is repeated five times. The highest value achieved is recorded, not the mean value (Sachs et al., 2009). The device calculates the expected MIP value based on the age and sex entered using the formula for males $120 - (0.41 \times \text{age})$ and for females $108 - (0.61 \times \text{age})$. Values <60 cmH_2O in adults under 40 years, <50 cmH_2O in adults between 40 and 80 years, and <40 cmH_2O in adults over 80 years indicate weakness of the of the diaphragm and extra-diaphragmatic inspiratory muscles [68,69].

The measurement of diaphragm thickness (mm) at the end of inspiration and expiration was performed with the ultrasound device Mindray DC-8 (Mindray Medical International Ltd., Shenzhen, Guandgong, China), with a linear probe frequency of 7.5–10.0 MHz with the patient in supine position in B-mode. The probe was placed above the apposition zone, between the eighth and ninth intercostal spaces, 0.5–2.0 cm below the costophrenic angle, between the anterior and middle axillary line on the right side. The thickness of the diaphragm was measured at the end of inspiration and at the end of expiration. The measurements are presented as a three-layered structure consisting of a hypoechoic inner muscle layer surrounded by two hyperechoic outer membranes (peritoneum and pleura). To objectively quantify the thickening of the diaphragm, at least three measurements are required and the data are presented as an average of the measurements. Here, 2.1 ± 0.4 (1.3–3) mm in men and 1.9 ± 0.4 (1.1–2.7) in women are cut-off values for diaphragm thickness (mm) at the end of inspiration and 2.8 ± 0.6 (1.7–3.9) in men and 2.5 ± 0.6 (1.3–3.7) in women for diaphragm thickness at the end of expiration [70,71].

2.7. Peripheral Muscle Strength Assessment

The peripheral muscle strength assessment includes the strength of forearm flexors (*m. biceps brachii*; MSUE; N) and of the leg extensors (*m. quadriceps*; MSLE; N). Both were measured using the digital dynamometer Pelican 1150 (Lafayette Instrument Company, Lafayette, LA, USA) in accordance with standard protocols [72]. The strength of the biceps brachii muscle was measured in a sitting position with the arm bent at the elbow by 90 degrees. The researcher placed the dynamometer on the distal part of the forearm and the patient flexed the arm at the elbow against the resistance of the researcher. The strength of the quadriceps muscle was measured in a sitting position with the knee bent at 90 degrees. The researcher placed the dynamometer on the distal part of the lower leg and the patient stretched their leg against the resistance of the researcher. The measurement was repeated three times and the mean value was recorded.

2.8. Statistical Analysis

All statistical analyses were performed using SPSS software (IBM SPSS Statistics for Windows, version 23.0. Armonk, NY, USA: IBM Corp.) with a significance level of $\alpha = 0.05$. The normality of the distribution of the data was checked using the Shapiro–Wilk test. Only seven variables had missing data (less than 5%), for which we performed a series of mean imputations. Patients were classified into tertiles of the DPI score using the visual binning method. Accordingly, 23 patients were classified into the first tertile of the DPI (DPI $\leq$ 11.2) and 24 patients in the second (DPI 11.3–20.4) and third (DPI $\geq$ 20.5). General characteristics, anthropometric measurements, body composition, and dietary habits were presented as the mean and standard deviation for continuous variables and as a percentage for categorical variables according to the tertiles of the DPI. Comparisons between tertiles were performed using a one-way analysis of variance (ANOVA) with a post hoc Bonferroni test for continuous variables and a chi-square test or Fisher's exact test for categorical variables. Associations between continuous dependent variables (upper and lower muscle strength, diaphragm thickness ate the end of inhalation and exhalation, MIP, FEV_1, FVC, FEV_1/FVC) and the tertiles of the DPI were observed using multivariate linear regression in crude and adjusted models. In the first model, we controlled for sex (categorical), age (continuous), number of diagnoses (continuous), GOLD stage (categorical), smoking (categorical), and daily energy intake (continuous). In the second model, we additionally controlled for body mass index (continuous), percentage of body fat (continuous), and the skeletal muscle index (continuous).

3. Results

A total of 71 patients with COPD with an average age of 66.5 ± 8.4 years took part in this study. The study population was almost equally divided between men (53.5%) and women (46.5%). According to the GOLD diagnostic protocol, most patients had GOLD stage 2 COPD. In addition to COPD, 30% of patients had one to three other dual diagnoses, of which hypertension (36.6%), emphysema (12.7%), and dyslipidemia (11.3%) were the most common. In addition, more than half of the patients were former smokers.

The average DPI in this study population was 18.7 ± 11.8. For further analysis, the study population was divided into tertiles according to the DPI. The descriptive statistics of the DPI for each tertile are shown in Figure 1. The average DPI of the patients in the first tertile was 7.3 ± 3.0, in the second 16.0 ± 3.0, and in the third 32.2 ± 8.8. The average contribution of the food groups to the DPI is shown in Figure 2. The foods from the whole grain group had the lowest contribution to the DPI in the first tertile and the contribution increased significantly ($p < 0.001$) until the last tertile. Conversely, the foods from the vegetable group contributed the most to the patients' DPI in the first tertile, with the contribution decreasing significantly ($p < 0.001$) by the third tertile.

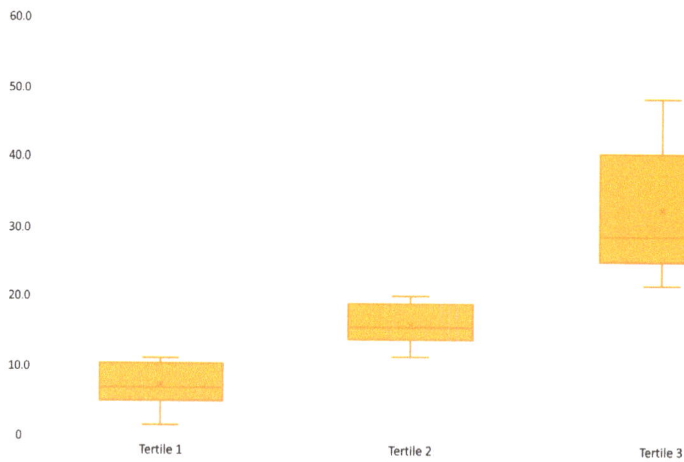

Figure 1. Descriptive statistics of the dietary phytochemical index across tertiles of patients with COPD (n = 71).

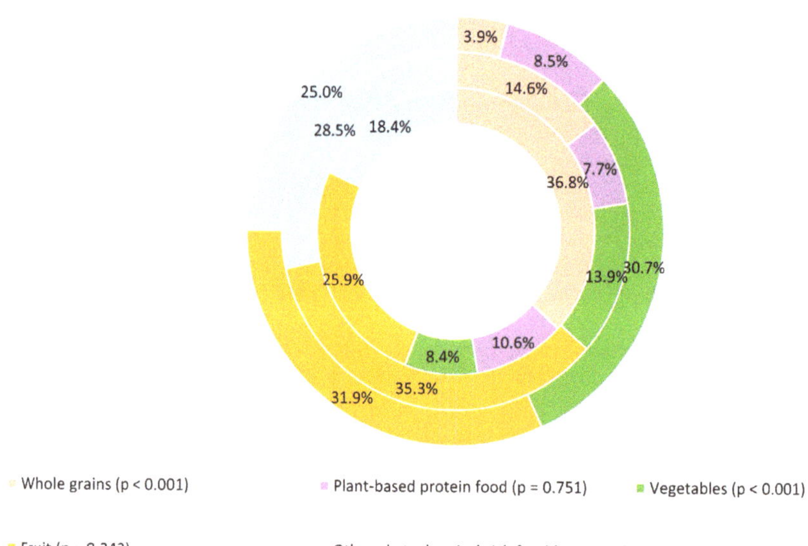

Figure 2. Relative contribution of the food groups to the daily DPI across the DPI tertiles. The external circle represents the first tertile, while the inner circles represent the next higher tertile. The differences between the tertiles of the DPI were tested using a one-way analysis of variance with the post hoc Bonferroni test ($p < 0.05$).

The differences in the general characteristics of the study population between the tertiles of the DPI are shown in Table 1. The only significant difference ($p = 0.044$) was observed between sexes, with more males (73.9%) in the first tertile of the DPI and more females (62.5%) in the third tertile of the DPI.

Table 1. General characteristics of patients with chronic obstructive pulmonary disease across the tertiles of the dietary phytochemical index [1].

Variables	Total ($n = 71$)	DPI Tertiles			p-Values [2]
		T1 (DPI ≤ 11.2)	T2 (DPI 11.3–20.4)	T3 (DPI ≥ 20.5)	
Age (yr.)	66.5 ± 8.4	68.3 ± 8.6	65.9 ± 7.5	65.5 ± 9.0	0.461
Sex (%)					
Male	53.5	73.9	50.0	37.5	0.044
Female	46.5	26.1	50.0	62.5	
GOLD stage (%)					
1	23.9	17.4	29.2	25.0	0.835
2	42.3	39.1	41.7	45.8	
3	23.9	26.1	25.0	20.8	
4	9.9	17.4	4.2	8.3	
Number of diagnoses (%)					
1	30.0	26.1	21.7	41.7	0.111
2	30.0	30.4	34.8	25.0	
3	17.1	4.3	30.4	16.7	
4	20.0	34.8	8.7	16.7	
5	1.4	4.3	0.0	0.0	
6	1.4	0.0	4.3	0.0.	
Smoking (%)					
No	1.4	0.0	0.0	1.4	0.869
Yes	42.3	39.1	41.7	42.3	
Former	56.3	60.9	58.3	56.3	

DPI—dietary phytochemical index; T—tertile; [1] data are shown as mean ± standard deviation or percentage, depending on the type of variable. [2] Differences between tertiles of the DPI were tested using one-way analysis of variance with the post hoc Bonferroni test for continuous variables and chi-square test/Fisher's exact test for categorical variables ($p < 0.05$).

Assessment of anthropometry and body composition revealed that the majority of patients had a normal weight status (43.7%), with an average body fat percentage of 27.5% ± 9.1%. According to the skeletal muscle index, the majority of patients (83.1%) had normal appendicular muscle mass. No differences were found in the anthropometric measurements and body composition of the patients across the tertiles of the DPI (Table 2).

The dietary habits of patients with COPD according to the tertiles of the DPI are shown in Table 3. On average, patients had a daily energy intake of 1529 ± 405 kcal, with patients in the lowest and highest tertiles having a significantly lower ($p = 0.034$) energy intake than patients in the second tertile. The proportion of proteins, carbohydrates, and fats in the daily energy intake did not differ between the patients across the DPI tertiles.

Table 2. Anthropometric measurements and body composition of patients with chronic obstructive pulmonary disease across the tertiles of the dietary phytochemical index [1].

Variables	Total (n = 71)	DPI Tertiles			p-Values [2]
		T1 (DPI ≤ 11.2)	T2 (DPI 11.3–20.4)	T3 (DPI ≥ 20.5)	
Weight (kg)	76.2 ± 17.5	77.6 ± 15.7	78.0 ± 21.6	73.0 ± 14.5	0.552
Height (cm)	171.4 ± 7.9	173.5 ± 7.9	17.8 ± 7.0	168.9 ± 8.3	0.134
BMI (kg/m^2)	25.8 ± 5.2	25.8 ± 4.9	26.2 ± 6.4	25.5 ± 4.3	0.900
BMI category (%)					
Underweight Normal Overweight Obesity	7.0 43.7 19.7 29.6	13.0 34.8 17.4 34.8	8.3 33.3 25.0 33.3	0.0 62.5 16.7 20.8	0.295
Fat-free mass (kg)	54.4 ± 11.0	57.0 ± 10.5	55.0 ± 12.0	51.5 ± 10.1	0.225
Body fat (%)	27.5 ± 9.1	25.9 ± 9.1	27.8 ± 9.6	28.9 ± 8.8	0.532
SMI (kg/m^2)	7.4 ± 1.3	7.6 ± 1.3	7.7 ± 1.4	7.1 ± 1.0	0.224
SMI category					
Reduced Normal	16.9 83.1	30.4 69.6	12.5 87.5	16.9 83.1	0.152

DPI—dietary phytochemical index; T—tertile; BMI—body mass index; SMI—skeletal muscle index; [1] data are shown as mean ± standard deviation or percentage, depending on the type of variable. [2] Differences between tertiles of the DPI were tested using one-way analysis of variance with the post hoc Bonferroni test for continuous variables and chi-square test/Fisher's exact test for categorical variables ($p < 0.05$).

Table 3. Dietary habits of patients with chronic obstructive pulmonary disease across the tertiles of the dietary phytochemical index [1].

Variables	Total (n = 71)	DPI Tertiles			p-Values [2]
		T1 (DPI ≤ 11.2)	T2 (DPI 11.3–20.4)	T3 (DPI ≥ 20.5)	
Energy (kcal)	1529 ± 405	1457 ± 359 [a]	1701 ± 417 [b]	1425 ± 393 [a]	0.034
Protein (% kcal)	16.2 ± 3.0	15.5 ± 2.3	15.7 ± 2.8	17.2 ± 3.5	0.087
Carbohydrate (% kcal)	41.2 ± 7.9	39.1 ± 6.2	42.2 ± 9.7	42.2 ± 7.1	0.289
Total fat (% kcal)	43.1 ± 6.9	45.5 ± 6.5	42.4 ± 7.6	41.5 ± 6.0	0.113

DPI—dietary phytochemical index; T—tertile; [1] data are shown as mean ± standard deviation or percentage, depending on the type of variable. [2] Differences between tertiles of the DPI were tested using one-way analysis of variance with the post hoc Bonferroni test (differences are indicated with a and b) for continuous variables ($p < 0.05$).

The association between respiratory function and muscle strength with the DPI is shown in Table 4. No associations were found in unadjusted analyses. After adjustment for sex, age, number of diagnoses, smoking, GOLD stage, and daily energy intake, multivariate linear regression reveals that the DPI is associated with FEV_1 (p-trend < 0.001), FVC (p-trend = 0.001), FEV_1/FVC (p-trend < 0.001), and MSUE (p-trend < 0.001). Furthermore, after additional adjustment for body mass index, percent body fat, and the skeletal muscle index, the association between the DPI and FEV1 (p-trend < 0.001), FVC (p-trend = 0.002), FEV_1/FVC (p-trend < 0.001), and MSUE (p-trend = 0.002) remained unchanged, while a positive association between the DPI and MIP (p-trend = 0.026) and an inverse association between diaphragm thickness at the end of inhalation (p-trend = 0.012) and end of exhalation (p-trend = 0.013) emerged.

Table 4. Multivariate linear regression of the association between muscle strength and respiratory function of patients with chronic obstructive pulmonary disease with the dietary phytochemical index [1].

Variables	DPI Tertiles			p-Trend
	T1 (DPI ≤ 11.2)	T2 (DPI 11.3–20.4)	T3 (DPI ≥ 20.5)	
FEV_1 (%)				
Crude [2]	Reference	11.07 (−1.52–23.66)	10.40 (−2.19–23.00)	0.150
Model 1 [3]		2.97 (−3.62–9.56)	4.02 (−2.29–10.32)	<0.001
Model 2 [4]		3.70 (−3.19–10.77)	4.35 (−2.12–10.82)	<0.001
FVC (%)				
Crude	Reference	8.08 (−2.83–18.98)	6.11 (−4.93–17.16)	0.309
Model 1		3.27 (−6.13–12.68)	5.76 (−3.24–14.77)	0.001
Model 2		5.78 (−3.97–15.52)	6.84 (−2.19–15.87)	0.002
FEV_1/FVC				
Crude	Reference	0.06 (−0.04–0.16)	0.06 (−0.04–0.16)	0.406
Model 1		0.01 (−0.06–0.08)	0.001 (−0.07–0.07)	<0.001
Model 2		0.004 (−0.07–0.08)	−0.002 (−0.07–0.07)	<0.001
MIP (cmH_2O)				
Crude	Reference	3.21 (−9.22–15.65)	1.25 (−11.18–13.69)	0.873
Model 1		1.39 (−11.65–14.44)	4.69 (−7.79–17.19)	0.056
Model 2		−1.09 (−14.25–12.06)	3.97 (−8.23–16.16)	0.026
Diaphragm thickness—inhalation (mm)				
Crude	Reference	−0.20 (−0.54–0.15)	−0.32 (−0.66–0.02)	0.172
Model 1		−0.19 (−0.44–0.26)	−0.13 (−0.47–0.20)	0.053
Model 2		−0.15 (−0.494–0.19)	−0.12 (−0.44–0.20)	0.012
Diaphragm thickness—exhalation (mm)				
Crude	Reference	−0.12 (−0.40–0.17)	−0.27 (−0.55–0.02)	0.182
Model 1		0.01 (−0.29–0.31)	−0.11 (−0.40–0.18)	0.061
Model 2		−0.09 (−0.39–0.21)	−0.13 (−0.40–0.15)	0.013
MSUE (N)				
Crude	Reference	29.80 (−2.67–62.27)	6.81 (−25.32–38.94)	0.165
Model 1		43.48 (13.67–73.29)	22.59 (−5.95–51.13)	<0.001
Model 2		42.92 (11.49–74.34)	23.66 (−5.48–52.80)	0.002
MSLE (N)				
Crude	Reference	8.08 (−20.93–37.09)	14.33 (−14.68–43.34)	0.616
Model 1		9.50 (−22.44–41.45)	20.51 (−10.07–51.09)	0.252
Model 2		12.61 (−21.08–46.29)	22.29 (−8.65–53.84)	0.387

DPI—dietary phytochemical index; T—tertile; MIP—maximum inspiratory pressure; FEV_1—forced expiratory volume in the first second; FVC—forced vital capacity; MSUE—upper muscle strength; MSLE—lower muscle strength; [1] data are shown as unstandardized β coefficients and the 95% confidence interval. [2] Crude values of multivariate linear regression with the DPI as the independent variable ($p < 0.05$). [3] Model 1: adjusted for sex, age, number of diagnoses, smoking, GOLD stage, and daily energy intake. [4] Model 2: adjusted for sex, age, number of diagnoses, smoking, daily energy intake, body mass index, percent body fat, and the skeletal muscle index.

4. Discussion

To our knowledge, this cross-sectional study is the first to observe an association between respiratory function and muscle strength and comprehensive intake of phytochemicals, estimated by the DPI, in patients with COPD. In terms of respiratory function, we observed a relationship between FEV_1, FVC, FEV_1/FVC, MIP, and the DPI and an inverse relationship between diaphragm thickness during inhalation and exhalation. We also observed a positive relationship between upper muscle strength and the DPI. Associations were significant only after controlling for covariates.

COPD is one of the chronic diseases with a high mortality rate, whose prevalence has been increasing for decades [3–5]. The different outcomes of COPD, such as emphysema, chronic bronchitis, asthma, cough, expectoration, wheezing, etc., can significantly affect the patient's quality of life [73,74]. Malnutrition is one of the most important comorbidities in patients with COPD, which can worsen the above-mentioned consequences and the quality of life [2,75,76]. Indeed, nutritional support to treat malnutrition in patients with COPD can improve quality of life [77–79]. Moreover, the dietary patterns that are described as healthy ones and imply consumption of whole grains, fish, fruit, and vegetables may lower the risk of COPD [10,80–82]. The existing results on the effect of dietary patterns on respiratory capacity are inconclusive. Several prospective studies have shown that healthy dietary patterns can increase FEV_1 and FVC [81,83,84]. On the other hand, Ardestani et al. [14] found that COPD patients adhered to the DASH diet less well than the control group and that there is no correlation between adherence to the DASH diet and FEV_1 or FVC. The possible explanations for the potential benefits of this diet are seen in the higher intake of vitamins and phytochemicals with antioxidant potential as well as in the intake of dietary fiber. Patients with COPD have higher levels of oxidative stress compared to healthy people [85,86]. The published literature indicates that vitamin C, vitamin E, vitamin A, carotenoids, and phenols may have a positive effect on COPD and respiratory capacity [25,87,88].

To date, over 100,000 different phytochemicals have been identified in food and drinks [36]. Daily intake of phytochemicals cannot be observed in a comprehensive way due to the lack of data on their quantity in food and drinks. However, it has been shown that a variety of phytochemicals in a complex mixture, such as in food, have a stronger antioxidant effect than the intake of a single phytochemical. Therefore, we chose the DPI as an indirect measure of the intake of phytochemicals through the consumption of phytochemical-rich food. Namely, the DPI is calculated as percentages of energy intake from the phytochemical-rich food in daily energy intake. The phytochemical-rich food includes fruit, vegetables, whole grains, legumes, seeds, nuts, olives, olive oil, herbs, spices, coffee, tea, soy products, cocoa, beer, and wine [41]. In line with the results of previous studies on the benefits of consuming certain phytochemicals in people with COPD [25,27], we hypothesized that the synergistic effect of phytochemicals would affect respiratory function. Therefore, we hypothesized that patients with a higher DPI would have better respiratory function (FVC, FEV_1, and FEV_1/FVC), which was confirmed by the results of our study. Although we do not know the diversity of phytochemical content in the patients' diets, these results suggest that dietary patterns consisting of the consumption of foods high in phytochemicals may have a positive impact on COPD outcomes. Therefore, promoting the consumption of phytochemical-rich food could be one of the educational nutritional strategies in COPD rehabilitation programs. However, future randomized controlled studies with a precise dietary plan on the amount of the various phytochemicals are required to determine consumption recommendations.

Measurements of FEV_1, FVC, and their ratio are the gold standard for the diagnosis of COPD [62]; however, we also measured inspiratory muscle strength and function with the MIP and diaphragm thickness at the end of inhalation (T min) and end of exhalation (T max). These respiratory muscles are important for alveolar ventilation and their impairment can worsen COPD outcomes in patients [89,90]. The pathophysiological process of COPD can lead to a shortening of the diaphragm by reducing the fiber-contracting protein and promoting oxidative stress [91,92]. To our knowledge, this study is the first to examine inspiratory muscle strength and function in relation to dietary habits. We hypothesized that patients with a higher DPI would have a larger layer of diaphragm due to the antioxidant capacity of the phytochemicals. In addition, antioxidants could reduce fatigue during exercise and promote the muscle fiber adaptation process in athletes [93]. Therefore, we hypothesized that higher consumption of foods high in phytochemicals may be associated with better MIP measurements. The results show that the DPI was inversely associated with diaphragm thickness at the end of inhalation and exhalation after adjustment for sex, smoking, GOLD stage, number of diagnoses, daily energy intake, body mass index, percent body fat, and the skeletal muscle index. Diaphragm thickness was lower in patients in the third tertile than in the second tertile of the DPI. Since there is no available literature on the relationship between dietary factors and respiratory muscle function and strength, we cannot assume that only the consumption of phytochemicals causes these findings. However, it seems interesting to point out that patients in the second tertile had, on average, a higher energy intake than patients in the other tertiles, and the average energy intake of patients in the second tertile was in line with the European Food Safety Authority recommendation for energy for adults aged 60-69 years with a physical activity level of 1.4 [94]. On this point, we recommend that future studies focus on this topic. Meanwhile, the present study showed a positive relationship between the DPI and MIP after adjustment for covariates. This suggests that increased consumption of foods high in phytochemicals may have a positive effect on respiratory muscle strength. Inspiratory muscle strength and function is generally higher in men and non-smokers, while it declines with age [95]. In addition, in the available literature malnutrition is associated with lower inspiratory muscle strength and function [90,96–98]. In the present study, the age and presence of smokers are similar across the tertile, while there are significantly more men in the first tertile and significantly more women in the third tertiles. The majority of patients in our study had an adequate body mass index and skeletal muscle index.

The results of the existing literature linked the strength of the inspiratory and peripheral muscles in patients with COPD [99]. Malnutrition and reduction in muscle mass is common in patients with COPD [1,2,4]. Two recent randomized clinical trials have shown that protein supplementation can increase peripheral muscle strength in patients with COPD [100,101]. However, to our knowledge, no other dietary component or dietary pattern has been observed in relation to peripheral muscle strength in patients with COPD. In terms of the peripheral muscle strength, we hypothesized that a higher intake of phytochemical-rich food could reduce the oxidative stress, consequently reducing muscle fatigue and damage to the skeletal muscle [93,102]. Accordingly, we examined the relationship between the DPI and MSUE and MSLE, where a positive relationship emerged only for MSUE and was higher in the second tertile than in the third tertile after controlling for the covariates in the analysis. One possible explanation for the extent of the correlation could lie in the higher energy intake of the patients in the second tertiles. However, since we did not observe a direct correlation, we cannot draw any conclusions. In addition, in the present study, we found no difference between the tertiles of the DPI with respect to the contribution of protein to energy intake.

To our knowledge, this is the first study to estimate the DPI in patients with COPD, with an average value of 18.7 $\pm$ 11.8 in the total study population ($\leq$11.2 DPI in the first tertile, 11.3–20.4 DPI in the second and $\geq$20.5 DPI in the third). Furthermore, the DPI has not been estimated in the healthy adult population in Croatia, nor in the adult population with chronic non-communicable diseases, but only in school-age children, in whom the median DPI was 11.8 (7.7–16.2) [103]. However, the DPI has been used in cross-sectional and case–control studies and has been associated with health outcomes in several chronic non-communicable diseases. In the last five years, for example, it has been associated with outcomes, disease severity, or the odds ratio of [42] various cancers [45–49], metabolic syndrome [52], skeletal disorders [53,54], cardiovascular diseases [56–58], nutritional status [59,60], and non-alcoholic fatty liver disease [61]. Younger adults (mean age 36.1 years) with migraine headaches had a DPI of up to 17.99 in the first tertile, 17.99–25.93 in the second tertile, and more than 25.93 in the third tertile [42]. Men aged 57.17 $\pm$ 8.04 years with benign prostatic hyperplasia had an average DPI of 25 $\pm$ 11 and men aged 65.5 $\pm$ 13.0 years with prostate cancer had a DPI of 20.4 $\pm$ 9.9, which was significantly lower in both studies compared to the healthy control group [45,46]. Patients with colorectal cancer (58.2 $\pm$ 10.4 years) had a mean DPI of 19.8 $\pm$ 16.0 [47], while the DPI in patients with glioma (aged 20 to 75 years) ranged from 21 (lowest tertile) to 30 (highest tertile) [48]. The highest DPIs were observed in women with breast cancer (62.4 ± 10.8 years), with an average DPI of 54.76 ± 12.96 [49]. In all studies, the cancer was newly diagnosed or no more than 6 months old, and a lower cancer rate was associated with a higher DPI. With regard to skeletal diseases, premenopausal (DPI range from 7.45 to 23.33 by quartile) and postmenopausal (DPI range from 8.00 to 22.04 by quartile) women with a higher DPI had a lower risk of osteoporosis [53], and patients (49.2 ± 8.2 years) with knee osteoarthritis (mean DPI 28.5 ± 7.2) had a lower DPI than the control group [54]. In addition, patients in the highest quartiles/tertiles of the DPI had a lower risk of metabolic syndrome (age 20–75 years; mean DPI 23.13 ± 9.95) and stroke (mean age 64.8 years; DPI range by tertiles from 21 to 29) [52,56]. In terms of nutritional status, the participant (44.7 ± 10.8 years; mean DPI 26.23 ± 9.48) who manifested a metabolically unhealthy overweight/obesity phenotype had a lower DPI [59]. However, general obesity was not associated with the DPI in men (33.7 ± 24.7) and women (36.2 ± 26.8), and only some of the indicators such as waist circumference in women and waist-to-hip ratio in men were associated with the DPI [60]. The study in which a lower DPI was observed concerned patients with non-alcoholic fatty liver disease. Here, the DPI was 17.4 ± 8.7, but the odds ratio decreased significantly across the DPI tertiles [61]. In our study, the observed DPI was 5 or more units less than in the aforementioned studies. This difference could influence the direction and strength of the relationship between the DPI and respiratory function, inspiratory muscle strength and function, or peripheral muscle strength in the present study. In addition, our patients were not newly diagnosed with COPD, but had a history of 6 to 30 years. It must be emphasized that studies on the DPI in patients with chronic non-communicable diseases have used different dietary methods (FFQ, dietary records, or 24 h recalls), which may influence the estimation of the DPI.

If we look at the contribution of the different phytochemical-rich food groups to the DPI, we can see that the whole grain group contributes 10 times less to the DPI in the first tertile than in the third tertile, which is the opposite for the vegetable group. The food groups that contributed most to the DPI in the first tertile were fruit, vegetables, and other phytochemical-rich foods; in the second tertile, fruit, other phytochemical-rich foods, and whole grains; and in the third tertile, whole grains, fruit, and other phytochemical-rich foods. The phytochemical-rich food group in our study consisted of herbs, spices, coffee, tea, soy products, cocoa, beer and wine, and olive oil. According to the available literature, only one study in the last five years has shown the contribution of food group to the DPI [104]. In younger adults (18–35 years) with diabetes mellitus type 1, fruit contributed over 50% and vegetables over 20% to the DPI, but the authors did not present differences in the contribution of food groups between tertiles of patients. In this study, an association was found between the DPI and a lower risk of hypoglycemia and low high-density lipoprotein cholesterol, but not with other cardiometabolic risk factors [104]. The other studies in which the results of differences in food group consumption between tertiles or quartiles of the DPI were presented as daily energy intake (kcal/day), contribution to daily energy intake (% kcal/day), or amount (g/day). It is therefore difficult to identify similarities and differences between the populations studied. However, it must be emphasized that fruit and vegetable intake increases across tertiles/quartiles along with whole grain intake, except in the study of women with breast cancer, where fruit and vegetable intake was similar across quartiles [42,45,47–49,54,56,58,60,61]. We hypothesized that patients in higher tertiles of the DPI would have a higher intake of fruits, vegetables, and whole grains, which could impact better health outcomes in COPD. The hypothesis was based on the knowledge that whole grains are a good source of fiber, and it has been found that people who have higher intake of fiber per day have a lower risk of COPD [80,82,105]. However, the present study did not examine the total fiber intake, but only the energy from whole grains and their products. Furthermore, the present study did not examine the combined fruit and vegetable intake in grams per day. Fruit and vegetable intake was one variable of the DPI, and its contribution to the DPI was presented separately. A higher intake of fruit and vegetables may be beneficial for COPD patients, but the effects of their independent consumption on COPD risk or outcomes are inconsistent [80,83,105–107]. In addition, certain fruits and vegetables appear to have a different impact on COPD outcomes [21,108]. It must also be emphasized that we did not observe the consumption of other food groups such as cured or processed meat or fish, which could alter the effects on COPD outcomes [11,82,109,110]. Therefore, future work should take a broader dimension and, in addition to the intake of foods that contribute to the intake of phytochemicals, also investigate other nutritional parameters to assess the full contribution of these foods.

When interpreting the results, we must be aware that this is a cross-sectional study with limited ability to observe a causal relationship between the DPI and COPD outcomes. The sample size and pattern may influence the results of this study. Even though we had a sample that allows the observation of the association between the DPI and COPD outcomes, the sample is small and consists mainly of middle-aged men. The present study population was not newly diagnosed patients with COPD, but patients who have been suffering from COPD for 6 to 30 years. In addition, the majority of our patients had an adequate BMI and a normal SMI. Moreover, the energy intake of the participants in our sample was low, whereas energy intake and energy intake from photochemical-rich foods are the main variables of the DPI. Energy intake was observed using 24 h recalls, which may be biased by the cognitive abilities of elderly patients. To compensate for the potential bias due to daily variation in food intake, we collected three 24 h recalls on non-consecutive days [111]. In addition, the patients did not know exactly on which day they would be interviewed for the 24 h recalls in order to minimize the change in their daily routine and eating habits. However, we did not account for potential seasonal variation. One of the major strengths of the present study was the assessment of objective measures using spirometry, which is the gold standard of the COPD diagnostic protocol [62]. Also, except for respiratory function, we objectively measured the strength and function of inspiratory muscles and the strength of the peripheral muscles, which are important factors in the progression of COPD and mortality [89,90].

5. Conclusions

In conclusion, we found a relation between respiratory function, inspiratory muscle strength and function, and peripheral muscle strength with the intake of phytochemicals observed with the dietary phytochemical index. However, our results suggest that phytochemical intake may be inversely associated with diaphragm thickness. It is desirable that future research include a prospective cohort study and controlled clinical trials to investigate the long-term effects of phytochemical intake in patients with COPD and to determine the benefits of increased intake of foods rich in phytochemicals for nutritional therapy in these patients. However, the insights of this study support the promotion of the consumption of foods high in phytochemicals in a nutritional education program as part of COPD rehabilitation.

Author Contributions: Conceptualization, A.R., S.B.M. and I.R.; methodology, A.R., A.I., S.B.M. and I.R.; software, A.I.; formal analysis, A.I.; investigation, A.R. and S.B.M.; data curation, A.I.; writing—original draft preparation, A.R. and A.I.; writing—review and editing, A.R. and A.I.; visualization, A.I.; supervision, I.R. All authors have read and agreed to the published version of the manuscript.

Funding: This research received no external funding.

Institutional Review Board Statement: This study was conducted in accordance with the Declaration of Helsinki and approved by the Ethics Committee of the School of Medicine, University of Zagreb (reference number: 251-59-10106-23-111/203, class: 641-01/23-02/01, date: 17 November 2023).

Informed Consent Statement: Informed consent was obtained from all subjects involved in this study.

Data Availability Statement: The data presented in this study are available on request from the corresponding author, as they are required for the further analysis of the dissertation.

Acknowledgments: The authors would like to thank the medical staff of the Special Hospital for Pulmonary Diseases for their cooperation and support in collecting data for this study. In addition, the authors would like to thank volunteer Antonija Karić, graduate student in Nutrition at the Faculty of Food Technology and Biotechnology, University of Zagreb, for her assistance in dietary assessment.

Conflicts of Interest: The authors declare no conflicts of interest.

References

1. Celli, B.; Fabbri, L.; Criner, G.; Martinez, F.J.; Mannino, D.; Vogelmeier, C.; Montes de Oca, M.; Papi, A.; Sin, D.D.; Han, M.K.; et al. Definition and nomenclature of chronic obstructive pulmonary disease: Time for its revision. *Am. J. Respir. Crit. Care Med.* **2022**, *206*, 1317–1325. [CrossRef] [PubMed]
2. Mannino, D.M.; Buist, A.S. Global burden of COPD: Risk factors, prevalence, and future trends. *Lancet* **2007**, *370*, 765–773. [CrossRef] [PubMed]
3. May, S.M.; Li, J.T.C. Burden of chronic obstructive pulmonary disease: Healthcare costs and beyond. *Allergy Asthma Proc.* **2015**, *36*, 4–10. [CrossRef]
4. Safiri, S.; Carson-Chahhoud, K.; Noori, M.; Nejadghaderi, S.A.; Sullman, M.J.M.; Ahmadian Heris, J.; Ansarin, K.; Mansournia, M.A.; Collins, G.S.; Kolahi, A.-A.; et al. Burden of chronic obstructive pulmonary disease and its attributable risk factors in 204 countries and territories, 1990–2019: Results from the Global Burden of Disease Study 2019. *BMJ* **2022**, *378*, e069679. [CrossRef]
5. Halpin, D.M.G.; Celli, B.R.; Criner, G.J.; Frith, P.; López Varela, M.V.; Salvi, S.; Vogelmeier, C.F.; Chen, R.; Mortimer, K.; Montes de Oca, M.; et al. The GOLD Summit on chronic obstructive pulmonary disease in low- and middle-income countries. *Int. J. Tuberc. Lung Dis.* **2019**, *23*, 1131–1141. [CrossRef]
6. Rochester, C.L.; Vogiatzis, I.; Holland, A.E.; Lareau, S.C.; Marciniuk, D.D.; Puhan, M.A.; Spruit, M.A.; Masefield, S.; Casaburi, R.; Clini, E.M.; et al. An Official American Thoracic Society/European Respiratory Society Policy Statement: Enhancing implementation, use, and delivery of pulmonary rehabilitation. *Am. J. Respir. Crit. Care Med.* **2015**, *192*, 1373–1386. [CrossRef]
7. Vermeeren, M.A.P.; Creutzberg, E.C.; Schols, A.M.W.J.; Postma, D.S.; Pieters, W.R.; Roldaan, A.C.; Wouters, E.F.M. Prevalence of nutritional depletion in a large out-patient population of patients with COPD. *Respir. Med.* **2006**, *100*, 1349–1355. [CrossRef] [PubMed]
8. Bell, K.; Lawson, J.; Penz, E.; Cammer, A. Systematic review of tailored dietary advice and dietitian involvement in the treatment of chronic obstructive pulmonary disease (COPD). *Respir. Med.* **2024**, *225*, 107584. [CrossRef]
9. Keogh, E.; Mark Williams, E. Managing malnutrition in COPD: A review. *Respir. Med.* **2021**, *176*, 106248. [CrossRef]
10. Parvizian, M.K.; Dhaliwal, M.; Li, J.; Satia, I.; Kurmi, O.P. Relationship between dietary patterns and COPD: A systematic review and meta-analysis. *ERJ Open Res.* **2020**, *6*, 168–2019. [CrossRef]
11. Zhai, H.; Wang, Y.; Jiang, W. Fruit and vegetable intake and the risk of chronic obstructive pulmonary disease: A dose-response meta-analysis of observational studies. *BioMed Res. Int.* **2020**, *2020*, 3783481. [CrossRef] [PubMed]
12. Zheng, P.-F.; Shu, L.; Si, C.-J.; Zhang, X.-Y.; Yu, X.-L.; Gao, W. Dietary patterns and chronic obstructive pulmonary disease: A meta-analysis. *COPD J. Chronic Obstr. Pulm. Dis.* **2016**, *13*, 515–522. [CrossRef] [PubMed]
13. Gutiérrez-Carrasquilla, L.; Sánchez, E.; Hernández, M.; Polanco, D.; Salas-Salvadó, J.; Betriu, À.; Gaeta, A.M.; Carmona, P.; Purroy, F.; Pamplona, R.; et al. Effects of mediterranean diet and physical activity on pulmonary function: A cross-sectional analysis in the ILERVAS Project. *Nutrients* **2019**, *11*, 329. [CrossRef] [PubMed]
14. Ardestani, M.E.; Onvani, S.; Esmailzadeh, A.; Feizi, A.; Azadbakht, L. Adherence to Dietary Approaches to Stop Hypertension (DASH) dietary pattern in relation to chronic obstructive pulmonary disease (COPD): A case–control study. *J. Am. Coll. Nutr.* **2017**, *36*, 549–555. [CrossRef]
15. Fischer, A.; Johansson, I.; Blomberg, A.; Sundström, B. Adherence to a mediterranean-like diet as a protective factor against COPD: A nested case-control study. *COPD J. Chronic Obstr. Pulm. Dis.* **2019**, *16*, 272–277. [CrossRef]
16. Wen, J.; Gu, S.; Wang, X.; Qi, X. Associations of adherence to the DASH diet and the Mediterranean diet with chronic obstructive pulmonary disease among US adults. *Front. Nutr.* **2023**, *10*, 1031071. [CrossRef]
17. Trichopoulou, A.; Martínez-González, M.A.; Tong, T.Y.; Forouhi, N.G.; Khandelwal, S.; Prabhakaran, D.; Mozaffarian, D.; de Lorgeril, M. Definitions and potential health benefits of the Mediterranean diet: Views from experts around the world. *BMC Med.* **2014**, *12*, 112. [CrossRef]
18. Challa, H.J.; Ameer, M.A.; Uppaluri, K. *DASH Diet to Stop Hypertension*; StatPearls Publishing: Treasure Island, FL, USA, 2020.
19. Meteran, H.; Thomsen, S.F.; Miller, M.R.; Hjelmborg, J.; Sigsgaard, T.; Backer, V. Self-reported intake of fruit and vegetables and risk of chronic obstructive pulmonary disease: A nation-wide twin study. *Respir. Med.* **2018**, *144*, 16–21. [CrossRef] [PubMed]
20. Boeing, H.; Bechthold, A.; Bub, A.; Ellinger, S.; Haller, D.; Kroke, A.; Leschik-Bonnet, E.; Müller, M.J.; Oberritter, H.; Schulze, M.; et al. Critical review: Vegetables and fruit in the prevention of chronic diseases. *Eur. J. Nutr.* **2012**, *51*, 637–663. [CrossRef]
21. Kaluza, J.; Larsson, S.C.; Orsini, N.; Linden, A.; Wolk, A. Fruit and vegetable consumption and risk of COPD: A prospective cohort study of men. *Thorax* **2017**, *72*, 500–509. [CrossRef]
22. Ahmad, A.; Shameem, M.; Husain, Q. Altered oxidant-antioxidant levels in the disease prognosis of chronic obstructive pulmonary disease. *Int. J. Tuberc. Lung Dis.* **2013**, *17*, 1104–1109. [CrossRef] [PubMed]

23. Okubo, H.; Shaheen, S.O.; Ntani, G.; Jameson, K.A.; Syddall, H.E.; Aihie Sayer, A.; Dennison, E.M.; Cooper, C.; Robinson, S.M. Processed meat consumption and lung function: Modification by antioxidants and smoking. *Eur. Respir. J.* **2014**, *43*, 972–982. [CrossRef] [PubMed]
24. Keranis, E.; Makris, D.; Rodopoulou, P.; Martinou, H.; Papamakarios, G.; Daniil, Z.; Zintzaras, E.; Gourgoulianis, K.I. Impact of dietary shift to higher-antioxidant foods in COPD: A randomised trial. *Eur. Respir. J.* **2010**, *36*, 774–780. [CrossRef]
25. Zhai, T.; Li, S.; Hu, W.; Li, D.; Leng, S. Potential micronutrients and phytochemicals against the pathogenesis of chronic obstructive pulmonary disease and lung cancer. *Nutrients* **2018**, *10*, 813. [CrossRef] [PubMed]
26. Hikichi, M.; Mizumura, K.; Maruoka, S.; Gon, Y. Pathogenesis of chronic obstructive pulmonary disease (COPD) induced by cigarette smoke. *J. Thorac. Dis.* **2019**, *11*, S2129–S2140. [CrossRef]
27. Rahman, I. Review: Antioxidant therapeutic advances in COPD. *Ther. Adv. Respir. Dis.* **2008**, *2*, 351–374. [CrossRef]
28. Manochkumar, J.; Singh, A.; Efferth, T.; Ramamoorthy, S. Untapping the protective role of carotenoids against respiratory diseases. *Phytomedicine* **2022**, *104*, 154286. [CrossRef]
29. Mustra Rakic, J.; Wang, X.-D. Role of lycopene in smoke-promoted chronic obstructive pulmonary disease and lung carcinogenesis. *Arch. Biochem. Biophys.* **2020**, *689*, 108439. [CrossRef]
30. Santus, P.; Sola, A.; Carlucci, P.; Fumagalli, F.; Di Gennaro, A.; Mondoni, M.; Carnini, C.; Centanni, S.; Sala, A. Lipid peroxidation and 5-lipoxygenase activity in chronic obstructive pulmonary disease. *Am. J. Respir. Crit. Care Med.* **2005**, *171*, 838–843. [CrossRef]
31. Garcia-Larsen, V.; Potts, J.F.; Omenaas, E.; Heinrich, J.; Svanes, C.; Garcia-Aymerich, J.; Burney, P.G.; Jarvis, D.L. Dietary antioxidants and 10-year lung function decline in adults from the ECRHS survey. *Eur. Respir. J.* **2017**, *50*, 1602286. [CrossRef]
32. Culpitt, S. V Inhibition by red wine extract, resveratrol, of cytokine release by alveolar macrophages in COPD. *Thorax* **2003**, *58*, 942–946. [CrossRef] [PubMed]
33. Donnelly, L.E.; Newton, R.; Kennedy, G.E.; Fenwick, P.S.; Leung, R.H.F.; Ito, K.; Russell, R.E.K.; Barnes, P.J. Anti-inflammatory effects of resveratrol in lung epithelial cells: Molecular mechanisms. *Am. J. Physiol. Cell. Mol. Physiol.* **2004**, *287*, L774–L783. [CrossRef] [PubMed]
34. Shishodia, S.; Potdar, P.; Gairola, C.G.; Aggarwal, B.B. Curcumin (diferuloylmethane) down-regulates cigarette smoke-induced NF- B activation through inhibition of I B kinase in human lung epithelial cells: Correlation with suppression of COX-2, MMP-9 and cyclin D1. *Carcinogenesis* **2003**, *24*, 1269–1279. [CrossRef] [PubMed]
35. Meja, K.K.; Rajendrasozhan, S.; Adenuga, D.; Biswas, S.K.; Sundar, I.K.; Spooner, G.; Marwick, J.A.; Chakravarty, P.; Fletcher, D.; Whittaker, P.; et al. Curcumin Restores Corticosteroid Function in Monocytes Exposed to Oxidants by Maintaining HDAC2. *Am. J. Respir. Cell Mol. Biol.* **2008**, *39*, 312–323. [CrossRef] [PubMed]
36. Leitzmann, C. Characteristics and health benefits of phytochemicals. *Complement. Med. Res.* **2016**, *23*, 69–74. [CrossRef]
37. Monjotin, N.; Amiot, M.J.; Fleurentin, J.; Morel, J.M.; Raynal, S. Clinical evidence of the benefits of phytonutrients in human healthcare. *Nutrients* **2022**, *14*, 1712. [CrossRef]
38. Liu, R.H. Health-promoting components of fruits and vegetables in the diet. *Adv. Nutr.* **2013**, *4*, 384S–392S. [CrossRef]
39. Bohn, T.; McDougall, G.J.; Alegría, A.; Alminger, M.; Arrigoni, E.; Aura, A.; Brito, C.; Cilla, A.; El, S.N.; Karakaya, S.; et al. Mind the gap—Deficits in our knowledge of aspects impacting the bioavailability of phytochemicals and their metabolites—A position paper focusing on carotenoids and polyphenols. *Mol. Nutr. Food Res.* **2015**, *59*, 1307–1323. [CrossRef]
40. Li, Z.; Forester, S.; Jennings-Dobbs, E.; Heber, D. Perspective: A comprehensive evaluation of data quality in nutrient databases. *Adv. Nutr.* **2023**, *14*, 379–391. [CrossRef]
41. McCarty, M.F. Proposal for a dietary "phytochemical index". *Med. Hypotheses* **2004**, *63*, 813–817. [CrossRef]
42. Amani Tirani, S.; Balali, A.; Kazemi, M.; Askari, G.; Khorvash, F.; Arab, A. The predictive role of the dietary phytochemical index in relation to the clinical and psychological traits of migraine headaches. *Sci. Rep.* **2024**, *14*, 6886. [CrossRef] [PubMed]
43. Park, Y.; Park, K. Phytochemical index and the risk of gastritis/gastric ulcer among Korean adults: A prospective cohort study. *Nutrients* **2024**, *16*, 2514. [CrossRef] [PubMed]
44. Hatami, A.; Ahmadi-Khorram, M.; Keykhaei, F.; Hashemi, M.; Javid, R.; Hashempour, M.; Esfehani, A.J.; Nematy, M. Dietary acid load as well as dietary phytochemical index, and association with multiple sclerosis: Results from a case–control study. *BMC Nutr.* **2024**, *10*, 93. [CrossRef] [PubMed]
45. Mousavi, S.N.; Nouri, M.; Yousefi Rad, E.; Kazemi, R.; Birjandi, M.; Coe, S.; Saboori, S. Association between dietary phytochemical index and risk of benign prostatic hyperplasia: A case-control study. *J. Health Popul. Nutr.* **2024**, *43*, 35. [CrossRef] [PubMed]
46. Mahmoodi, M.; Mohammadi, F.; Rajabzadeh-Dehkordi, M.; Jalilpiran, Y.; Makhtoomi, M.; Nouri, M.; Faghih, S. The association between healthy diet indicator and phytochemical index with prostate cancer odds ratio: A case-control study. *J. Health Popul. Nutr.* **2024**, *43*, 116. [CrossRef]
47. Bentyaghoob, S.; Dehghani, F.; Alimohammadi, A.; Shateri, Z.; Kahrizsangi, M.A.; Nejad, E.T.; Nouri, M.; Rashidkhani, B. Oxidative balance score and dietary phytochemical index can reduce the risk of colorectal cancer in Iranian population. *BMC Gastroenterol.* **2023**, *23*, 183. [CrossRef]
48. Rigi, S.; Shayanfar, M.; Mousavi, S.M.; Mohammad-Shirazi, M.; Sharifi, G.; Esmaillzadeh, A. Dietary phytochemical index in relation to risk of glioma: A case-control study in Iranian adults. *Nutr. J.* **2021**, *20*, 31. [CrossRef]
49. Ghoreishy, S.M.; Aminianfar, A.; Benisi-Kohansal, S.; Azadbakht, L.; Esmaillzadeh, A. Association between dietary phytochemical index and breast cancer: A case–control study. *Breast Cancer* **2021**, *28*, 1283–1291. [CrossRef]

50. Darabi, Z.; Vasmehjani, A.A.; Salehi-Abargouei, A.; Mirzaei, M.; Hosseinzadeh, M. Dietary phytochemical index and psychological disorders in a large sample of Iranian adults: A population-based study. *J. Health Popul. Nutr.* **2023**, *42*, 126. [CrossRef]
51. Darooghegi Mofrad, M.; Siassi, F.; Guilani, B.; Bellissimo, N.; Azadbakht, L. Association of dietary phytochemical index and mental health in women: A cross-sectional study. *Br. J. Nutr.* **2019**, *121*, 1049–1056. [CrossRef]
52. Vasmehjani, A.A.; Darabi, Z.; Nadjarzadeh, A.; Mirzaei, M.; Hosseinzadeh, M. The relation between dietary phytochemical index and metabolic syndrome and its components in a large sample of Iranian adults: A population-based study. *BMC Public Health* **2021**, *21*, 1587. [CrossRef] [PubMed]
53. Yoo, H.; Park, K. Association between phytochemical index and osteoporosis in women: A prospective cohort study in Korea. *Nutrients* **2023**, *15*, 1605. [CrossRef]
54. Amirkhizi, F.; Ghoreishy, S.M.; Hamedi-Shahraki, S.; Asghari, S. Higher dietary phytochemical index is associated with lower odds of knee osteoarthritis. *Sci. Rep.* **2022**, *12*, 9059. [CrossRef] [PubMed]
55. Mehranfar, S.; Jalilpiran, Y.; Ejtahed, H.-S.; Seif, E.; Shahrestanaki, E.; Mahdavi-Gorabi, A.; Esmaeili-Abdar, M.; Larijani, B.; Qorbani, M. Association of dietary phytochemical index with cardiometabolic risk factors. *Int. J. Vitam. Nutr. Res.* **2022**, *93*, 559–576. [CrossRef] [PubMed]
56. Rigi, S.; Mousavi, S.M.; Shakeri, F.; Keshteli, A.H.; Benisi-Kohansal, S.; Saadatnia, M.; Esmaillzadeh, A. Dietary phytochemical index in relation to risk of stroke: A case-control study. *Nutr. Neurosci.* **2022**, *25*, 2239–2246. [CrossRef]
57. Golzarand, M.; Bahadoran, Z.; Mirmiran, P.; Sadeghian-Sharif, S.; Azizi, F. Dietary phytochemical index is inversely associated with the occurrence of hypertension in adults: A 3-year follow-up (the Tehran Lipid and Glucose Study). *Eur. J. Clin. Nutr.* **2015**, *69*, 392–398. [CrossRef]
58. Gamba, M.; Pano, O.; Raguindin, P.F.; Roa-Diaz, Z.M.; Muka, T.; Glisic, M.; Franco, O.H.; Marques-Vidal, P. Association between total Dietary Phytochemical Intake and cardiometabolic health outcomes—Results from a 10-year follow-up on a middle-aged cohort population. *Nutrients* **2022**, *15*, 4793. [CrossRef]
59. Pourreza, S.; Mirzababaei, A.; Naeini, F.; Naghshi, S.; Mirzaei, K. Association of dietary phytochemical index with metabolically unhealthy overweight/obesity phenotype among Iranian women: A cross-sectional study. *Front. Nutr.* **2022**, *9*, 959341. [CrossRef]
60. Asgari, E.; Jayedi, A.; Dehghani Firouzabadi, F.; Noruzi, Z.; Farazi, M.; Djafarian, K.; Shab-Bidar, S. Association of the dietary phytochemical index with general and central obesity in a sample of Iranian adults. *J. Funct. Foods* **2021**, *83*, 104546. [CrossRef]
61. Salehi-sahlabadi, A.; Teymoori, F.; Mokhtari, E.; Taghiyar, M.; Hekmatdoost, A.; Mirmiran, P. Dietary phytochemical index and the risk of non-alcoholic fatty liver disease: A case-control study among Iranian adults. *Complement. Ther. Med.* **2022**, *71*, 102881. [CrossRef]
62. Venkatesan, P. GOLD COPD report: 2024 update. *Lancet Respir. Med.* **2024**, *12*, 15–16. [CrossRef] [PubMed]
63. Kaić-Rak, A.; Antonić, K. *Tablice o Sastavu Namirnica i Pića*; Zavod za zaštitu zdravlja SR Hrvatske: Zagreb, Croatia, 1990.
64. van Klaveren, J.D.; Goedhart, P.W.; Wapperom, D.; van der Voet, H. A European tool for usual intake distribution estimation in relation to data collection by EFSA. *EFSA Support. Publ.* **2012**, *9*, 300E. [CrossRef]
65. World Health Organization The Global Health Observatory—Body Mass Index. Available online: https://www.who.int/data/gho/data/themes/topics/topic-details/GHO/body-mass-index (accessed on 17 September 2024).
66. Cederholm, T.; Barazzoni, R.; Austin, P.; Ballmer, P.; Biolo, G.; Bischoff, S.; Compher, C.; Correia, I.; Higashiguchi, T.; Holst, M.; et al. ESPEN guidelines on definitions and terminology of clinical nutrition. *Clin. Nutr.* **2017**, *36*, 49–64. [CrossRef] [PubMed]
67. Moore, V.C. Spirometry: Step by step. *Breathe* **2012**, *8*, 232–240. [CrossRef]
68. Sachs, M.C.; Enright, P.L.; Hinckley, K.D.; Jiang, R.; Barr, R.G. Performance of maximum inspiratory pressure tests and maximum inspiratory pressure reference equations for 4 race/ethnic groups. *Respir. Care* **2009**, *54*, 1321–1328.
69. Rodrigues, A.; Da Silva, M.L.; Berton, D.C.; Cipriano, G.; Pitta, F.; O'Donnell, D.E.; Neder, J.A. Maximal inspiratory pressure: Does the choice of reference values matter? *Chest* **2017**, *152*, 32–39. [CrossRef]
70. Carrillo-Esper, R.; Perez-Calatayud, A.A.; Arch-Tirado, E.; Diaz-Carrillo, M.A.; Garrido-Aguirre, E.; Tapia-Velazco, R.; Pena-Perez, C.A.; Los Monteros, I.E.; Meza-Marquez, J.M.; Flores-Rivera, O.I.; et al. Standardization of sonographic diaphragm thickness evaluations in healthy volunteers. *Respir. Care* **2016**, *61*, 920–924. [CrossRef]
71. Boussuges, A.; Rives, S.; Finance, J.; Chaument, G.; Vallee, N.; Risso, J.-J.; Bregeon, F. Ultrasound assessment of diaphragm thickness and thickening: Reference values and limits of normality when in a seated position. *Front. Med.* **2021**, *8*, 742703. [CrossRef]
72. Filipec, M.; Lončarić Kelečić, A.; Jurinić, A. *Dinamometrija*; Libertas međunarodno sveučilište: Zagreb, Croatia, 2020.
73. Anandan, J.; Dwivedi, D.P.; Govindaraj, V. Clinical phenotypes of COPD and their impact on quality of life: A cross-sectional study. *Respir. Med.* **2023**, *220*, 107452. [CrossRef]
74. Zhou, Y.; Ampon, M.; Abramson, M.; James, A.; Maguire, G.P.; Wood-Baker, R.; Johns, D.; Marks, G.B.; Reddel, H.K.; Toelle, B.G. Respiratory symptoms, disease burden, and quality of life in Australian adults according to GOLD spirometry grades: Data from the BOLD Australia Study. *Int. J. Chronic Obstr. Pulm. Dis.* **2023**, *18*, 2839–2847. [CrossRef]
75. Deng, M.; Lu, Y.; Zhang, Q.; Bian, Y.; Zhou, X.; Hou, G. Global prevalence of malnutrition in patients with chronic obstructive pulmonary disease: Systemic review and meta-analysis. *Clin. Nutr.* **2023**, *42*, 848–858. [CrossRef] [PubMed]
76. Fekete, M.; Fazekas-Pongor, V.; Balazs, P.; Tarantini, S.; Szollosi, G.; Pako, J.; Nemeth, A.N.; Varga, J.T. Effect of malnutrition and body composition on the quality of life of COPD patients. *Physiol. Int.* **2021**, *108*, 238–250. [CrossRef] [PubMed]

77. Collins, P.F.; Elia, M.; Stratton, R.J. Nutritional support and functional capacity in chronic obstructive pulmonary disease: A systematic review and meta-analysis. *Respirology* **2013**, *18*, 616–629. [CrossRef]
78. Lattanzi, G.; Lelli, D.; Antonelli Incalzi, R.; Pedone, C. Effect of macronutrients or micronutrients supplementation on nutritional status, physical functional capacity and quality of life in patients with COPD: A systematic review and meta-analysis. *J. Am. Nutr. Assoc.* **2024**, *43*, 473–487. [CrossRef]
79. Fekete, M.; Csípő, T.; Fazekas-Pongor, V.; Bálint, M.; Csizmadia, Z.; Tarantini, S.; Varga, J. The possible role of food and diet in the quality of life in patients with COPD—A state-of-the-art review. *Nutrients* **2023**, *15*, 3902. [CrossRef] [PubMed]
80. Hirayama, F.; Lee, A.H.; Binns, C.W.; Zhao, Y.; Hiramatsu, T.; Tanikawa, Y.; Nishimura, K.; Taniguchi, H. Do vegetables and fruits reduce the risk of chronic obstructive pulmonary disease? A case–control study in Japan. *Prev. Med.* **2009**, *49*, 184–189. [CrossRef]
81. Shaheen, S.O.; Jameson, K.A.; Syddall, H.E.; Aihie Sayer, A.; Dennison, E.M.; Cooper, C.; Robinson, S.M. The relationship of dietary patterns with adult lung function and COPD. *Eur. Respir. J.* **2010**, *36*, 277–284. [CrossRef]
82. Varraso, R.; Fung, T.T.; Hu, F.B.; Willett, W.; Camargo, C.A. Prospective study of dietary patterns and chronic obstructive pulmonary disease among US men. *Thorax* **2007**, *62*, 786–791. [CrossRef]
83. Tabak, C.; Smit, H.A.; Heederik, D.; Ocké, M.C.; Kromhout, D. Diet and chronic obstructive pulmonary disease: Independent beneficial effects of fruits, whole grains, and alcohol (the MORGEN study). *Clin. Exp. Allergy* **2001**, *31*, 747–755. [CrossRef]
84. Shin, M.-K.; Kwak, S.H.; Park, Y.; Jung, J.Y.; Kim, Y.S.; Kang, Y.A. Association between dietary patterns and chronic obstructive pulmonary disease in Korean adults: The Korean genome and epidemiology study. *Nutrients* **2021**, *13*, 4348. [CrossRef]
85. Rahman, I. Oxidative stress and redox regulation of lung inflammation in COPD. *Eur. Respir. J.* **2006**, *28*, 219–242. [CrossRef] [PubMed]
86. Lin, Y.-C.; Wu, T.-C.; Chen, P.-Y.; Hssieh, L.-Y.; Yeh, S.-L. Comparison of plasma and intake levels of antioxidant nutrients in patients with chronic obstructive pulmonary disease and healthy people in Taiwan: A case-control study. *Asia Pac. J. Clin. Nutr.* **2010**, *19*, 393–401. [PubMed]
87. Sargeant, L.A.; Jaeckel, A.; Wareham, N. Interaction of vitamin C with the relation between smoking and obstructive airways disease in EPIC Norfolk. *Eur. Respir. J.* **2000**, *16*, 397. [CrossRef]
88. Tabak, C.; Arts, I.C.W.; Smith, H.A.; Heederik, D.; Kromhout, D. Chronic obstructive pulmonary disease and intake of catechins, flavonols, and flavones. *Am. J. Respir. Crit. Care Med.* **2001**, *164*, 61–64. [CrossRef]
89. Donaldson, A.V.; Maddocks, M.; Martolini, D.; Pokley, M.I.; Man, W.D.-C. Muscle function in COPD: A complex interplay. *Int. Int. J. Chronic Obstr. Pulm. Dis.* **2012**, *7*, 523–535.
90. Cao, Y.; Li, P.; Wang, Y.; Liu, X.; Wu, W. Diaphragm dysfunction and rehabilitation strategy in patients with chronic obstructive pulmonary disease. *Front. Physiol.* **2022**, *13*, 872277. [CrossRef] [PubMed]
91. Similowski, T.; Yan, S.; Gauthier, A.P.; Macklem, P.T.; Bellemare, F. Contractile properties of the human diaphragm during chronic hyperinflation. *N. Engl. J. Med.* **1991**, *325*, 917–923. [CrossRef]
92. Ottenheijm, C.A.C.; Heunks, L.M.A.; Sieck, G.C.; Zhan, W.-Z.; Jansen, S.M.; Degens, H.; de Boo, T.; Dekhuijzen, P.N.R. Diaphragm dysfunction in chronic obstructive pulmonary disease. *Am. J. Respir. Crit. Care Med.* **2005**, *172*, 200–205. [CrossRef]
93. Supruniuk, E.; Górski, J.; Chabowski, A. Endogenous and exogenous antioxidants in skeletal muscle fatigue development during exercise. *Antioxidants* **2023**, *12*, 501. [CrossRef]
94. European Food Safety Authority Nutrient Recommendations. Available online: https://efsa.gitlab.io/multimedia/drvs/index.htm (accessed on 12 February 2021).
95. Chen, H.I.; Kuo, C.S. Relationship between respiratory muscle function and age, sex, and other factors. *J. Appl. Physiol.* **1989**, *66*, 943–948. [CrossRef]
96. Smargiassi, A.; Inchingolo, R.; Tagliaboschi, L.; Di Marco Berardino, A.; Valente, S.; Corbo, G.M. Ultrasonographic assessment of the diaphragm in chronic obstructive pulmonary disease patients: Relationships with pulmonary function and the influence of body composition—A pilot study. *Respiration* **2014**, *87*, 364–371. [CrossRef] [PubMed]
97. Nishimura, Y.; Tsutsumi, M.; Nakata, H.; Tsunenari, T.; Maeda, H.; Yokoyama, M. Relationship between respiratory muscle strength and lean body mass in men with COPD. *Chest* **1995**, *107*, 1232–1236. [CrossRef] [PubMed]
98. Lista-Paz, A.; Langer, D.; Barral-Fernández, M.; Quintela-del-Río, A.; Gimeno-Santos, E.; Arbillaga-Etxarri, A.; Torres-Castro, R.; Vilaró Casamitjana, J.; Varas de la Fuente, A.B.; Serrano Veguillas, C.; et al. Maximal respiratory pressure reference equations in healthy adults and cut-off points for defining respiratory muscle weakness. *Arch. Bronconeumol.* **2023**, *59*, 813–820. [CrossRef] [PubMed]
99. Malaguti, C.; Napolis, L.M.; VillaÇa, D.; Neder, J.A.; Nery, L.E.; Corso, S.D. Relationship between peripheral muscle structure and function in patients with chronic obstructive pulmonary disease with different nutritional status. *J. Strength Cond. Res.* **2011**, *25*, 1795–1803. [CrossRef] [PubMed]
100. Møgelberg, N.; Tobberup, R.; Møller, G.; Godtfredsen, N.S.; Nørgaard, A.; Andersen, J.R. High-protein diet during pulmonary rehabilitation in patients with chronic obstructive pulmonary disease. *Dan. Med. J.* **2022**, *69*, A03220185. [PubMed]
101. Ahmadi, A.; Eftekhari, M.H.; Mazloom, Z.; Masoompour, M.; Fararooei, M.; Eskandari, M.H.; Mehrabi, S.; Bedeltavana, A.; Famouri, M.; Zare, M.; et al. Fortified whey beverage for improving muscle mass in chronic obstructive pulmonary disease: A single-blind, randomized clinical trial. *Respir. Res.* **2020**, *21*, 216. [CrossRef]
102. Taherkhani, S.; Valaei, K.; Arazi, H.; Suzuki, K. An overview of physical exercise and antioxidant supplementation influences on skeletal muscle oxidative stress. *Antioxidants* **2021**, *10*, 1528. [CrossRef]

103. Rumbak, I.; Ilić, A.; Škorvaga, P.; Brečić, R.; Colić Barić, I.; Bituh, M. Dietary Phytochemical Index in School-Age Children: Sociodemographic and Lifestyle-Related Factors. *Proceedings* **2023**, *91*, 243.
104. Delshad Aghdam, S.; Siassi, F.; Nasli Esfahani, E.; Qorbani, M.; Rajab, A.; Sajjadpour, Z.; Bashiri, A.; Aghayan, M.; Sotoudeh, G. Dietary phytochemical index associated with cardiovascular risk factor in patients with type 1 diabetes mellitus. *BMC Cardiovasc. Disord.* **2021**, *21*, 293. [CrossRef]
105. Butler, L.M.; Koh, W.-P.; Lee, H.-P.; Yu, M.C.; London, S.J. Dietary fiber and reduced cough with phlegm. *Am. J. Respir. Crit. Care Med.* **2004**, *170*, 279–287. [CrossRef]
106. Walda, I.; Tabak, C.; Smit, H.; Räsänen, L.; Fidanza, F.; Menotti, A.; Nissinen, A.; Feskens, E.; Kromhout, D. Diet and 20-year chronic obstructive pulmonary disease mortality in middle-aged men from three European countries. *Eur. J. Clin. Nutr.* **2002**, *56*, 638–643. [CrossRef] [PubMed]
107. Miedema, I.; Feskens, E.J.M.; Heederik, D.; Kromhout, D. Dietary determinants oflong-term uncidence of chronic nonspecific lung diseases. *Am. J. Epidemiol.* **1993**, *138*, 37–45. [CrossRef] [PubMed]
108. Butland, B.K. Diet, lung function, and lung function decline in a cohort of 2512 middle aged men. *Thorax* **2000**, *55*, 102–108. [CrossRef]
109. Varraso, R.; Fung, T.T.; Barr, R.G.; Hu, F.B.; Willett, W.; Camargo, C.A. Prospective study of dietary patterns and chronic obstructive pulmonary disease among US women. *Am. J. Clin. Nutr.* **2007**, *86*, 488–495. [CrossRef]
110. Tabak, C.; Feskens, E.; Heederik, D.; Kromhout, D.; Menotti, A.; Blackburn, H. Fruit and fish consumption: A possible explanation for population differences in COPD mortality (The Seven Countries Study). *Eur. J. Clin. Nutr.* **1998**, *52*, 819–825. [CrossRef] [PubMed]
111. Lee, R.D.; Neiman, D.C. *Nutritional Assessment*, 6th ed.; McGraw-Hill: Boston, MA, USA, 2003; ISBN 9780077475222.

nutrients MDPI

Article

Metabolite Profiling of *Allium hookeri* Leaves Using UHPLC-qTOF-MS/MS and the Senomorphic Activity of Phenolamides

Thi-Phuong Doan, Mi Zhang, Jin-Pyo An, Jorge-Eduardo Ponce-Zea, Van-Hieu Mai, Byeol Ryu, Eun-Jin Park and Won-Keun Oh *

Research Institute of Pharmaceutical Sciences, College of Pharmacy, Seoul National University, Seoul 08826, Republic of Korea; phuongdoan@snu.ac.kr (T.-P.D.); mintazhang@snu.ac.kr (M.Z.); ntopjp77@gmail.com (J.-P.A.); jepz210689@snu.ac.kr (J.-E.P.-Z.); maihieu@snu.ac.kr (V.-H.M.); estrella56@snu.ac.kr (B.R.); eunjin_p@snu.ac.kr (E.-J.P.)

* Correspondence: wkoh1@snu.ac.kr; Tel.: +82-2-880-7872

Abstract: The plant *Allium hookeri*, a member of the *Allium* genus, has a rich history of culinary and medicinal use. Recent studies have unveiled its potent antioxidant and anti-inflammatory properties. While research on *A. hookeri* has demonstrated its neuroprotective and anti-neuroinflammatory effects, the specific bioactive compounds responsible for these effects remain unidentified in prior research. This study utilized an untargeted metabolomic approach, employing HRESI-qTOF MS/MS-based molecular networking, to comprehensively profile the chemical composition of metabolites in *A. hookeri* and identify new compounds within the plant. As a result, ten compounds, comprising one novel flavonoid (**2**) and nine known compounds (**1** and **3–10**), were isolated and identified through NMR analysis. The inhibitory effects of all isolated compounds on the senescent cell-associated secretory phenotype (SASP), which is pivotal in neuroprotective actions, were evaluated. Biological activity testing revealed *N-trans*-feruloyltyramine (**7**) to be the most potent compound, effectively inhibiting SASP markers and contributing to the senomorphic activities of *A. hookeri*. These findings underscore the potential of phenolamides from *A. hookeri* as a promising source of bioactive compounds for mitigating senescence-associated diseases.

Keywords: *Allium hookeri*; *N-trans*-feruloyltyramine; senomorphic effect; SASP inhibitor

1. Introduction

The *Allium* genus, which is the largest within the Amaryllidaceae family, comprises over 900 species [1], including well-recognized vegetables like onion (*A. cepa*), garlic (*A. sativum*), chives (*A. schoenoprasum*), leeks (*A. ampeloprasum* var. *porrum*), and rakkyo (*A. chinense*) [2]. *Allium hookeri* Thwaites, commonly known as hooker chive or wide-leaf chives, represent a herbaceous plant indigenous to regions such as India, Sri Lanka, Myanmar, Bhutan, southwestern China [3,4], and Nepal [5]. Its recent expansion has extended into the southern areas of Korea beginning in 2012 [6–8]. Due to the distinctive flavor characteristic of the *Allium* genus, both the leaves and fleshy roots of *A. hookeri* are used as vegetables, holding particular significance for the locals and serving as spices or supplementary foods [5,9]. Traditionally, the roots have been utilized by local communities in India for treating coughs, colds, burns, injuries, eruptions of the skin, and wound healing [5,10]. The leaves of *A. hookeri* are also employed for medicinal purposes, including the treatment of stomach ulcers, fever reduction, and blood pressure management [5,10]. Extensive studies on the roots of *A. hookeri* have unveiled regulatory effects against asthmatic changes [11], as well as antioxidant, neuroprotective [8,12,13], antimicrobial [14], anti-diabetic [15,16], immunomodulatory [17], anti-inflammatory [18,19], and bone-forming activities [20]. Additionally, the leaves of *A. hoookeri* also exhibited anti-obesity [21], anti-inflammatory, and immunomodulating effects [17]. The phytochemical profile of *A. hookeri* includes organosulphur compounds [22], flavonoids [23], fatty acids, phenolic, and polyphenols [12,14,23,24], and essential oils [25]. Despite the numerous reported activities of *A. hookeri*, only a few studies have established a direct link between compounds and their biological activities, such as fatty acids, phenolic and polyphenolic compounds with antimicrobial activity [14] and phenolic compounds with antioxidant properties [12].

The aging of the global population is becoming an increasingly significant medical concern. While life expectancy has increased over the past century, the additional years gained have not necessarily translated into a state of good health, especially for individuals aged 60 years and older [26]. In response to the challenges posed by population aging, the World Health Organization (WHO) has formulated a definition of healthy aging, describing it as a process of developing and maintaining functional abilities that contribute to well-being in older age [27]. Furthermore, the United Nations has designated the period from 2021 to 2030 as the UN Decade of Healthy Ageing [26]. The "hallmarks" of aging refer to the accumulation of damage, including genomic instability, telomere attrition, epigenetic alterations, the loss of proteostasis, mitochondrial dysfunctions, deregulated nutrient sensing, cellular senescence, stem cell exhaustion, and altered intercellular communication [28]. Among these hallmarks, cellular senescence, characterized by irreversible cell cycle arrest, the expression of senescence-associated beta-galactosidase (SA-β-gal), and the senescence-associated secretory phenotype (SASP) [29], plays a significant role in complex biological processes related to aging and age-related disorders [30]. Cellular senescence also plays a crucial role in the wound-healing process, involving inflammation, new tissue formation, and tissue remodeling as a physiological response to tissue injury [31]. While senescent fibroblasts contribute positively to wound healing by limiting any excess collagen deposition through the SASP, which includes collagen-degrading matrix metalloproteinases (MMPs) [32], their persistent presence in chronic wounds impedes closure. This persistence is marked by senescence indicators, oxidative stress, and proinflammatory cytokines in fibroblasts, highlighting their role in chronic wound pathology [33,34]. As individuals age, senescent cells tend to accumulate in tissues and organs, thereby contributing to the development of age-related diseases or chronic wounds [30]. The removal of senescent cells from tissues and organs may represent a crucial strategy for preventing and treating age-related diseases, thereby increasing the health span [28]. Senotherapeutics achieve their effect by targeting the following two approaches: eliminating senescent cells (senolytics) or inhibiting senescent phenotypes such as SA-β-gal or SASP secretion (senomorphics) [28]. To date, numerous natural products, such as quercetin, fisetin, piperlongumine, and the curcumin analog, have been recognized as senolytic agents [35]. Additionally, natural senomorphics like rapamycin, resveratrol, kaempferol, apigenin, and epigallocatechin gallate (EGCG) have been documented [36], indicating the potential of natural products as a promising source for senotherapeutic drug discovery.

This study aimed to investigate the phytochemical constituents in *A. hookeri* leaves using an untargeted metabolomic approach, incorporating feature-based molecular networking (FBMN), along with the isolation and characterization of major nodes. Additionally, the research evaluated their senomorphic effects, potentially contributing to their ethnomedicinal use in wound healing and in vitro neuroprotection. This study also sought to identify the key compounds responsible for the senomorphic effects of *A. hookeri*, examining both lipopolysaccharides (LPS)-induced nitric oxide (NO) production and the bleomycin-induced senescence model.

2. Materials and Methods

2.1. Materials

Optical rotations were determined using a JASCO P-2000 polarimeter (JASCO International Co., Ltd., Tokyo, Japan). IR spectra were measured with a Nicolet 6700 FT-IR spectrometer (Thermo Electron Corp., Waltham, MA, USA). NMR data analysis was performed with a JNM-ECA 600 MHz spectrometer (Jeol Ltd., Tokyo, Japan) coupled with a 5 mm CPTCI cryoprobe (Bruker, Germany). For column chromatography, silica gel (Merck KGaA, Darmstadt, Germany, particle size 63–200 μm) and RP-18 (Merck KGaA, particle size 75 μm) were used. Sephadex LH-20 from Sigma-Aldrich (St. Louis, MO, USA) was also used. Thin-layer chromatography (TLC) was conducted using silica gel 60 F_{254} and RP-18 F_{254} plates from Merck KGaA, Darmstadt, Germany. High-performance liquid chromatography (HPLC) was carried out using a Gilson system with a UV detector (at 201 and 254 nm) and an Optima Pak C_{18} column (10 × 250 mm, particle size 5 μm, RS TECH Co., Ltd., Chungcheongbuk-do, Korea).

2.2. Plant Material

A. hookeri was purchased from the commercial stores in March 2019 and was authenticated by Professor W. K. Oh. The samples were dried at room temperature, and a voucher specimen (2019-SNU-12) was deposited in the herbarium at the College of Pharmacy, Seoul National University, Seoul, Republic of Korea.

2.3. UHPLC-qTOF-MS/MS Experiments

The chemical profiling of *A. hookeri* was performed using an Agilent 6530 Q-TOF mass spectrometer equipped with an Agilent 1260 Infinity UHPLC (Agilent Technologies, Santa Clara, CA, USA). The chromatographic analysis utilized a Waters Acquity UHPLC® BEH C18 (100 mm × 2.1 mm, 1.7 μm) maintained at 40 °C, and LC-MS/MS analyses were conducted in the fast data-dependent acquisition (DDA) mode. The chromatographic separation was operated with the gradient of acetonitrile (contained 0.1% formic acid, B)/H_2O (contained 0.1% formic acid, A) as follows: 0–20 min, 10–90% B; 20.1–22 min, 100% B; and 22.1–24.0 min, 10% B. Electrospray ionization (ESI) conditions included an untargeted MS scan from 100 to 1500 m/z in positive and negative ion modes. The instrumental parameters were set as follows: sheath gas temperature, 350 °C; gas flow, 10 L/min; nebulizer pressure, 30 psig. The scan source parameters encompassed the VCap (4000 V), nozzle voltage (1000 V), fragmentor (180 V), skimmer (65 V), and octopole RF peak voltages (750 V) with a collision energy of 50 eV.

2.4. Sample Preparation of A. hookeri for MS/MS Analysis

The fresh leaves of *A. hooker* (5 g) underwent sonication at room temperature for 1.5 h using 20 mL of 70% EtOH (3 times) at room temperature. The combined total extracts were then dried under a vacuum pump and then sequentially chromatographed using Sep-Pak® Plus Short C18 (360 mg Sorbent per Cartridge, 55–105 μm, Waters Corporation, Milford, MA, USA), eluting with H_2O, 25%, 50%, 75%, 90%, and 100% MeOH/H_2O. All the samples were dried and diluted to a final concentration of 2.0 mg/mL with HPLC-grade MeOH for further analysis. Following drying, all samples were diluted at a concentration of 2.0 mg/mL using HPLC-grade MeOH for subsequent analysis. Prior to injection into the mass spectrometer, all samples underwent filtration through a 0.20 μm membrane filter (Advantec, Tokyo Roshi Kaisha, Japan), with each sample injection consisting of 2 μL.

2.5. Extraction and Isolation

The air-dried leaves of *A. hookeri* were cut into small pieces and extracted with 70% EtOH using sonication for 90 min (three times) at room temperature. The resulting combined extract was then suspended in water and applied to a Diaion HP-20 column chromatography (CC). Elution was achieved using a MeOH/H_2O gradient, resulting in the separation of the extract into the following three different fractions: H1 (50% MeOH), H2 (75% MeOH), H3 (100% MeOH). Fraction H3 was further subjected to normal-phase silica gel CC, eluting with an elution gradient of EtOAc/MeOH (2:1, 1:1, to 0:1) to obtain four fractions (N1-N4). Fraction N2, exhibiting the target peaks corresponding to flavones and amides, was further chromatographed on a reverse-phase C_{18} column with a mobile phase of 50–100% MeOH in water to provide 18 sub-fractions (R1-R18). Sub-fraction R2 was then processed through a Sephadex LH-20 column, with elution achieved using 100% MeOH and yielding ten fractions (L1-L10). Fraction L2 was subjected to purification via an HPLC system equipped with an RP C_{18} column, ultimately resulting in the isolation of compound **4** (5.6 mg); fraction L5 provided compound **2** (10.0 mg). Fraction L4 was further processed through an MPLC column, separating it into ten sub-fractions (M1-M10). After the purification of sub-fraction M3 through the HPLC system, compounds **1** (20.0 mg), **3** (5.0 mg), and **7** (3.8 mg) were obtained. Similarly, compounds **9** (4.3 mg) and **10** (8.5 mg) were yielded from sub-fraction M5 through the HPLC system, while sub-fraction M7 contained compounds **5** (12.5 mg), **6** (3.8 mg), and **8** (5.2 mg).

Physicochemical Properties of Isolated Compounds

Apigenin-7-*O*-glucuronide (**1**): pale yellow amorphous powder; $[\alpha]_D^{25} = -32.1$ (*c* 0.1, MeOH); IR (KBr) ν_{max} 3298, 2908, 2818, 1736, 1662, 1607, 1498, 1443, 1349, 1299, 1250, 1175, 1105, 1086, 1061, 1026, 833, 763, 679, 629 cm^{-1}; ^{1}H NMR (pyridine-d_5, 600 MHz) and ^{13}C NMR (pyridine-d_5, 150 MHz): Figures S14 and S15; HRESIMS found *m/z* 477.0899 $[M + H]^+$ (calcd for $C_{21}H_{19}O_{11}$ at 477.0927, *m/z* error—5.87 ppm).

Apigenin-7-*O*-[α-L-rhamnopyranosyl(1→2)]β-D-glucuronic acid methyl ester (**2**): pale yellow amorphous powder; $[\alpha]_D^{25} = -13.4$ (*c* 0.1, MeOH); UV (MeOH) λ_{max} (log ε) 203 (−0.91), 253 (−0.67), 347 (−0.55); IR (KBr) ν_{max} 3370, 2926, 2382, 2357, 2307, 1748, 1658, 1608, 1513, 1443, 1344, 1298, 1248, 1179, 1099, 949, 835, 679, 604 cm^{-1}; ^{1}H NMR (pyridine-d_5, 600 MHz) and ^{13}C NMR (pyridine-d_5, 150 MHz): Table 1; HRESIMS found *m/z* 605.1500 $[M - H]^-$ (calcd. for $C_{28}H_{29}O_{15}$ at 605.1506, *m/z* error—1.0 ppm).

Table 1. ^{1}H and ^{13}C NMR data of compound **2**.

Pos.	**2**	
	δ_C [a]	δ_H (*J* in Hz) [b]
2	165.5	
3	104.5	6.93, s
4	183.3	
5	158.3	
6	95.6	7.20, overlap.
7	163.7	
8	100.8	7.04, s
9	163.4	
10	107.4	
1′	122.4	
2′	129.5	7.85, d (5.1)
3′	117.4	7.19, overlap.
4′	163.3	
5′	117.4	
6′	129.5	
1″	100.0	6.03, d (7.3)
2″	77.8	4.65, t (7.8)
3″	78.7	4.47, t (8.8)
4″	73.3	4.52, t (8.8)
5″	77.5	4.88, d (8.5)
-C=O	170.4	
-$COOCH_3$	52.6	3.62, s
4′-OCH_3		
1‴	103.1	6.45, s
2‴	72.9	4.84, br s
3‴	73.2	4.58, d (7.7)
4‴	74.5	4.38, t (9.1)
5‴	70.6	4.80, m
6‴	19.4	1.85, d (6.0)

[a] Recorded in Pyridine-d_5 at 600 MHz, [b] Recorded in Pyridine-d_5 at 150 MHz.

Apigenin 7-*O*-glucuronide methyl ester (**3**): pale yellow amorphous powder; $[\alpha]_D^{25} = -19.8$ (*c* 0.1, MeOH); IR (KBr) ν_{max} 3725, 3630, 3600, 3316, 2926, 2387, 2352, 2312, 1752, 1618, 1588, 1523, 1468, 1363, 1339, 1248, 1174, 1044, 835, 684, 670, 645 cm^{-1}; ^{1}H NMR (DMSO-d_6, 600 MHz) and ^{13}C NMR (DMSO-d_6, 150 MHz): Figures S17 and S18; HRESIMS found *m/z* 461.1055 $[M + H]^+$ (calcd. for $C_{22}H_{21}O_{11}$ at 461.1084, *m/z* error—6.29 ppm).

Chrysoeriol-7-*O*-*β*-D-glucuronide (**4**): pale yellow amorphous powder; $[\alpha]_D^{25} = +30.7$ (*c* 0.1, MeOH); UV (MeOH) λ_{max} (log *ε*) 252 (−1.95), 350 (−1.85); IR (KBr) ν_{max} 3730, 3620, 3595, 3300, 2946, 2387, 2307, 1748, 1613, 1503, 1418, 1333, 1174, 1039, 689, 670, 645 cm^{-1}; ^{1}H NMR (DMSO-d_6, 500 MHz) and ^{13}C NMR (DMSO-d_6, 125 MHz): Figures S22 and S23; HRESIMS found *m/z* 477.1032 $[M + H]^+$ (calcd. for $C_{22}H_{21}O_{12}$ at 477.1033, *m/z* error—0.2 ppm).

Chrysoeriol-7-*O*-*β*-D-glucuronic acid methyl ester (**5**): pale yellow amorphous powder; $[\alpha]_D^{25} = -64.7$ (*c* 0.1, MeOH); UV (MeOH) λ_{max} (log *ε*) 203 (−0.90), 252 (−0.67), 348 (−0.52); IR (KBr) ν_{max} 3725, 3700, 3625, 3595, 3306, 2966, 2387, 2362, 2342, 2307, 1748, 1513, 1418, 1363, 1333, 1049, 1034, 1014, 689, 674, 649, 615 cm^{-1}; ^{1}H NMR (DMSO-d_6, 600 MHz) and ^{13}C NMR (DMSO-d_6, 150 MHz): Figures S27 and S28; HRESIMS found *m/z* 491.1193 $[M + H]^+$ (calcd. for $C_{23}H_{23}O_{12}$ at 491.1190, *m/z* error 0.61 ppm).

Paprazine (**6**): pale yellow amorphous powder; $[\alpha]_D^{25} = -18.1$ (*c* 0.1, MeOH); IR (KBr) ν_{max} 3717, 3696, 3627, 2972, 2386, 2351, 2302, 146, 1508, 1220, 1051, 818, 673 cm^{-1}; ^{1}H NMR (DMSO-d_6, 500 MHz) and ^{13}C NMR (DMSO-d_6, 125 MHz): Figures S31 and S32; HRESIMS found *m/z* 284.1281 $[M + H]^+$ (calcd. for $C_{17}H_{18}NO_3$ at 284.1287, *m/z* error—2.11 ppm).

N-trans-feruloyltyramine (**7**): pale yellow amorphous powder; $[\alpha]_D^{25} = -24.7$ (*c* 0.1, MeOH); IR (KBr) ν_{max} 3731, 3702, 3627, 3597, 3344, 2942, 2381, 2357, 2307, 1592, 1508, 1265, 1225, 1031, 823, 679 cm^{-1}; ^{1}H NMR (DMSO-d_6, 400 MHz) and ^{13}C NMR (DMSO-d_6, 100 MHz): Figures S35 and S36; HRESIMS found *m/z* 314.1381 $[M + H]^+$ (calcd. for $C_{18}H_{20}NO_4$ at 314.1392, *m/z* error—3.50 ppm).

N-trans-feruloyl-3-*O*-methyldopamine (**8**): pale yellow amorphous powder; $[\alpha]_D^{25} = -13.0$ (*c* 0.1, MeOH); UV (MeOH) λ_{max} (log *ε*) 240 (−1.60), 290 (−1.54), 318 (−1.49); IR (KBr) ν_{max} 3737, 3726, 3702, 3627, 3592, 3305, 2972, 2938, 2381, 2357, 2312, 1752, 1602, 1508, 1269, 1220, 1126, 1036, 689, 669 cm^{-1}; ^{1}H NMR (DMSO-d_6, 600 MHz) and ^{13}C NMR (DMSO-d_6, 150 MHz): Figures S40 and S41; HRESIMS found *m/z* 344.1427 $[M + H]^+$ (calcd. for $C_{19}H_{21}NO_5$ at 344.1420, *m/z* error 2.03 ppm).

5,7,4′-Trimethoxyflavone (**9**): pale yellow amorphous powder; $[\alpha]_D^{25} = -49.1$ (*c* 0.1, MeOH); UV (MeOH) λ_{max} (log *ε*) 230 (−0.85), 265 (−0.62), 328 (−0.56); IR (KBr) ν_{max} 3349, 2942, 2351, 1642, 1607, 1518, 1458, 1424, 1349, 1255, 1220, 1181, 1160, 1126, 1091, 1051, 1026, 837, 673 cm^{-1}; ^{1}H NMR (DMSO-d_6, 600 MHz) and ^{13}C NMR (DMSO-d_6, 150 MHz): Figures S45 and S46; HRESIMS found *m/z* 313.1084 $[M + H]^+$ (calcd. for $C_{18}H_{17}O_5$ at 313.1076, *m/z* error 2.6 ppm).

Diosgenin-3-*O*-[[*β*-D-glucopyranosyl(1→4)]-*α*-L-rhamnopyranosyl(1→4)]-[*α*-L-rhamn opyranosyl(1→2)]]*β*-D-glucopyranoside (**10**): pale yellow amorphous powder; $[\alpha]_D^{25} = -39.4$ (*c* 0.1, MeOH); IR (KBr) ν_{max} 3414, 2933, 2898, 2362, 2312, 1542, 1458, 1378, 1309, 1135, 1036, 907, 828, 673, 645 cm^{-1}; ^{1}H NMR (pyridine-d_5, 500 MHz) and ^{13}C NMR (pyridine-d_5, 125 MHz): Figures S49 and S50; HRESIMS found *m/z* 1031.5406 $[M + H]^+$ (calcd. for $C_{28}H_{29}O_{15}$ at 1031.5427, *m/z* error—2.04 ppm).

2.6. Cell Culture

RAW264.7 cells were generously supplied by Prof. S. H. Sung (Seoul National University, Seoul, Republic of Korea) and were cultured in HyClone Dulbecco's modified Eagle's medium (DMEM) from, (Cytiva, Logan, UT, USA). The culture conditions included incubation at 37 °C in 5% CO_2 and supplementation with 10% fetal bovine serum (FBS), 100 units/mL of penicillin, and 100 μg/mL of streptomycin. Subculturing was conducted every 48 h.

2.7. LPS-Induced NO Production and Cell Viability

The cells were seeded at a density of 5×10^4 cells/well in 96-well plates and allowed to incubate overnight. Once the cells adhered to the wells, lipopolysaccharide (LPS, 1 μg/mL) was added, both with and without the addition of the isolated compounds. After the treatment of the tested compounds, the Griess reagent method was employed to access the nitrate levels, which consisted of a 1:1 ratio of solution A (1% sulfanilamide) and solution B (5% phosphoric acid with 0.1% naphthyl ethylenediamine-HCl). A microplate reader (VersaMax, Molecular Devices, LLC., San Jose, CA, USA) was used to measure the absorbance at 540 nm. A standard nitrite was used to evaluate the nitrite levels in the samples. Cell viability was assessed using a 3-(4,5-dimethyl-2-thiazolyl)-2,5-diphenyl-2H-tetrazolium bromide (MTT) assay. In short, 3T3-L1 adipocytes were seeded and cultured in DMEM with 10% FBS on 96-well plates. After 24 h of incubation, the cells were treated with the test compounds, which were dissolved in a serum-free medium for one day. Subsequently, 20 μL of the 2 mg/mL MTT solution (Sigma) was added to each well and left to incubate in the dark for 4 h. After discarding the supernatant, formazan was dissolved in DMSO, and the absorbance was measured at 550 nm using a microplate reader (VersaMax, Molecular Devices, LLC., San Jose, CA, USA).

2.8. Bleomycin-Induced Senescence Model

The A549 human lung carcinoma epithelial cell line, resembling the type II epithelial-like cell line, was procured from the Korean Cell Line Bank (Seoul, Republic of Korea). The cells were cultured in an RPMI 1640 medium (Welgene, Deajeon, Republic of Korea) supplemented with 10% FBS (Gibco), 100 U of penicillin, and 100 mg/mL of streptomycin (Hyclone). For experiments involving bleomycin-induced senescence, A549 cells were exposed to 5 mg/mL of bleomycin sulfate (Tokyo Chemical Industry Co., Ltd., Tokyo, Japan) for 4 days in a growth medium. To evaluate the senomorphic effect, cells were co-treated with 5 mg/mL of bleomycin and the indicated compounds for 6 days. Then, RNA was extracted to compare the aging-related markers after bleomycin-induced senescence.

Senescence-Associated β-Galactosidase Staining

Cells were subjected to staining with the Senescence β-Glactosidase Staining Kit (#9860, Cell Signaling Technology, Denver, MA, USA) according to the provided guidelines. Following the staining process, the cell samples were examined under an Olympus ix70 microscope (Olympus Corporation, Tokyo, Japan).

2.9. RNA Extraction and Quantitative Real-Time Polymerase Chain Reaction (qRT-PCR)

Human dermal fibroblast (HDF) cells were seeded in a 6-well plate at a density of 80,000 per well. After a 3-day treatment, 250 μL of the TRIzol reagent (Invitrogen, Waltham, MA, USA) was added to each well for total RNA extraction. Subsequently, 1 μg of the total RNA, along with the M-MLV Reverse Transcriptase kit (Bioneer, Daejeon, Republic of Korea), were used for cDNA synthesis in a 20 μL reaction, which was later diluted to 100 μL and utilized as a template in the following real-time qPCR reactions. Real-time qPCR was conducted using the AccuPower® 2X GreenStar™ qPCR Master Mix (Bioneer), and all reactions were executed in triplicate with the expression levels of the markers normalized to the expression level of 18s ribosomal RNA.

2.10. Statistical Analyses

The data underwent analysis through GraphPad PRISM 5 software (GraphPad Software, Inc., La Jolla, CA, USA) and are expressed as the mean ± standard deviation (SD) derived from triplicate experiments. To substantiate comparisons among the group means, an analysis of variance (ANOVA) was applied, followed by Tukey's multiple comparison test for post hoc analysis. Statistical significance was established at a threshold of $p < 0.05$.

3. Results

3.1. Feature-Based Molecular Networking of the *A. hookeri* Leaf Extract

The mass data of the total extract and three fractions (H1–H3) were analyzed using MassHunter software, and the results are shown in Figure S1 (Supplementary Materials) for the positive mode. For the molecular networking analysis, the feature-based molecular networking (FBMN) generated from the GNPS platform was visualized using Cytoscape, as shown in Figure S2 (Supplementary Materials) for the full network and Figure 1A for the clusters of interest.

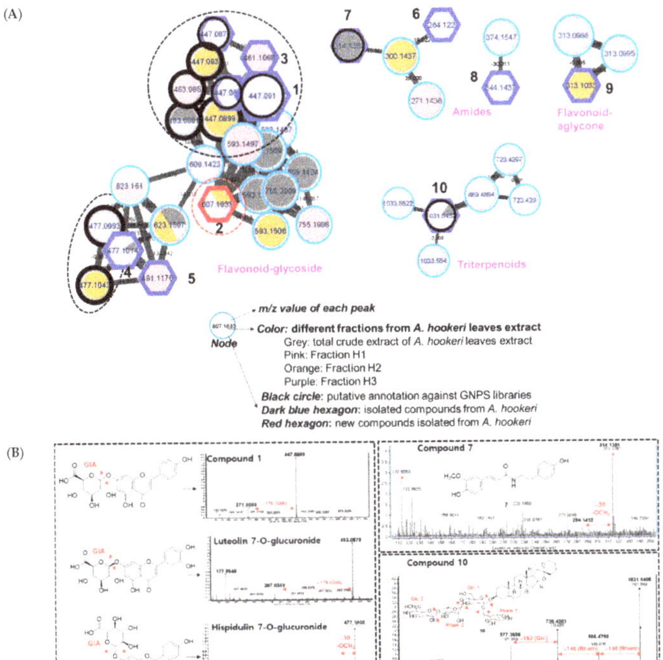

Figure 1. (**A**) Molecular networking of the crude extract, EtOAc, and *n*-BuOH fractions from the leaves of *Allium hookeri* using HRESI-qTOF-MS/MS data recorded in the positive mode. The black frame was assigned using GNPS, and the blue frame for the accuracy of the MN was confirmed by isolating compounds (**1**–**10**) from each cluster and confirming their structures to the physicochemical properties of reported compounds using spectroscopic methods. The red frame shows the new compound **2**, which was first identified from this plant. (**B**) An analysis of the cluster of interest related to flavonoid–glycoside suggested by molecular networking.

As shown in Figure 1A, four clusters of interest were identified, including flavonoid-glycosides, amides, and triterpenoids. In the flavonoid–glycoside cluster, three compounds were annotated using the GNPS platform against the online database of GNPS, namely, apigenin-7-*O*-glucuronide (*m/z* 447 Da), (2*S*,3*S*,4*S*,5*R*,6*S*)-6-[2-(3,4-dihydroxyphenyl)-5-hydroxy-4-oxochromen-7-yl]oxy-3,4,5-trihydroxyoxane-2-carboxylic acid (*m/z* 463 Da), and (2*S*,3*S*,4*S*,5*R*,6*S*)-3,4,5-trihydroxy-6-[5-hydroxy-2-(4-hydroxyphenyl)-6-methoxy-4-oxochromen-7-yl]oxyoxane-2-carboxylic acid (*m/z* 477 Da). The amide cluster displayed the presence of moupinamide (*N-trans*-feruloyltyramine) (*m/z* 314 Da), while the triterpenoid group was suggested to contain the compound β-D-glucopyranoside (3β,22β,25*R*)-26-(β-D-glucopyranosyloxy)-22-hydroxyfurost-5-en-3-yl *O*-6-deoxy-α-L-mannopyranosyl-(1$\rightarrow$2)-*O*-[6-deoxy-α-L-mannopyranosyl-(1$\rightarrow$4)] (*m/z* 1031 Da). The mass data for each putative compound were analyzed in detail to understand their fragmentation pattern, which is exhibited in Figure 1B. Among these annotated compounds, compounds **1**, **7**, and **10** were isolated to confirm their structures.

Compound **1**, observed within the flavonoid–glycoside cluster at an *m/z* value of 447.0899 Da (Figure 1A), was characterized as apigenin-7-*O*-glucuronide via a comparison against GNPS library matching. Additionally, its identification was corroborated via nuclear magnetic resonance (NMR) spectroscopy, referencing previously documented data from the literature [37]. The mass fragmentation analysis of compound **1** and the other identified nodes (black circle) within the flavonoid–glycoside cluster revealed the consistent presence of a glucuronic acid moiety, as evidenced by distinct *m/z* differences of 176 Da in their primary fragments (Figure 1B). A node of *m/z* 461.1068 Da was not assigned against GNPS libraries. However, this node was clustered in the same group as compound **1**, and the mass difference of 14 Da suggests that an additional methoxy (-OCH_3) replaced a hydroxy group. Compound **3** was then isolated, and the structure was confirmed as the apigenin 7-*O*-glucuronide methyl ester via NMR spectra compared to the literature [38] and mass fragmentation analysis (Figure 2A). Similarly, compound **4**, which shared the same *m/z* value but had a different retention time to the annotated compound (2*S*,3*S*,4*S*,5*R*,6*S*)-3,4,5-trihydroxy-6-[5-hydroxy-2-(4-hydroxyphenyl)-6-methoxy-4-oxochromen-7-yl]oxyoxane-2-carboxylic acid was further confirmed by its mass fragments and NMR data to be chrysoeriol-7-*O*-*β*-D-glucuronide [39]. The mass data of compound **5** (*m/z* 491 Da) showed a loss of 191 Da, which is characteristic of a methyl-GlA, a methoxy (30 Da), and a hydroxy (17 Da). Additionally, a mass difference of 14 Da compared to compound **4** indicated that **5** had an additional methyl group attached in the GlA unit to form the methyl GlA ester. Compound **5** was also purified, and the structure was confirmed using NMR and comparing it to the reference, confirming it to be the chrysoeriol-7-*O*-*β*-D-glucuronic acid methyl ester [40]. Compound **9**, situated within a flavonoid–aglycone cluster (Figure 1A) and exhibiting an observed *m/z* value of 313.1084 Da, was conclusively identified as 5,7,4′-trimethoxyflavone. This determination was based on its NMR spectroscopic data, which sufficiently matches the literature report [41] and is further supported by mass fragmentation analysis, which revealed the presence of a fragment with an *m/z* of 287 Da $[M-OCH_3]^+$, as shown in Figure 2A.

An analysis of the fragmentation of **7** suggested that it contained a methoxy unit due to the observation of a *m/z* 30 Da (-OCH_3) loss. Following isolation, NMR elucidation, and comparison with the literature, **7** was identified to be the same as the GNPS assignment of *N*-*trans*-feruloyltyramine [42]. Compound **6** (*m/z* 284 Da) was located in the same cluster as **7** and showed a 30 Da mass difference, indicating the absence of the methoxy group compared to **7**. Compound **6** was isolated, and its NMR confirmed the structure to be paprazine [43]. Compound **8** (*m/z* 344 Da) suggested the presence of an additional methoxy compared to **7**. The NMR of **8** was analyzed and compared with previous reports to identify it as *N*-trans-feruloyl-3-*O*-methyldopamine [43].

In the triterpenoid cluster, compound **10** (*m/z* 1031 Da) was suggested to be diosgenin-3-*O*-[[*β*-D-glucopyranosyl(1→4)]-*α*-L-rhamnopyranosyl(1→4)]-[*α*-L-rhamnopyranosyl(1→2)]] *β*-D-glucopyranoside. The mass fragmentation analysis agreed with the presence of two rhamose (Rham) units, as evidenced by the mass loss at *m/z* 146 Da. It also contained two glucose (Glc) moieties, as indicated by the mass loss at *m/z* 162 Da. After isolation, NMR analysis, and comparison to previous reports, the structure of **10** was confirmed to be annotated [44]. Within this cluster, two nodes with *m/z* values of 1033 Da were observed, differing by two hydrogens from compound **10** yet sharing identical fragments, including those at 577, 739, and 885 Da. The mass loss analysis of these nodes indicates the presence of 2 Glc (−162 Da), 1 Rham (−146 Da), and Arabinose (Ara, −148 Da). This information allows for two possible structural configurations, as displayed in Figure S4A (Supplementary Materials). Similarly, a node at 869.4894 Da within the same cluster displayed fragments indicative of mass losses corresponding to two Rham (146 Da) and a Glc (162 Da). Compared to compound **10**, this node exhibited a mass difference of 162 Da, suggesting the presence of an additional Glc. Consequently, this structure can be assigned to one of nine potential configurations, as illustrated in Figure S4B (Supplementary Materials). Furthermore, within this cluster, two nodes were identified at *m/z* 723.4238 and 723.4296 Da (with retention times of 8.15 and 13.36 min, respectively), indicating a 308 Da mass difference [= 162 (Glc) + 146 (Rham)] in comparison to compound **10**. The mass fragmentation analysis of these two peaks was conducted and searched in SciFinder, revealing 19 possible structural candidates (Figure S4C,D, Supplementary Materials). These predicted compounds vary in their absolute configurations, which cannot be discerned solely through mass analysis.

(A)

(B)

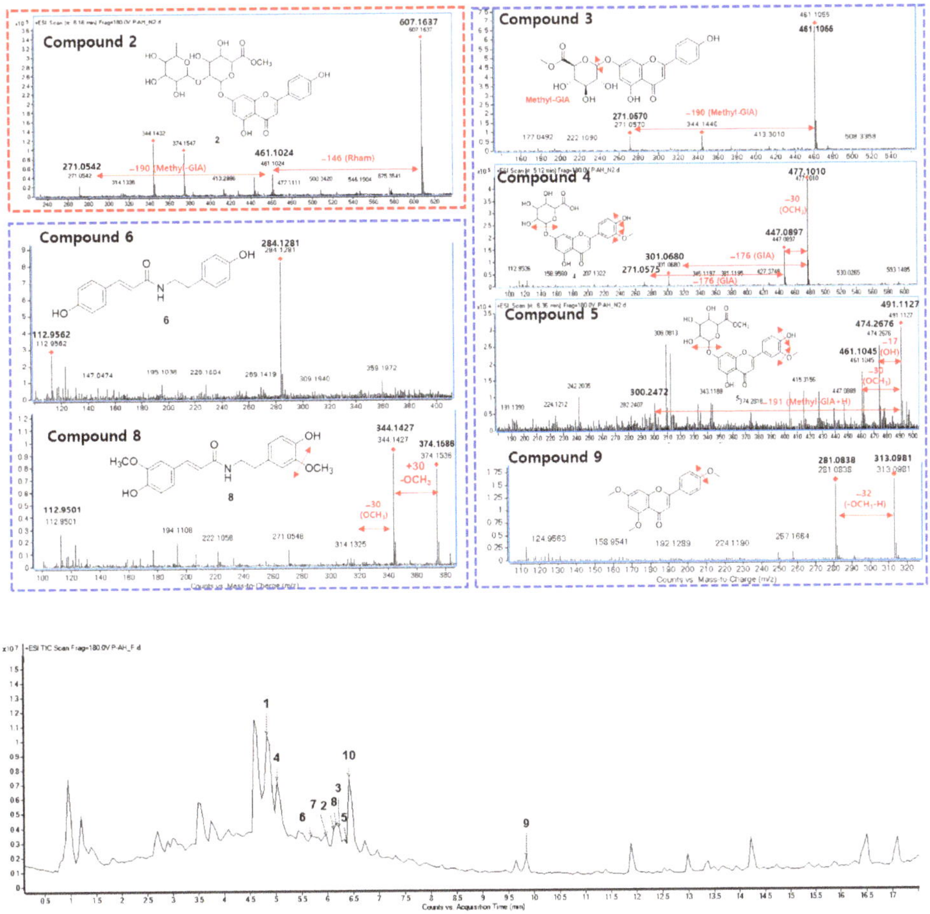

Figure 2. (**A**) Fragmentation analysis of isolated compounds. (**B**) Chemical profiling of isolated compounds in the *A. hookeri* leaf extract. Total ion chromatography (TIC) of *Allium hookeri* leaves recorded with HRESI-qTOF-MS/MS (positive mode). Compounds **1**–**10** were marked in the feature-based molecular networking displayed in Figure 1, and their structures are shown in Figure 3.

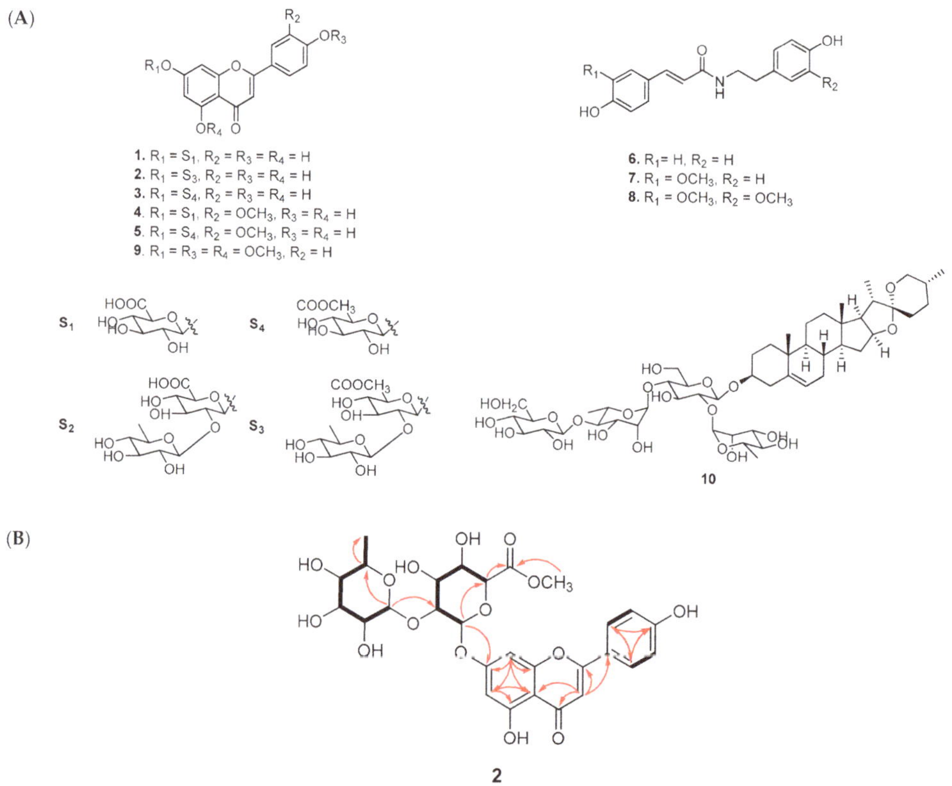

Figure 3. (A) Chemical structures of compounds 1–10 from *A. hookeri*. (B) Key COSY (bold) and HMBC (red arrows) correlations of the new compound 2 isolated from *A. hookeri*.

3.2. Isolation and Structural Elucidation of New Compound 2

The crude extract was further applied to various column chromatography methods to isolate ten compounds, comprising one new compound (**2**) and nine known compounds (**1**, **3–10**), as shown in Figure 1. The chemical structures of known compounds were confirmed via mass analysis and a comparison with previous reports, as mentioned above.

Compound **2** was obtained as a pale yellow powder with an established molecular formula of $C_{28}H_{30}O_{15}$ based on its negative HRESIMS at 605.1500 $[M-H]^-$ (calcd for $C_{28}H_{29}O_{15}$ at 605.1506). In the FBMN, compound **2** was observed in a cluster of flavonoid–glycosides, suggesting that the structure of **2** has the same skeleton. As shown in Figure 3, the mass fragmentation of **2** indicated that it contained one Rham (*m/z* 146 Da) and one methyl-GlA (*m/z* 190 Da) unit. The ^{1}H NMR spectrum of **2** showed five aromatic proton signals at δ_H 7.85 (2H, d, J = 5.1 Hz), 7.20 (overlap), 7.19 (2H, overlap), 7.04 (1H, s), one olefinic proton at δ_H 6.93 ppm, two anomeric signals at δ_H 5.44 (1H, d, J = 7.5 Hz) and 5.11 (1H, d, J = 1.8 Hz), six oxygenated protons [δ_H 4.65, t (7.8); 4.47, t (8.8); 4.52, t (8.8); 4.88, d (8.5); 4.84, br s; 4.58, d (7.7); 4.38, t (9.1); 4.80, m], one methoxy group (δ_H 3.90, s) and one methyl group [δ_H 1.18, d, (6.3)]. The ^{13}C NMR data of **2** displayed 28 carbon signals, including one ketone (δ_C 183.3), an ester carbon (δ_C 170.4), 14 aromatic signals (δ_C 100.8–165.5), two anomeric carbons (δ_C 100.0, 95.6), eight carbons bearing oxygen (δ_C 70.6–78.7), and one methyl (δ_C 19.4). The HMBC data of **2** confirmed the presence of a flavone moiety via the correlations in the two aromatic rings (Figure 3B). The glucuronic acid attached to C-7 of the flavone moiety was revealed by the cross-peaks from H-1′ (δ_H 6.03, d, J = 7.3 Hz) to C-7 (δ_C 163.7). The methoxy group attached to C-3′ was confirmed by the correlation from the methoxy proton signal (δ_H 3.89, s) to aromatic carbon at δ_C 148.8 ppm. The rhamnose sugar moiety was identified by the presence of a methyl group (δ_H 1.18, d, (6.0)/δ_C 18.0 ppm) and its correlation with carbon signals of sugar at δ_C 69.4 and 73.0 ppm. The position of rhamnose moiety was represented by the correlation from H-1‴ (δ_H 6.45 ppm) to C-2″ (δ_C 77.8 ppm). The absolute configuration of the sugar unit was determined following acid hydrolysis and compared with the authentic sugar. The retention time of the sugar derivative in **2** was consistent with that of authentic sugar. Therefore, the structure of **2** was identified, as shown in Figure 3, and named apigenin-7-*O*-[α-L-rhamnopyranosyl(1→2)]β-D-glucuronic acid methyl ester.

3.3. Bio-Activity of Isolated Compounds from *A. hookeri*

In our assay system, senescent human dermal fibroblast (HDF) or lung fibroblast (IMR-90) cells were induced by replicative exhaustion. SA-β-gal activity and SASP secretion were used to evaluate senomorphic activity. Positive SA-β-gal staining and overexpression of SASP factors such as IL-6, IL-8, and IL-1α were confirmed in replicative senescent HDF cells. Drugs that reduced SA-β-gal staining or inhibited expression of these SASP factors are thought to be senomorphic candidates.

Ten isolated compounds (**1**–**10**) from *A. hookeri* were evaluated for their capacity in reducing NO production. The cell viability of these compounds was tested at 5 and 20 μM on LPS-induced NO production in RAW 264.7 cells compared to quercetin, a positive control. As a result, no compounds showed any cytotoxicity up to 20 μM (Figure 4A), and among them, compound **6** showed the best effect in reducing NO production (Figure 4B). In addition, compounds **6**–**8** shared similar structures, so their senomorphic effects in bleomycin (BLM)-senescent A549 cells were further evaluated. Two SASP markers, IL-6 and IL-8, were used to test senomorphic activity. As shown in Figure 5A,B, compounds **6**–**8** reduced the expression of both IL-6 and IL-8 in stress-induced senescent A549 cells that were exposed to 5 μM of BML after 6 days of treatment. The dose-dependent manner of each compound was also tested, and compounds **6**–**8** were found to have senomorphic effects by decreasing the expression of IL-6 and IL-8 (Figure 5B). After 6 days of treatment, the SA-β-gal staining was significantly reduced by 10 μM without any detected toxicity for all three compounds (Figure 5C). Furthermore, the SASP inhibitory activities of **6**–**8** in replicative senescent HDF cells were tested. The compounds were treated at 10 μM on replicative senescent HDF cells, which were confirmed to be senescent through positive SA-β-gal staining (Figure S52, Supplementary Materials) and upregulated SASP makers, including IL-1α and IL-8. After 72 h of treatment, compounds **6**–**8** significantly reduced the expression of IL-1α and IL-8 (Figure 6A,B). Among them, compound **7** showed the best effect in replicative senescent HDF cells in a dose-dependent manner. As a result, compound **7** showed senomorphic activities in replicative senescent HDF cells at 5 and 10 μM by significantly reducing the expression levels of both IL-1α and IL-8 (Figure 6C,D).

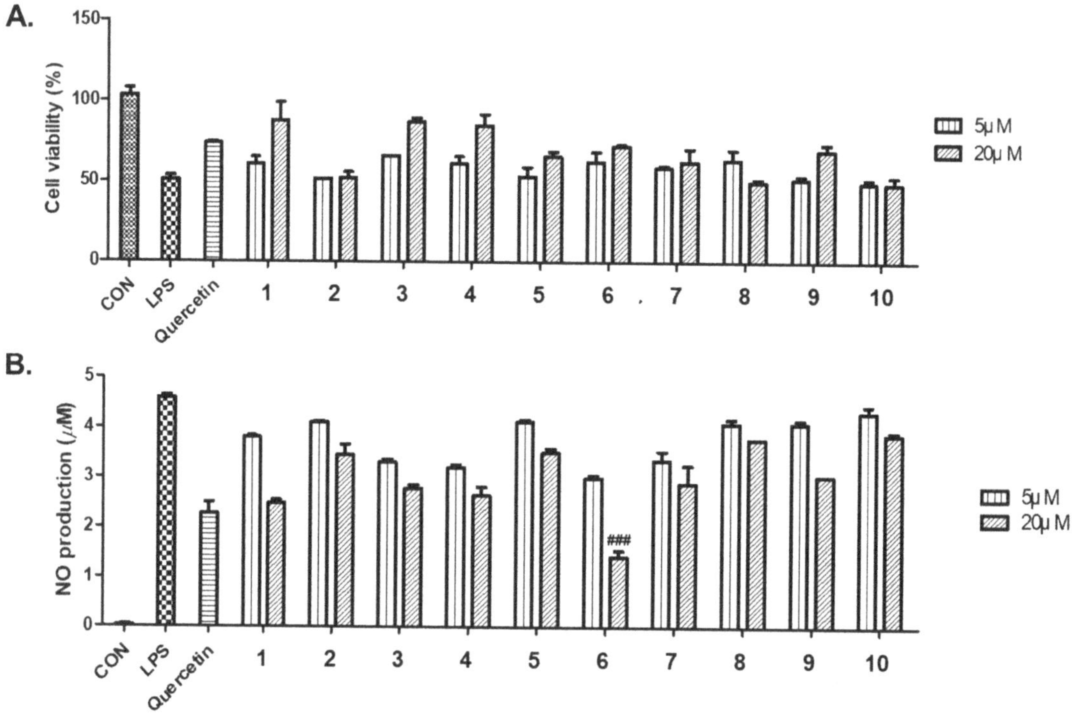

Figure 4. (**A**) The cell viability of compounds **1–10** from *A. hookeri* was measured using the EZ-Cytox cell viability assay. (**B**) The inhibitory effects of compounds **1–10** on LPS-induced NO production in RAW 264.7 cells compared to quercetin used as a positive control. Cell viability results indicate the relative cell viability compared to the untreated group (100%). NO assay data reflect the levels of NO production, calculated by utilizing the absorbance values at 540 nm and referencing a nitrite standard curve (white bar, untreated control group; black bar, LPS-treated control group); ### $p < 0.05$ compared to the LPS-treated control group.

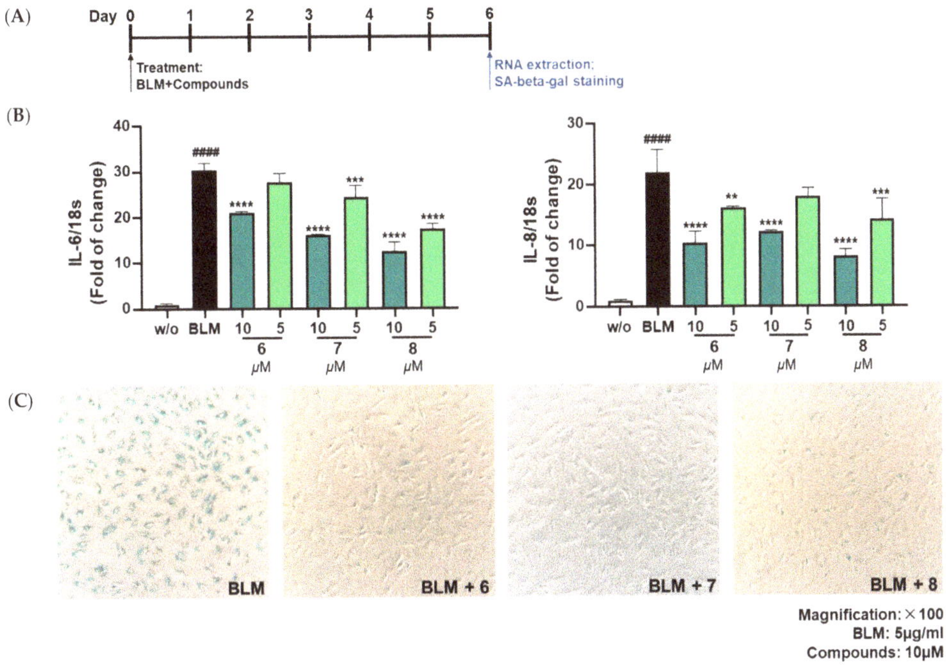

Figure 5. Senomorphic effects in BLM-senescent A549 cells of compounds **6–8** from *A. hookeri*. (**A**) A549 cells were exposed to 5 μg/mL of bleomycin (BML) and co-treated with the indicated compounds for 6 days. Then, the cells were analyzed via RNA extraction or SA-β-gal staining. (**B**) Compounds **6–8** were tested in a dose-dependent manner, and all three compounds showed senomorphic effects by decreasing the expression of IL-6 and IL-8 in stress-induced senescent cells. (**C**) After 6 days of treatment, SA-β-gal staining was significantly reduced by 10 μM in all these compounds, and no severe toxicity was detected. Data are presented as the mean ± SDs (n = 3) with one-way ANOVA with Dunnett's multiple comparisons were performed at ** $p < 0.01$, *** $p < 0.001$ and **** $p < 0.0001$ compared to the control samples; *t*-test, #### $p < 0.0001$.

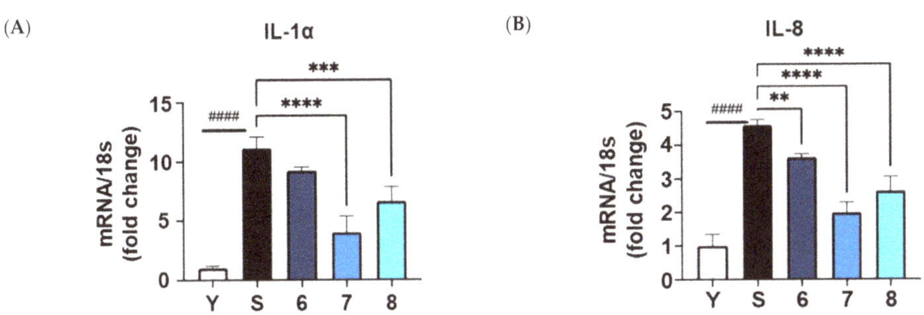

Figure 6. *Cont.*

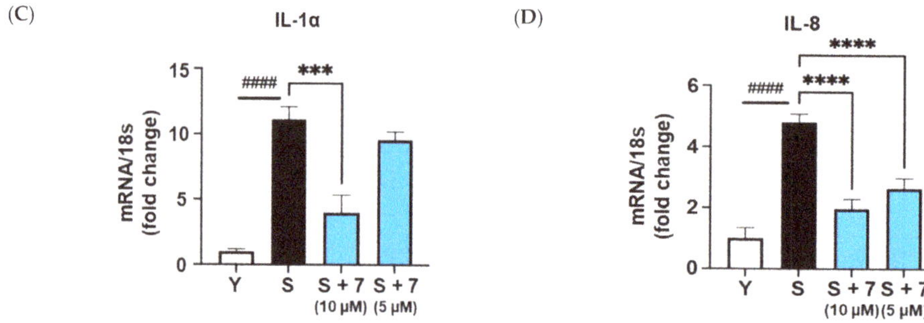

Figure 6. SASP inhibitor in replicative senescent HDF cells of compounds **6–8** from *A. hookeri*. In total, 10 μM of compounds **6–8** were treated on replicative senescent HDF, which was confirmed via positive SA-β-gal staining (Figure S43) and upregulated SASP factors such as IL-1α and IL-8. (**A**,**B**) compounds **6–8** significantly reduced the expression of IL-1α or IL-8 after 72 h of treatment, and compound **7** showed the best effect among them. (**C**,**D**) Compound **7** was tested and found to have a senomorphic effect in replicative senescent HDF cells in a dose-dependent manner. Data are presented as the mean ± SDs (n = 3) with one-way ANOVA with Dunnett's multiple comparisons at ** $p < 0.01$, *** $p < 0.001$ and **** $p < 0.0001$ compared to the control samples; *t*-test, #### $p < 0.0001$.

4. Discussion

In this study, a new compound (**2**) was identified, alongside nine known compounds (**1**, **3–10**), isolated from *A. hookeri*. The application of the feature-based molecular networking (FBMN) strategy not only provided a detailed chemical profile of metabolites in this extensively studied plant but also proved effective in isolating a novel compound from *A. hookeri*, thereby enriching its chemical diversity.

The senomorphic effects of all the isolated phytochemicals, characterized by a reduction in SASP markers, including IL-6, IL-8, IL-1α, and SA-β-gal, staining were evaluated. The results indicate that *N-trans*-feruloyltyramine (**7**) exhibits the most promising SASP-inhibitory activity among the isolated compounds. Notably, cellular senescence is integral to the wound-healing process, with the persistent presence of senescence-associated secretory phenotypes (SASP) marked by indicators of senescence, oxidative stress, and proinflammatory cytokines in fibroblasts, highlighting their involvement in the chronic wound pathology [33,34]. Consequently, the inhibition of SASP markers could potentially contribute to wound healing, aligning with the traditional use of *A. hookeri*. Furthermore, this is the first report of the senomorphic activity of *N-trans*-feruloyltyramine, which has previously been demonstrated to possess a wide range of biological effects, such as protection against scopolamine-induced cholinergic dysfunction on the cortex and hippocampus [45] and β-amyloid peptide-induced neurotoxicity [46], the inhibition of melanin biosynthesis [47], antioxidant, cytotoxic activities, and protection against H_2O_2-induced oxidative damage [48].

Of particular interest, the active compounds (**6–8**) had a similar skeleton to avenanthramide C (Avn C), with the only difference being the phenyl ethyl moieties of **6–8** and the unit of benzoic acid of avenanthramide C. Avenanthramide C has recently been extensively studied for its protective effects against pediatric pneumonia [49], allergic inflammation [50], its senomorphic effect [51], and ability to restore impaired plasticity and cognition in a mice model of Alzheimer's disease [52]. The in vitro results from these studies suggested that Avn C reduces cytokines, including IL-4 [50], IL-6 [50,51], IL-8 [51], TNF-α [50,51], and SASP [51]. These findings are consistent with the present study's data, which demonstrate the potential of phenolamides from *A. hookeri* to inhibit SASP in senescent cells and contribute to their senomorphic activities. Hence, its natural amide skeleton could be a promising analog for developing drugs to treat age-related diseases.

This study leveraged advanced analytical techniques, specifically UHPLC-qTOF-MS/MS-based molecular networking, to rapidly elucidate the secondary metabolite profile of hooker chive (*A. hookeri*), a plant of nutritional and medicinal significance. This approach facilitated the identification of a novel compound within the plant. Furthermore, the senomorphic activity of *A. hookeri* was elucidated for the first time, with particular attention given to the active skeleton, phenolamides, and the principal compound, *N-trans*-feruloyltyramine. This revelation establishes a link between the traditional uses of the plant and its in vitro physiological effects. Nevertheless, this study is not without limitations. Firstly, the chemical profiling of *A. hookeri* relied on putative constructions derived from GNPS libraries, which may have omitted certain well-established compounds that were not present in shared repositories or that were misaligned due to the structural isomers inherent in natural products. Secondly, the investigation has yet to unveil the mechanistic basis underlying the senomorphic effects exerted by the lead compound.

5. Conclusions

In summary, the study employed HRESI-qTOF-MS/MS-based molecular networking to the phytochemical profile of *A. hookeri* leaves, revealing flavonoid–glycosides, flavonoid–aglycones, triterpenoids, and phenolamides. Subsequently, ten compounds, comprising one new flavonoid (apigenin-7-*O*-[α-L-rhamnopyranosyl(1→2)]β-D-glucuronic acid methyl ester) and nine known ones, were isolated and identified through NMR analysis. An evaluation of these compounds demonstrated their impact on the senescent cell-associated secretory phenotype (SASP), with *N-trans*-feruloyltyramine (**7**) emerging as the most potent inhibitor. This underscores its crucial role in *A. hookeri*'s senomorphic activities, suggesting the potential of phenolamides as valuable bioactive compounds for combating senescence-associated diseases.

Supplementary Materials: The following supporting information can be downloaded at: https://www.mdpi.com/article/10.3390/nu15245109/s1, Figure S1. Total ion chromatography (TIC) using HR-ESI -qTOF-MS/MS of *A. hookeri* leaf extract and its fractions in positive mode. Figure S2. Total ion chromatography (TIC) of *A. hookeri* leaf extract and Sep-Pak fractions (0–100% MeOH/H_2O) using HR-ESI -qTOF-MS/MS in positive mode, Figure S3. Feature-based molecular networking of fractions and crude extract from leaves of *Allium hookeri* using HRESI-qTOF-MS/MS. Mass data was recorded in positive mode, Figure S4. Chemical structures of putative identification of components from leaves of *Allium hookeri* using HRESI-qTOF-MS/MS-based molecular networking, Figure S5. Mass/mass fragmentation of triterpenoid cluster in FBMN, Figure S6. HRESIMS data of compound **2**, Figure S7. IR(KBr) spectrum of compound **2**, Figure S8. ^{1}H NMR spectrum of compound **2** (600 MHz, pyridine-d_5), Figure S9. ^{13}C NMR spectrum of compound **2** (150 MHz, pyridine-d_5), Figure S10. HSQC spectrum of compound **2**, Figure S11. HMBC spectrum of compound **2**, Figure S12. The COSY spectrum of compound **2**, Figure S13. HRESIMS/MS of compound **1**, Figure S14. IR(KBr) spectrum of compound **1**, Figure S15. ^{1}H NMR spectrum of compound **1** (400 MHz, DMSO-d_6), Figure S16. HRESIMS/MS of compound **3**, Figure S17. IR(KBr) spectrum of compound **3**, Figure S18. ^{1}H NMR spectrum of compound **3** (600 MHz, DMSO-d_6), Figure S19. ^{13}C NMR spectrum of compound **3** (150 MHz, DMSO-d_6), Figure S20. HRESIMS data of compound **4**, Figure S21. UV spectrum of compound **4**, Figure S22. IR(KBr) spectrum of compound **4**, Figure S23. ^{1}H NMR spectrum of compound **4** (500 MHz, DMSO-d_6), Figure S24. ^{13}C NMR spectrum of compound **4** (125 MHz, DMSO-d_6), Figure S25. HRESIMS data of compound **5**, Figure S26. UV spectrum of compound **5**, Figure S27. IR(KBr) spectrum of compound **5**, Figure S28. ^{1}H NMR spectrum of compound **5** (600 MHz, DMSO-d_6), Figure S29. ^{13}C NMR spectrum of compound **5** (150 MHz, DMSO-d_6), Figure S30. HRESIMS data of compound **6**, Figure S31. IR(KBr) spectrum of compound **6**, Figure S32. ^{1}H NMR spectrum of compound **6** (500 MHz, DMSO-d_6), Figure S33. ^{13}C NMR spectrum of compound **6** (125 MHz, DMSO-d_6), Figure S34. HRESIMS data of compound **7**, Figure S35. IR(KBr) spectrum of compound **7**, Figure S36. ^{1}H NMR spectrum of compound **7** (400 MHz, DMSO-d_6), Figure S37. ^{13}C NMR spectrum of compound **7** (100 MHz, DMSO-d_6), Figure S38. HRESIMS data of compound **8**, Figure S39. UV spectrum of compound **8**, Figure S40. IR(KBr) spectrum of compound **8**, Figure S41. ^{1}H NMR spectrum of compound **8** (600 MHz, DMSO-d_6), Figure S42. ^{13}C NMR spectrum of compound **8** (150 MHz, DMSO-d_6), Figure S43. HRESIMS/MS data of compound **9**, Figure S44. UV spectrum of compound **9**, Figure S45. IR(KBr) spectrum of compound **9**, Figure S46. ^{1}H NMR spectrum of compound **9** (600 MHz, DMSO-d_6), Figure S47. ^{13}C NMR spectrum of compound

9 (150 MHz, DMSO-d_6), Figure S48. HRESIMS/MS data of compound **10**, Figure S49. IR(KBr) spectrum of compound **10**, Figure S50. ^{1}H NMR spectrum of compound **10** (500 MHz, pyridine-d_5), Figure S51. ^{13}C NMR spectrum of compound **10** (125 MHz, pyridine-d_5), Figure S52. Inhibitory effects of fractions and single compounds from *A. hookeri* on BLM-induced senescence system in RAW 264.7 cells using nitric oxide (NO) assay kit, Figure S53. SA-β-gal-positive senescent cells on replicative senescent HDF cell, Table S1. Putative identification of components from leaves of *Allium hookeri* using HRESI-qTOF-MS/MS-based molecular networking.

Author Contributions: Conceptualization and Methodology, T.-P.D., J.-P.A. and M.Z.; Investigation, T.-P.D., M.Z. and E.-J.P.; Resources, J.-E.P.-Z. and V.-H.M.; Data curation, T.-P.D., M.Z. and B.R.; Writing—original draft preparation, T.-P.D. and M.Z.; Writing—review and editing, T.-P.D. and W.-K.O.; Visualization, T.-P.D. and M.Z.; Supervision, Project administration, and Funding acquisition, W.-K.O. All authors have read and agreed to the published version of the manuscript.

Funding: This research was supported by grants from the Basic Science Research Program (NRF-2022R1A2C2005061) and (RS-2023-00218616) through the National Research Foundation of Korea (NRF), funded by the Ministry of Science and ICT in Korea.

Institutional Review Board Statement: Not applicable.

Informed Consent Statement: Not applicable.

Data Availability Statement: Data available in a publicly accessible repository.

Conflicts of Interest: The authors declare no conflict of interest.

References

1. The World Flora Online *Allium* L. Available online: https://wfoplantlist.org/plant-list/taxon/wfo-4000001260-2023-06?page=1 (accessed on 21 November 2023).
2. Sabiu, S.; Madende, M.; Ajao, A.A.; Aladodo, R.A.; Nurain, I.O.; Ahmad, J.B. The Genus Allium (Amaryllidaceae: Alloideae): Features, Phytoconstituents, and Mechanisms of Antidiabetic Potential of Allium Cepa and Allium Sativum. In *Bioactive Food as Dietary Interventions for Diabetes*; Elsevier: Amsterdam, The Netherlands, 2019; pp. 137–154.
3. Ren, F.; Wang, L.; Zhuo, W.; Chen, D.; Huang, H.; Zhang, L. Complete Chloroplast Genome of the Rare Medicinal Vegetable *Allium hookeri*. *Mitochondrial DNA Part B* **2022**, *7*, 6–7. [CrossRef] [PubMed]
4. Deka, B.; Manna, P.; Borah, J.C.; Talukdar, N.C. A Review on Phytochemical, Pharmacological Attributes and Therapeutic Uses of *Allium hookeri*. *Phytomed. Plus* **2022**, *2*, 100262. [CrossRef]
5. Ayam, V. *Allium hookeri*, Thw. Enum. A Lesser Known Terrestrial Perennial Herb Used as Food and Its Ethnobotanical Relevance in Manipur. *AJFAND* **2011**, *11*, 5389–5412. [CrossRef]
6. Bae, G.-C.; Bae, D.-Y. The Anti-Inflammatory Effects of Ethanol Extract of *Allium hookeri* Cultivated in South Korea. *Korea J. Herbol.* **2012**, *27*, 55–61. [CrossRef]
7. Park, E.-K.; Noh, J.-G.; Lee, M.-J.; Nam, S.-Y.; Hong, E.-Y.; Lee, C.-H. Effects of Shading Rates on Growth and Yield of *Allium hookeri* Cultivation at Greenhouse in Middle Area of Korea. *Prot. Hortic. Plant Fact.* **2016**, *25*, 320–327. [CrossRef]
8. Choi, J.-H.; Lee, E.-B.; Jang, H.-H.; Cha, Y.-S.; Park, Y.-S.; Lee, S.-H. *Allium hookeri* Extracts Improve Scopolamine-Induced Cognitive Impairment via Activation of the Cholinergic System and Anti-Neuroinflammation in Mice. *Nutrients* **2021**, *13*, 2890. [CrossRef] [PubMed]
9. Sharma, G.; Gohil, R.N.; Kaul, V. Cytological Status of *Allium hookeri* Thwaites (2n = 22). *Genet. Resour. Crop Evol.* **2011**, *58*, 1041–1050. [CrossRef]
10. Kala, C.P. Ethnomedicinal Botany of the Apatani in the Eastern Himalayan Region of India. *J. Ethnobiol. Ethnomed.* **2005**, *1*, 11. [CrossRef]
11. Bok, S.; Seo, J.; Bae, C.; Kang, B.; Cho, S.; Park, D. *Allium hookeri* Root Extract Regulates Asthmatic Changes through Immunological Modulation of Th1/Th2-related Factors in an Ovalbumin-induced Asthma Mouse Model. *Mol. Med. Rep.* **2019**, *20*, 3215–3223. [CrossRef]
12. Jun, H.-I.; Jang, H.; Ahn, D.; Kim, D.K.; Yang, J.H.; Yun, B.S.; Kim, Y.S. Isolation and Characterization of Phenolic Compound from *Allium hookeri* Root for Potential Use as Antioxidant in Foods. *Food Sci. Biotechnol.* **2015**, *24*, 2031–2034. [CrossRef]
13. Rho, S.H.; You, S.; Kim, G.-H.; Park, H.J. Neuroprotective Effect of *Allium hookeri* against H2O2-Induced PC12 Cell Cytotoxicity by Reducing Oxidative Stress. *Food Sci. Biotechnol.* **2020**, *29*, 1519–1530. [CrossRef] [PubMed]
14. Kim, J.E.; Seo, J.H.; Bae, M.S.; Bae, C.S.; Yoo, J.C.; Bang, M.A.; Cho, S.S.; Park, D.H. Antimicrobial Constituents from *Allium hookeri* Root. *Nat. Prod. Commun.* **2016**, *11*, 237–238. [CrossRef]
15. Roh, S.S.; Kwon, O.J.; Yang, J.H.; Kim, Y.S.; Lee, S.H.; Jin, J.S.; Jeon, Y.D.; Yokozawa, T.; Kim, H.J. *Allium hookeri* Root Protects Oxidative Stress-Induced Inflammatory Responses and β-Cell Damage in Pancreas of Streptozotocin-Induced Diabetic Rats. *BMC Complement. Altern. Med.* **2016**, *16*, 63. [CrossRef]

16. Park, S.H.; Bae, U.J.; Choi, E.K.; Jung, S.J.; Lee, S.H.; Yang, J.H.; Kim, Y.S.; Jeong, D.Y.; Kim, H.J.; Park, B.H.; et al. A Randomized, Double-Blind, Placebo-Controlled Crossover Clinical Trial to Evaluate the Anti-Diabetic Effects of *Allium hookeri* Extract in the Subjects with Prediabetes. *BMC Complement. Med. Ther.* **2020**, *20*, 211. [CrossRef] [PubMed]
17. Lee, Y.; Hyen Lee, S.; Sun Jeong, M.; Kim, J.B.; Hee Jang, H.; Choe, J.; Kim, D.W.; Lillehoj, H.S. In Vitro Analysis of the Immunomodulating Effects of *Allium hookeri* on Lymphocytes, Macrophages, and Tumour Cells. *J. Poult. Sci.* **2017**, *54*, 142–148. [CrossRef]
18. Jang, J.Y.; Lee, M.J.; You, B.R.; Jin, J.S.; Lee, S.H.; Yun, Y.R.; Kim, H.J. *Allium hookeri* Root Extract Exerts Anti-Inflammatory Effects by Nuclear Factor-KB down-Regulation in Lipopolysaccharide-Induced RAW264.7 Cells. *BMC Complement. Altern. Med.* **2017**, *17*, 126.
19. Kim, H.; Rho, S.H.; Lim, J.; Park, H.J.; Jeong, H. Protective Effect of Linoleic Acid against Inflammatory Reactions by Mast Cell via Caspase-1 Cascade Pathways. *J. Food Biochem.* **2019**, *43*, e12932. [CrossRef]
20. Park, H.; Jeong, J.; Hyun, H.; Kim, J.; Kim, H.; Oh, H.; Choi, J.; Hwang, H.; Oh, D.; Kim, J.; et al. Effects of a Hot-Water Extract of *Allium hookeri* Roots on Bone Formation in Human Osteoblast-Like MG-63 Cells In Vitro and in Rats In Vivo. *Planta Med.* **2016**, *82*, 1410–1415. [CrossRef]
21. Park, S.; No, K.; Lee, J. Anti-Obesity Effect of *Allium hookeri* Leaf Extract in High-Fat Diet-Fed Mice. *J. Med. Food* **2018**, *21*, 254–260. [CrossRef]
22. Yang, M.H.; Kim, N.H.; Heo, J.D.; Rho, J.R.; Ock, K.J.; Shin, E.C.; Jeong, E.J. Comparative Evaluation of Sulfur Compounds Contents and Antiobesity Properties of *Allium hookeri* Prepared by Different Drying Methods. *Evid.-Based Complement. Altern. Med.* **2017**, *2017*, 2436927. [CrossRef]
23. Hwang, J.S.; Lee, B.H.; An, X.; Jeong, H.R.; Kim, Y.E.; Lee, I.; Lee, H.; Kim, D.O. Total Phenolics, Total Flavonoids, and Antioxidant Capacity in the Leaves, Bulbs, and Roots of *Allium hookeri*. *Korean J. Food Sci. Technol.* **2015**, *47*, 261–266. [CrossRef]
24. Park, S.Y.; Je, J.Y.; Ahn, C.B. Phenolic Composition and Hepatoprotective Activities of *Allium hookeri* Against Hydrogen-Peroxide-Induced Oxidative Stress in Cultured Hepatocytes. *J. Food Biochem.* **2016**, *40*, 284–293. [CrossRef]
25. Li, R.; Wang, Y.F.; Sun, Q.; Hu, H. Bin Chemical Composition and Antimicrobial Activity of the Essential Oil from *Allium hookeri* Consumed in Xishuangbanna, Southwest China. *Nat. Prod. Commun.* **2014**, *9*, 863–864. [PubMed]
26. Thiyagarajan, J.A.; Mikton, C.; Harwood, R.H.; Gichu, M.; Gaigbe-Togbe, V.; Jhamba, T.; Pokorna, D.; Stoevska, V.; Hada, R.; Steffan, G.S.; et al. The UN Decade of Healthy Ageing: Strengthening Measurement for Monitoring Health and Wellbeing of Older People. *Age Ageing* **2022**, *51*, afac147. [CrossRef] [PubMed]
27. Beard, J.R.; Officer, A.; de Carvalho, I.A.; Sadana, R.; Pot, A.M.; Michel, J.-P.; Lloyd-Sherlock, P.; Epping-Jordan, J.E.; Peeters, G.M.E.E.G.; Mahanani, W.R.; et al. The World Report on Ageing and Health: A Policy Framework for Healthy Ageing. *Lancet* **2016**, *387*, 2145–2154. [CrossRef] [PubMed]
28. Boccardi, V.; Mecocci, P. Senotherapeutics: Targeting Senescent Cells for the Main Age-Related Diseases. *Mech. Ageing Dev.* **2021**, *197*, 111526. [CrossRef] [PubMed]
29. Sun, Y.; Coppé, J.P.; Lam, E.W.F. Cellular Senescence: The Sought or the Unwanted? *Trends Mol. Med.* **2018**, *24*, 871–885. [CrossRef] [PubMed]
30. van Deursen, J.M. The Role of Senescent Cells in Ageing. *Nature* **2014**, *509*, 439–446. [CrossRef]
31. Huang, W.; Hickson, L.J.; Eirin, A.; Kirkland, J.L.; Lerman, L.O. Cellular Senescence: The Good, the Bad and the Unknown. *Nat. Rev. Nephrol.* **2022**, *18*, 611–627. [CrossRef]
32. Jun, J.-I.; Lau, L.F. The Matricellular Protein CCN1 Induces Fibroblast Senescence and Restricts Fibrosis in Cutaneous Wound Healing. *Nat. Cell Biol.* **2010**, *12*, 676–685. [CrossRef]
33. Thompson, E.L.; Pitcher, L.E.; Niedernhofer, L.J.; Robbins, P.D. Targeting Cellular Senescence with Senotherapeutics: Development of New Approaches for Skin Care. *Plast. Reconstr. Surg.* **2022**, *150*, 12S–19S. [CrossRef] [PubMed]
34. Vande Berg, J.S.; Rose, M.A.; Haywood-Reid, P.L.; Rudolph, R.; Payne, W.G.; Robson, M.C. Cultured Pressure Ulcer Fibroblasts Show Replicative Senescence with Elevated Production of Plasmin, Plasminogen Activator Inhibitor-1, and Transforming Growth Factor-β1. *Wound Repair Regen.* **2005**, *13*, 76–83. [CrossRef] [PubMed]
35. Li, W.; Qin, L.; Feng, R.; Hu, G.; Sun, H.; He, Y.; Zhang, R. Emerging Senolytic Agents Derived from Natural Products. *Mech. Ageing Dev.* **2019**, *181*, 1–6. [CrossRef] [PubMed]
36. Luís, C.; Maduro, A.T.; Pereira, P.; Mendes, J.J.; Soares, R.; Ramalho, R. Nutritional Senolytics and Senomorphics: Implications to Immune Cells Metabolism and Aging—From Theory to Practice. *Front. Nutr.* **2022**, *9*, 958563. [CrossRef] [PubMed]
37. Lee, Y.; Kim, H.M.; Kim, J.H.; Lee, J.-H.; Zhang, K.X.; Gao, E.M.; Jeon, J.-S.; Syed, A.S.; Son, R.H.; Kim, J.-Y.; et al. Chemical Constituents of the *Ajuga Multiflora* Bunge and Their Protective Effects on Dexamethasone-Induced Muscle Atrophy in C_2C_{12} Myotubes. *Nat. Prod. Res.* **2023**, *37*, 1978–1985. [CrossRef]
38. Lehbili, M.; Alabdul Magid, A.; Kabouche, A.; Voutquenne-Nazabadioko, L.; Abedini, A.; Morjani, H.; Gangloff, S.C.; Kabouche, Z. Antibacterial, Antioxidant and Cytotoxic Activities of Triterpenes and Flavonoids from the Aerial Parts of *Salvia Barrelieri* Etl. *Nat. Prod. Res.* **2018**, *32*, 2683–2691. [CrossRef]
39. Myagchilov, A.V.; Gorovoi, P.G.; Sokolova, L.I. Flavonoids from Serratula Komarovii Iljin (the Asteraceae Family). *Russ. J. Bioorg. Chem.* **2021**, *47*, 1418–1423. [CrossRef]
40. Yanting, L.R.J.B.X.Z. Chrysoeriol-7-O-Beta-D Glucuronic Acid Methyl Ester and Extraction Method and Application Thereof. Patent CN107446009A, 8 December 2017.

41. Sutthanut, K.; Sripanidkulchai, B.; Yenjai, C.; Jay, M. Simultaneous Identification and Quantitation of 11 Flavonoid Constituents in Kaempferia Parviflora by Gas Chromatography. *J. Chromatogr. A* **2007**, *1143*, 227–233. [CrossRef]
42. van Zadelhoff, A.; Vincken, J.P.; de Bruijn, W.J.C. Facile Amidation of Non-Protected Hydroxycinnamic Acids for the Synthesis of Natural Phenol Amides. *Molecules* **2022**, *27*, 2203. [CrossRef]
43. Zheng, Y.; Su, B.; Wang, Y.; Wang, H.; Liao, H.; Liang, D. New Tyramine- and Aporphine-Type Alkamides with NO Release Inhibitory Activities from *Piper puberulum*. *J. Nat. Prod.* **2021**, *84*, 1316–1325. [CrossRef]
44. Chen, S.; Snyder, J.K. Diosgenin-Bearing, Molluscicidal Saponins from Allium Vineale: An NMR Approach for the Structural Assignment of Oligosaccharide Units. *J. Org. Chem.* **1989**, *54*, 3679–3689. [CrossRef]
45. Thangnipon, W.; Ngampramuan, S.; Suthprasertporn, N.; Jantrachotechatchawan, C.; Tuchinda, P.; Nobsathian, S. Protective Roles of N-Trans-Feruloyltyramine Against Scopolamine-Induced Cholinergic Dysfunction on Cortex and Hippocampus of Rat Brains. *Siriraj Med. J.* **2021**, *73*, 413–422. [CrossRef]
46. Thangnipon, W.; Suwanna, N.; Kitiyanant, N.; Soi-ampornkul, R.; Tuchinda, P.; Munyoo, B.; Nobsathian, S. Protective Role of N-Trans-Feruloyltyramine against β-Amyloid Peptide-Induced Neurotoxicity in Rat Cultured Cortical Neurons. *Neurosci. Lett.* **2012**, *513*, 229–232. [CrossRef] [PubMed]
47. Efdi, M.; Ohguchi, K.; Akao, Y.; Nozawa, Y.; Koketsu, M.; Ishihara, H. N-Trans-Feruloyltyramine as a Melanin Biosynthesis Inhibitor. *Biol. Pharm. Bull.* **2007**, *30*, 1972–1974. [CrossRef] [PubMed]
48. Gao, X.; Wang, C.; Chen, Z.; Chen, Y.; Santhanam, R.K.; Xue, Z.; Ma, Q.; Guo, Q.; Liu, W.; Zhang, M.; et al. Effects of N-Trans-Feruloyltyramine Isolated from Laba Garlic on Antioxidant, Cytotoxic Activities and H2O2-Induced Oxidative Damage in HepG2 and L02 cells. *Food Chem. Toxicol.* **2019**, *130*, 130–141. [CrossRef] [PubMed]
49. Pu, Z.; Shen, C.; Zhang, W.; Xie, H.; Wang, W. Avenanthramide C from Oats Protects Pyroptosis through Dependent ROS-Induced Mitochondrial Damage by PI3K Ubiquitination and Phosphorylation in Pediatric Pneumonia. *J. Agric. Food Chem.* **2022**, *70*, 2339–2353. [CrossRef] [PubMed]
50. Dhakal, H.; Yang, E.-J.; Lee, S.; Kim, M.-J.; Baek, M.-C.; Lee, B.; Park, P.-H.; Kwon, T.K.; Khang, D.; Song, K.-S.; et al. Avenanthramide C from Germinated Oats Exhibits Anti-Allergic Inflammatory Effects in Mast Cells. *Sci. Rep.* **2019**, *9*, 6884. [CrossRef]
51. Lim, J.S.; Lee, D.Y.; Kim, H.S.; Park, S.C.; Park, J.T.; Kim, H.S.; Oh, W.K.; Cho, K.A. Identification of a Novel Senomorphic Agent, Avenanthramide C, via the Suppression of the Senescence-Associated Secretory Phenotype. *Mech. Ageing Dev.* **2020**, *192*, 111355. [CrossRef]
52. Ramasamy, V.S.; Samidurai, M.; Park, H.J.; Wang, M.; Park, R.Y.; Yu, S.Y.; Kang, H.K.; Hong, S.; Choi, W.-S.; Lee, Y.Y.; et al. Avenanthramide-C Restores Impaired Plasticity and Cognition in Alzheimer's Disease Model Mice. *Mol. Neurobiol.* **2020**, *57*, 315–330. [CrossRef]

nutrients

MDPI

Article

Improvement of Cognitive Function by Fermented *Panax ginseng* C.A. Meyer Berries Extracts in an AF64A-Induced Memory Deficit Model

Eun-Jung Yoon [1,†], Jeong-Won Ahn [2,†], Hyun-Soo Kim [2], Yunseo Choi [1], Jiwon Jeong [1], Seong-Soo Joo [2,3,*] and Dongsun Park [1,*]

1 Laboratory of Animal Physiology and Medicine, Department of Biology Education, Republic of Korea National University of Education, Cheongju 28173, Chungbuk, Republic of Korea; ejyoon@knue.ac.kr (E.-J.Y.); jwone@knue.ac.kr (J.J.)
2 College of Life Science, Gangneung-Wonju National University, 7 Jukheon-gil, Gangneung 25457, Gangwon, Republic of Korea; 0000@gwnu.ac.kr (J.-W.A.); k4609@gwnu.ac.kr (H.-S.K.)
3 Huscion MAJIC R&D Center, 331 Pangyo-ro, Seongnam 13488, Gyeonggi, Republic of Korea
* Correspondence: ssj66@gwnu.ac.kr (S.-S.J.); dvmdpark@knue.ac.kr (D.P.); Tel.: +82-33-640-2856 (S.-S.J.); +82-43-230-3652 (D.P.)
† These authors contributed equally to this work.

Abstract: This study investigated the potential therapeutic properties of fermented ginseng berry extract (GBE) for Alzheimer's disease (AD). Fermented GBE was examined for its ginsenoside content and physiological properties, which have been suggested to have neuroprotective effects and improve cognitive function. The results showed that fermented GBE contains high levels of major active ginsenosides and exhibits antioxidant and acetylcholinesterase inhibitory activities. Post-fermented GBE demonstrated therapeutic potential in AF64A-induced damaged neural stem cells and an animal model of AD. These findings suggest that fermented GBE may hold promise as a candidate for developing new therapeutic interventions for memory deficits and cognitive disorders associated with AD and other neurodegenerative conditions. However, further studies are needed to evaluate the safety, tolerability, and efficacy of fermented GBE in human subjects and to determine its clinical applications. In conclusion, our study provides evidence that fermented GBE has potential as a natural product for the prevention and treatment of AD. The high levels of active ginsenosides and antioxidant and acetylcholinesterase inhibitory activities of fermented GBE suggest that it may be a promising therapeutic agent for improving cognitive function and reducing neurodegeneration.

Keywords: cognitive function; Alzheimer's disease; ginseng berry extracts; ginsenosides; nerve growth factor; brain-derived neurotrophic factor; neural stem cells; ICR mice

1. Introduction

Alzheimer's disease (AD) is a prevalent neurodegenerative disorder characterized by cognitive and memory impairments [1]. Key pathological features of AD include the accumulation of amyloid beta (Aβ) and tau protein, resulting in the formation of senile plaques and neurofibrillary tangles (NFTs) [2,3]. These etiological factors damage the cholinergic nervous system, leading to a loss of learning and memory [4–6]. AD is projected to become an increasingly significant public health issue due to the growing aging population, with estimates predicting one million cases by 2024 and three million cases by 2050 [7].

Although various therapeutic approaches are under investigation for AD, there is a need for more effective treatments and preventative measures due to an incomplete understanding of the pathophysiology [8–10]. Several therapeutic interventions have been explored, including acetylcholinesterase (AChE) inhibitors like donepezil and memantine [11], stem cells for cholinergic system regeneration [12], and therapeutic antibodies for causative agent removal [13]. However, their practical applications remain limited. Recently, there has been increasing interest in the application of natural extracts as potential therapeutic agents for AD. These agents include phenolic acids and flavonoids, which exhibit antioxidative [14], anti-neuroinflammatory [15], and anti-Aβ aggregation properties [16], as well as targeting tau protein [17] and cholinergic neurotransmission [18].

Various animal models have been used for drug screening in AD patients. Typical animal models of AD include spontaneously aging animals, transgenic animals, and chemically induced animal models. Among them, chemically induced animal models using amyloid beta (Aβ), cholinotoxin, and cholinergic antagonists are relatively economical. However, they have other disadvantages, such as short memory retention and sometimes requiring highly professional skills (e.g., intracerebroventricular injection). AF64A, a cholinergic toxin widely used in screening drugs for dementia treatment development, is internalized only into cholinergic neurons by the high-affinity choline transport system, causing alterations in the mRNA expression and activity of choline acetyltransferase (ChAT). This unique characteristic sets AF64A apart from other potential causes of AD [18–21]. Therefore, injection of AF64A decreases the release of acetylcholine (ACh), leading to cognitive impairments, including memory and learning deficits, which are characteristic of AD [18,22]. The AF64A-induced model stably maintains memory deficiency for 6 weeks, making it suitable for evaluating the therapeutic effects of drug candidates.

Ginseng berry extract (GBE) is a natural product that has shown potential in treating various diseases due to its ginsenoside content. Ginseng berries contain more ginsenosides than ginseng roots [23] and have been found to prevent atherogenesis [24], improve age-related diabetes [25], exhibit antioxidative effects as cosmetics [26], prevent scopolamine-induced memory deficits [27], and increase antitumor activity through regulation of the immune system [28]. Fermentation of natural products has also gained recent attention due to its ability to alter the chemical composition and biological activity of extracts [29]. Fermented foods offer several health benefits, such as antioxidant, antimicrobial, antifungal, anti-inflammatory, antidiabetic, and antiatherosclerotic activity, as components like vitamins, minerals, and biologically active peptides are altered, and non-nutrient substances are removed during fermentation [30–32]. Moreover, ginsenosides, including those found in fermented *Panax ginseng* extracts, are known to be absorbed in the gut when administered orally.

In this study, we hypothesized that the active ingredients would increase in fermented GBE compared to non-fermented GBE. To test this hypothesis, we compared the ginsenoside content and biological properties of fermented and non-fermented GBE. Specifically, we examined the antioxidative effects, AChE inhibitory activity, and neuroprotective effects, as these properties are known to be relevant to the pathophysiology of Alzheimer's disease. We also investigated the therapeutic effects of fermented GBE in human neural stem cells and an animal model of AD induced by AF64A. By evaluating the ginsenoside content and biological properties of fermented GBE, we aimed to determine whether it could hold potential as a therapeutic intervention for AD.

2. Materials and Methods

2.1. Sample Preparation

The preparation of GBE in this study followed the methodology described in earlier publications [33,34]. Fresh berries of *Panax ginseng* C.A. Meyer were collected from four-year-old plants in Yeoncheon-gun, Gyeonggi-do, Republic of Korea. The harvested berries were authenticated by Prof. Joo (Biopharmaceutical Lab, College of Life Science, Gangneung-Wonju National University, Republic of Korea), and a voucher specimen was deposited at the Herbarium of the College of Natural Science, Kangwon National University, Republic of Korea (#KWNU-98802). The collected berries underwent dehydration and seven steaming cycles at 100 °C for 2 h, each followed by 24 h drying periods at 50 °C. The fourth and seventh steam-dried berry products were mixed in equal amounts and then extracted twice using 65% ethanol (10-fold volume) for 4 h at room temperature, to prepare the GBE. The ensuing ethanol extracts were filtered using Hyundai Micro No. 2 filters (Hyundai micro, Seoul, Republic of Korea), then evaporated and lyophilized to yield the pre-fermented GBE. The fermentation process involved diluting the pre-fermented GBE with distilled water to 4 brix and fermenting with *Lactobacillus plantarum* (2.0×10^7 CFU/mL) for 48 h at 30 °C and 150 rpm. Post-fermentation, the extract was centrifuged at 8000× g for 1 h to remove any debris and *L. plantarum*. The supernatant was then collected, filtered, and lyophilized to produce the post-fermented GBE. This study involves a comparison between the pre-fermented and post-fermented GBE samples. All fermentation processes adhered to the procedures outlined in prior literature [35].

2.2. High-Performance Liquid Chromatography (HPLC) Analysis

The analysis of ginsenosides was conducted utilizing an Ultimate 3000 HPLC system (Thermo Fisher Scientific, Waltham, MA, USA), equipped with a diode array detector (DAD) [36]. For ginsenoside separation, a YMC-Triart C18 column (250 × 4.6 mm, 12 nm, S-5 μm, YMC, Tokyo, Japan) was employed, with the column temperature consistently maintained at 30 °C. A gradient elution program with solvent A (water) and solvent B (acetonitrile) was applied as follows: 0–10 min (20% B), 10–40 min (20–32% B), 40–55 min (32–50% B), 55–70 min (50–65% B), 70–72 min (65–90% B), 72–82 min (90% B), 82–84 min (90–20% B), and 84–90 min (20% B). This program was conducted at a flow rate of 1.6 mL/min. Detection was achieved at 203 nm, and the retention times and peak areas of the ginsenoside peaks were logged via Chromeleon software (version 7.2.10; Thermo Fisher Scientific, Waltham, MA, USA). Each peak was identified by comparing its retention times and UV spectra with those of the ginsenoside standard mixture (Biopurify Phytochemicals, Chengdu, China).

2.3. Determination of Polyphenol and Flavonoid Contents

The total polyphenol and flavonoid contents of the GBE were quantified using modified colorimetric methodologies. To assess total phenolic content, we employed a slightly altered Folin–Denis method, based on prior research [37]. In brief, we mixed 10 μL of a GBE sample (1 mg/mL) with 10 μL of 1 N Folin–Ciocalteu's phenol reagent (Sigma-Aldrich, St. Louis, MO, USA) and 170 μL of distilled water, incubating the mixture in the dark at room temperature for 5 min. Then, we added 10 μL of a 20% Na_2CO_3 solution and let the mixture incubate in the dark for another 20 min at room temperature. Using a microplate reader (Molecular Devices, San Jose, CA, USA), we measured the absorbance at 765 nm. We obtained a calibration curve using gallic acid (Sigma-Aldrich), expressing the total phenolic content as milligrams of gallic acid equivalents per gram of dry extract (mg GAE/g). To quantify flavonoid content, we used the aluminum chloride colorimetric method, based on prior research, with minor modifications [38]. Briefly, we combined 10 μL of GBE sample (1 mg/mL), 10 μL of a 10% $AlCl_3$ solution, 10 μL of 1 M potassium acetate, and 170 μL of distilled water. This mixture was incubated at room temperature for 30 min. We then measured the absorbance at 415 nm using a microplate reader and established a calibration curve using quercetin hydrate (TCI, Tokyo, Japan). The flavonoid content was expressed as milligrams of quercetin equivalents per gram of dry extract (mg QE/g).

2.4. Assessment of Lipid Peroxidation Levels

We evaluated lipid peroxidation by measuring the formation of malondialdehyde in brain tissue. In brief, we dissected the brain of a 7-week-old male ICR mouse immediately following intracardial perfusion. The brain tissue was homogenized in 10 volumes of cold phosphate-buffered saline (PBS) and centrifuged at 3000× g for 20 min at 4 °C to yield the supernatant. To stimulate lipid peroxidation, we combined 450 μL of the brain homogenate with 50 μM ferric chloride (25 μL), either in the presence or absence of pre- or post-fermented GBE (25 μL, 0–1000 μg/mL), and incubated the mixture for 30 min at 37 °C. We terminated the reaction by adding 500 μL of an 8.1% w/v sodium dodecyl sulfate solution and 1 mL of 20% acetic acid. After the supernatants cleared, we mixed

500 μL aliquots with an equal volume of a 0.8% *w/v* thiobarbituric acid solution and heated the Eppendorf tubes at 95 °C for 30 min. Following cooling on ice, we pipetted 100 μL of each sample into 96-well plates. We measured the absorbance at 532 nm using a microplate reader.

2.5. Evaluation of Antioxidant Scavenging Potential

The antioxidant scavenging potential of the pre- or post-fermented GBE was measured using the 1,1-diphenyl-2-picrylhydrazyl (DPPH) radical scavenging activity assay, following a method previously described [39]. Specifically, we added 10 μL of pre- or post-fermented GBE solution, at varying concentrations (0–1000 μg/mL) and dissolved in distilled water, to each well of a 96-well plate. Subsequently, we added 90 μL of a 0.2 mM DPPH solution, dissolved in methanol. Following a 10 min incubation period at room temperature, we measured the absorbance at 517 nm using a microplate reader. We calculated the DPPH radical scavenging activity using the following formula: % scavenging activity = (control absorbance − sample absorbance)/control absorbance × 100. We performed all sample analyses in triplicate.

2.6. Assessment of Hydroxyl Radical-Induced Oxidative Damage

The evaluation of hydroxyl radical-induced oxidative damage was executed through a metal-catalyzed reaction as described previously [40]. The target protein, bovine serum albumin (BSA), was prepared at a final concentration of 0.5 mg/mL in phosphate-buffered saline (PBS). This BSA solution was subjected to incubation both with and without 100 μM copper (Cu^{2+}) and 2.5 mM hydrogen peroxide (H_2O_2), in the presence or absence of pre- or post-fermented GBE at varying concentrations (0–1000 μg/mL). The control antioxidant utilized was ascorbate at 100 μM, directly dissolved in PBS. All reaction mixtures were housed in open tubes and placed in a shaking water bath maintained at a constant temperature of 37 °C. Following the completion of reactions, we separated each mixture using 10% sodium dodecyl sulfate–polyacrylamide gel electrophoresis (SDS–PAGE). Subsequent to separation, we stained the gel with a 0.1% Coomassie blue solution.

2.7. Determination of AChE Activity

The AChE activities were evaluated utilizing a modified Ellman's method, as previously described [41]. Briefly, the brain of an ICR mouse was dissected promptly following intracardial perfusion. The excised brain tissue was then homogenized in 20 volumes of cold phosphate-buffered saline (PBS), which contained a proteinase inhibitor cocktail (Sigma-Aldrich). For the measurement of AChE activity, the following components were mixed in a cuvette: 0.1 mL of the test sample, 2.5 mL of PBS, 0.1 mL of 10 mM 5,5′-dithio-bis-2-nitrobenzoic acid (Sigma-Aldrich), and 0.2 mL of brain homogenate. Subsequently, 0.1 mL of 75 mM acetylthiocholine iodide (Sigma-Aldrich) was added to the cuvette mixture. The enzymatic activity was recorded at 412 nm for a duration of 5 min, at 1 min intervals, using a microplate reader. The results were normalized and presented as a percentage of the control (vehicle) activity, using the formula: % activity = (sample activity/control activity) × 100. Each experiment was performed in triplicate.

2.8. Cell Culture and Maintenance

Human neural stem cells (F3) and choline acetyltransferase (ChAT)-overexpressing human neural stem cells (F3.ChAT) were cultured and maintained in a specialized medium. The culture medium consisted of Dulbecco's modified Eagle's medium (DMEM; Biowest, Nuaille', Cholet, France) fortified with antibiotics (100 IU/mL penicillin and 100 μg/mL streptomycin). The medium was further supplemented with 10% heat-inactivated fetal bovine serum (Biowest). Cell cultures were incubated at 37 °C in an environment maintained at 5% CO_2 and 95% air. For all experiments, cells were grown until they achieved a confluence of over 90% and were ensured to be within their first 20 passages to maintain optimal growth conditions and genetic stability.

2.9. Preparation and pH Adjustment of AF64A

AF64A was freshly prepared from acetyl-AF64A following a method described previously [40]. Acetyl-AF64A (Sigma-Aldrich) was rapidly dissolved in distilled water under constant stirring. The pH was initially adjusted to and maintained between 10.5 and 11.0 using a NaOH solution for a duration of 30 min. Following this, an HCl solution was added to decrease the pH to a range of 5.5–7.0. The final pH adjustment was made to 7.4 with the addition of a NaOH solution. The final concentration of AF64A was adjusted to 10.0 mM with the addition of distilled water. This stock solution was then further diluted with phosphate-buffered saline (PBS) to reach the desired working concentrations for the experiments.

2.10. Assessment of Cell Viability and Protective Effects of Pre- and Post-Fermented GBE

Cell viability following treatment with pre- or post-fermented GBE and AF64A was evaluated using the Cell Counting Kit-8 (CCK-8; Dojindo Laboratories, Japan). F3 and F3.ChAT cells were seeded at a density of 1×10^4 cells/well in a 96-well plate. After treatment with varying concentrations of pre- or post-fermented GBE (0–1000 μg/mL) and AF64A (0–1000 μM), 10 μL of CCK-8 was added to each well (containing 100 μL of culture medium) and the plate was incubated for 24 h at 37 °C. The number of viable cells was determined by measuring the absorbance at 450 nm using a microplate reader. The protective effects of pre- and post-fermented GBE against AF64A-induced cytotoxicity were assessed by measuring the release of lactate dehydrogenase (LDH) from F3 and F3.ChAT cells. LDH content in the culture supernatants was determined using a commercial LDH assay kit (Promega, Madison, WI, USA), which is based on a coupled enzymatic reaction that converts a tetrazolium salt into a red formazan product. The intensity of the formazan color, proportional to the number of lysed cells, was quantified by measuring the absorbance at 490 nm using a microplate reader. All experiments were conducted in triplicate.

2.11. Induction of Cognitive Deficits and Treatment in Mice

Six-week-old male ICR mice (SPF, certificate #211005) were obtained from Daehan Biolink (Daehan Biolink, Eumseong, Republic of Korea). The mice were kept in an environment with a constant temperature (23 ± 3 °C) and relative humidity (50 ± 10%), following a 12 h light/dark cycle. Standard rodent diets and purified water were available ad libitum. Following 1 week of acclimation to the laboratory conditions, the mice were randomly assigned to one of the following groups: Normal Control group (NC; $n = 7$), AF64A + Vehicle group (Veh; $n = 7$), AF64A + Donepezil group (Donepezil; $n = 7$), and AF64A + post-fermented GBE at 100 mg/kg (GBE100; $n = 7$), 200 mg/kg (GBE200; $n = 7$), and 400 mg/kg (GBE400; $n = 7$). Mice were anesthetized using ketamine (Yuhan Corporation, Seoul Republic of Korea) and rompun (Bayer Korea, Seoul, Republic of Korea) and positioned in a stereotaxic frame. To induce cognitive deficits, AF64A cholinotoxin was administered as previously described [18]. Following the skin incision, a fresh AF64A solution (3 nmol/3 μL/mouse) was infused into the right ventricle at the following stereotaxic coordinates from the bregma: posterior 0.6 mm, lateral 1.1 mm, and ventral 2.0 mm, at a flow rate of 0.5 μL/min. After a 2-week recovery period, either vehicle (0), 100, 200, and 400 mg/kg of GBE, or 2 mg/kg of donepezil, was orally administered once a day for 6 weeks (Figure 1). Prior to administration, mice were fasted for 4 h, with food and water provided ad libitum post-administration. Vehicle administration was performed concurrently with other study compounds for comparison purposes. All animal experiments were conducted following the Standard Operation Procedures of the Laboratory Animal Center at Chungbuk National University (CBNU, MFDS Approval #2), Republic of Korea. The protocol was approved by the Institutional Animal Care and Use Committee of CBNU (#CBNUA-1398-20-01).

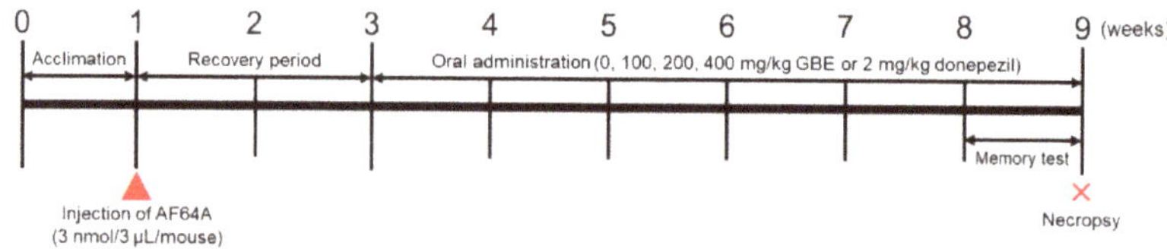

Figure 1. Schematic illustration of the experimental design. Six-week-old male ICR mice were randomly allocated into different groups: normal control group (NC; $n = 7$), AF64A + vehicle group (Veh; $n = 7$), AF64A + Donepezil group (Donepezil; $n = 7$), AF64A + post-fermented GBE 100 mg/kg group (GBE100; $n = 7$), AF64A + post-fermented GBE 200 mg/kg group (GBE200; $n = 7$), and AF64A + post-fermented GBE 400 mg/kg group (GBE400; $n = 7$). Two weeks following AF64A injection (3 nmol/3 μL/mouse), the mice were treated with GBE (100, 200, and 400 mg/kg) or donepezil (2 mg/kg) over a duration of 9 weeks. The doses of GBE and donepezil were administered orally and their frequencies varied as indicated by the arrows. Cognitive performance was evaluated at the beginning and during the 3rd and 9th weeks. The Morris water maze test was employed to evaluate spatial learning and memory, while the novel object recognition test was used to assess recognition memory.

2.12. Assessment of Passive Avoidance Memory Performance

The passive avoidance memory performance of mice was evaluated using a step-through Shuttle box (ENV-010MD; Med Associates, St. Albans, VT, USA). This evaluation was carried out daily for seven days, beginning 8 weeks after the AF64A injection. The Shuttle box apparatus comprises two compartments, one illuminated and the other dark. Both compartments are equipped with a steel-grid floor for the delivery of an electric shock. During the trials, mice were placed in the illuminated compartment, and the door to the dark compartment was opened. As the mice ventured into the dark compartment, they received an electric shock (0.4 mA for 2 s). After that, the latency time, defined as the time it took the mice to reenter the dark compartment after the light in the illuminated compartment was turned on, was recorded. A maximum latency time of 180 s was set as the cutoff for successful memory acquisition.

2.13. Assessment of Spatial Memory Using Morris Water Maze

The evaluation of spatial memory was conducted using a Morris water maze system (Smart v2.5; Panlab Technology, Barcelona, Spain), which was connected to a closed-circuit television (CCTV) system (Samsung, Changwon, Republic of Korea). The testing schedule aligned with the passive avoidance performance assessment and occurred 2 h later on the same day. The water maze trials utilized a circular water bath of 150 cm in diameter, filled with water to a depth of 27 cm. The water temperature was consistently maintained at 22 ± 2 °C. The bath was divided into four quadrants, with a hidden escape platform (10 cm in diameter, 25 cm in height) situated in the center of one of the quadrants. This platform was submerged 2 cm beneath the water's surface and was concealed using squid ink. Throughout the trials, the mice were trained to locate the concealed platform using various external cues. The positions of these cues remained constant for the duration of the experiments. The escape latency, defined as the time it took for the mice to find the platform during the trials, was recorded by tracking their movements via the CCTV monitor.

2.14. Quantitative Real-Time Polymerase Chain Reaction (PCR) Analysis

Total RNA was extracted from F3, F3.ChAT cells, and brain tissues using TRIzol Reagent (Invitrogen, Carlsbad, CA, USA), following the manufacturer's instructions. The real-time quantitative PCR was performed as described in prior literature. The housekeeping gene, glyceraldehyde 3-phosphate dehydrogenase (GAPDH), served as an internal standard to normalize the expression of target transcripts. Primers used to amplify the transcripts of choline transporter (CHT), choline acetyltransferase (ChAT), vesicular acetylcholine transporter (VAChT), nicotinic acetylcholine receptor (nAChR) α5 and β2, muscarinic1 acetylcholine receptor (m1AChR), nerve growth factor (NGF), and brain-derived growth factor (BDNF) are listed in Supplementary Table S1. Data from three independent assays, each conducted in triplicate, were analyzed using the comparative Ct method [42].

2.15. *Western Blot Analysis*

Both the F3 and F3.ChAT cells, as well as brain tissues, were homogenized in 10 volumes of Radioimmunoprecipitation Assay (RIPA) buffer (Thermo Fisher Scientific, Waltham, MA, USA), supplemented with protease (Sigma-Aldrich) and phosphatase (Sigma-Aldrich) inhibitors. The Western blotting procedure was performed as previously described [12]. Membranes were subjected to immunoblotting with the appropriate primary antibodies, which was followed by incubation with horseradish peroxidase-conjugated anti-rabbit and anti-mouse secondary antibodies (Jackson ImmunoResearch Laboratories, Inc., West Grove, PA, USA). The specific antibodies utilized in this study are detailed in Supplementary Table S2. Band densities were quantified using ImageJ software (NIH, Bethesda, MD, USA) and were normalized to the actin controls.

2.16. *Glial Fibrillary Acidic Protein (GFAP) Immunostaining of Brain Tissue*

The brain tissues of the mice were perfused with a 10% paraformaldehyde solution, followed by a 48 h post-fixation in the same solution. Tissues were then cryoprotected in a 30% sucrose solution for 72 h. Coronal cryosections, 1.0 mm posterior to the bregma and 30 μm thick, were prepared. For the immunohistochemical staining of astrocytic GFAP, brain cryosections were rinsed in Tris-buffered saline (TBS) and treated with 3% hydrogen peroxide for 5 min to block endogenous peroxidase activity. After rinsing with TBS and a blocking step with 5% BSA, the sections were incubated at 4 °C overnight with a GFAP-specific antibody (1:300; rabbit polyclonal, Chemicon, Temecula, CA, USA). This was followed by incubation with a secondary antibody conjugated with Alexa Fluor-594 (1:300; Molecular Probes, Eugene, OR, USA). The sections were counterstained with 4′,6-diamidino-2-phenylindole (DAPI, Sigma-Aldrich) to visualize cellular nuclei. GFAP staining was used in combination with DAPI staining to identify astrocytes based on their characteristic morphology and location within the brain tissue. Following staining, all samples were immediately evaluated and photographed using a fluorescence microscope (EVOS FL Auto2 Cell imaging system; Thermo Fisher Scientific, Waltham, MA, USA). The area of GFAP-positive cells was quantified using ImageJ software.

2.17. *Brain Acetylcholine Concentration Analysis*

To measure the concentration of acetylcholine, the mice's brains were weighed and homogenized in nine volumes of phosphate-buffered saline (PBS) that included a protease inhibitor cocktail (Sigma-Aldrich). The protease inhibitors were included to prevent the degradation of acetylcholine by acetylcholinesterase, ensuring an accurate measurement of its concentration. The brain tissue was rapidly collected and processed after the mice were sacrificed to reduce ischemic damage and inhibit post-mortem metabolism. After centrifugation at 13,500× *g* for 6 min at 4 °C, the supernatant's acetylcholine concentration was measured using the Amplex Red acetylcholine/acetylcholinesterase assay kit (Molecular Probes, Eugene, OR, USA) according to the manufacturer's instructions. In this assay, acetylcholinesterase hydrolyzes acetylcholine to produce choline, which is then oxidized into betaine and H_2O_2 by choline oxidase. H_2O_2 reacts with Amplex Red (7-dihydroxyphenoxazine) in the presence of horseradish peroxidase, generating the highly fluorescent compound, resorufin. The resulting fluorescence was measured using a fluorescence microplate reader (Molecular Devices) with an excitation range of 530–560 nm and emission detection at 590 nm. It is important to note that the control group's reported value of almost 1 mmol/g of tissue may vary, so it should be interpreted with caution.

2.18. Statistical Analyses

Statistical analyses were carried out using a one-way ANOVA, followed by Tukey's post hoc test. The normality of the data was not explicitly tested prior to applying ANOVA, but the assumption of normality was inferred through the visual inspection of histograms and normal probability plots where necessary. All analyses were carried out using the Statistical Package for the Social Sciences for Windows software (version 12.0; SPSS Inc., Chicago, IL, USA). Statistical significance was set at $p < 0.05$. All data are presented as the mean $\pm$ standard deviation (SD).

3. Results

3.1. Composition of Ginsenosides, Polyphenols, and Flavonoids in Pre- and Post-Fermented GBE

To investigate the effect of GBE fermentation, we analyzed the contents of pre- and post-fermented GBE using HPLC. As shown in Figure 2 and Supplementary Table S3, the pre-fermented GBE was primarily composed of Re, Rd, Rb1, Rb2, and Rc, while the post-fermented GBE exhibited significant increases in Rg3(S), Rg3(R), Rk1, and Rg5 compared to the pre-fermented GBE. Interestingly, the contents of total polyphenols and flavonoids also significantly increased after fermentation, from 24.26 $\pm$ 0.23 to 28.40 $\pm$ 0.10 mg GAE/g and from 3.95 $\pm$ 0.07 to 4.71 $\pm$ 0.12 mg QE/g, respectively.

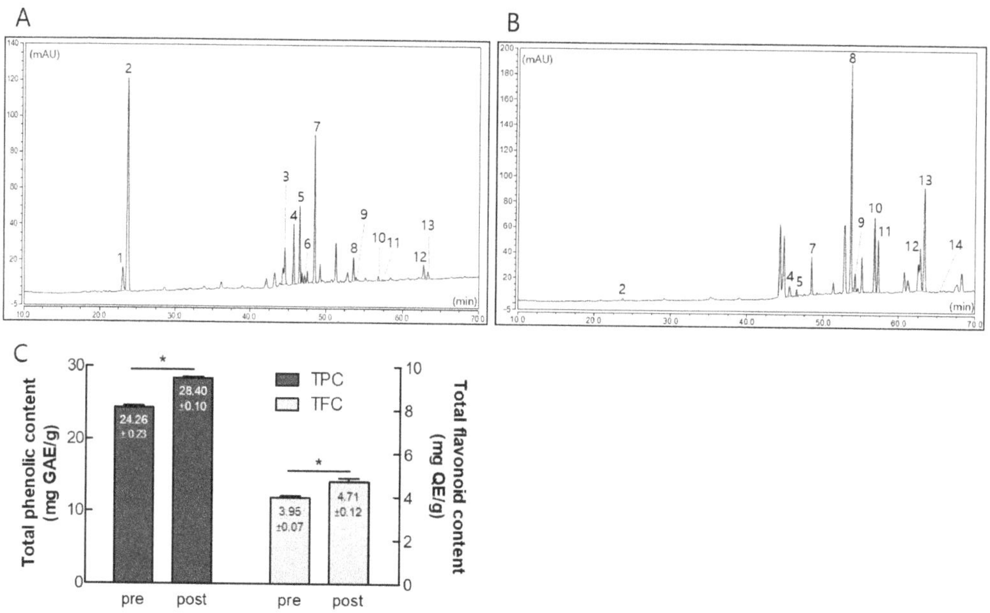

Figure 2. Contents of ginsenoside, total polyphenols, and flavonoids in pre- and post-fermented ginseng berry extract (GBE). (**A**,**B**) High-performance liquid chromatography (HPLC) chromatograms of ginsenosides in pre- (**A**) and post- (**B**) fermented GBE. Peaks were analyzed based on HPLC chromatograms of the ginsenoside standard mixture. (**C**) Total amounts of phenol (mg gallic acid equivalents per gram of dry extract) and flavonoid (mg quercetin equivalents per gram of dry extract) compounds. Data are presented as mean $\pm$ SD in triplicates. * $p < 0.05$, significantly different from pre-fermented GBE.

3.2. Comparative Physiological Properties of Pre- and Post-Fermented GBE

To investigate the physiological properties of pre- and post-fermented GBE, we analyzed their effects on TBARS, DPPH, AChE inhibitory effect, and hydroxyl radical-mediated oxidation using assays. As shown in Figure 3A, treatment with $FeCl_3$ (50 μM) resulted in a 2.4-fold increase in MDA production, which was reduced by both pre- and post-fermented GBE. The antioxidative effects of post-fermented GBE were significantly different at 125 μg/mL compared to pre-fermented GBE. Similarly, the radical scavenging activity (RSA) of post-fermented GBE was significantly increased at 250 μg/mL, while the RSA of pre-fermented GBE was only significant at 500 μg/mL (Figure 3B). In addition, the activity of AChE decreased with increasing concentrations of pre- and post-fermented GBE, significantly reducing from 16 μg/mL in pre-fermented GBE to 2 μg/mL in post-fermented GBE (Figure 3C). The inhibitory effect of AChE activity in post-fermented GBE was significantly different at 250 μg/mL compared to pre-fermented GBE. Both pre- and post-fermented GBE exhibited antioxidative effects in the hydroxyl radical-mediated oxidation assay at 125 μg/mL, with the effect of post-fermented GBE being generally superior to that of pre-fermented GBE (Figure 3D). Subsequent experiments were therefore conducted using post-fermented GBE.

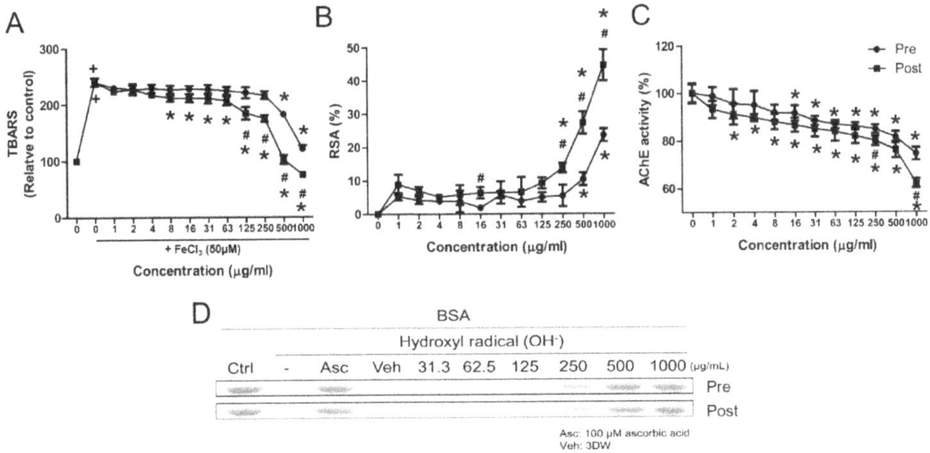

Figure 3. Physiological properties of pre- and post-fermented GBE. (**A**) Inhibitory activity on $FeCl_3$-induced lipid peroxidation (thiobarbituric acid reactive substances (TBARS) production), (**B**) 1,1-diphenyl-2-picrylhydrazyl (DPPH) radical-scavenging activity (RSA) in 10 min, (**C**) acetylcholinesterase (AChE) activity in brain tissue treated with pre- and post-fermented GBE, and (**D**) hydroxyl radical-mediated oxidation assay using H_2O_2 and BSA. All samples were analyzed in triplicate. Data are presented as mean ± SD in triplicates. + $p < 0.05$, significantly different from normal control; * $p < 0.05$, significantly different from vehicle; # $p < 0.05$, significantly different from pre-fermented GBE.

3.3. *Protective Effects of Post-Fermented GBE on AF64A-Induced Damage in F3 and F3.ChAT Cells*

To confirm the protective effect, the cytotoxicity of post-fermented GBE and AF64A was evaluated at various concentrations (0–1000 μM, respectively) on F3 and F3.ChAT cells. Overall, post-fermented GBE was almost non-toxic, but toxicity was observed at the highest concentration (1000 μg/mL) (Figure 4A). In the case of AF64A (Figure 4B), toxicity was observed at 63 μM, and the experiment was conducted at 100 μM, at which 80% of the F3 and F3.ChAT cells survived. The LDH assay showed that AF64A significantly increased the release of LDH from the F3 and F3.ChAT cells (Figure 4C,D); however, post-fermented GBE treatment significantly decreased it in a dose-dependent manner. However, treatment with donepezil (1 μM) as a reference drug did not show a protective effect.

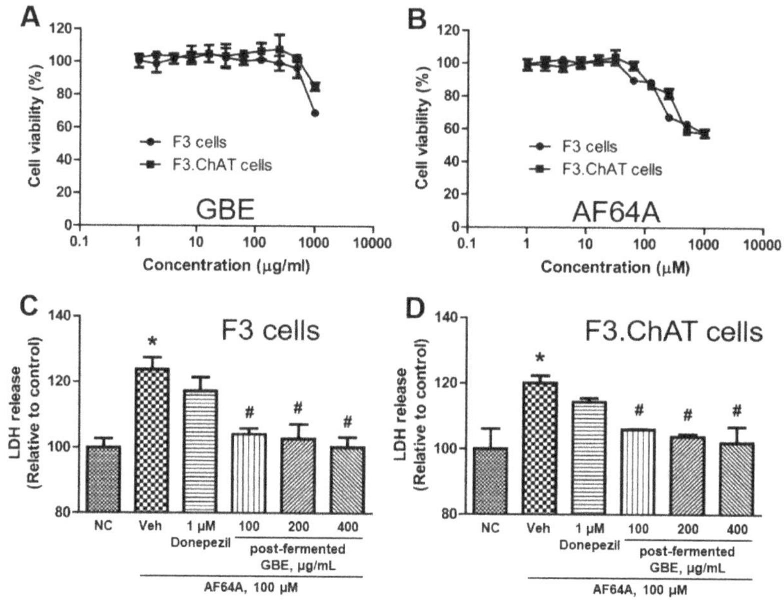

Figure 4. Cytotoxicity and protective effect of post-fermented GBE in F3 and F3.ChAT cells. (**A**,**B**) Cell viability of F3 and F3.ChAT cells was treated with various doses of post-fermented GBE (0 to 1000 μg/mL) (**A**) and various doses of AF64A (0 to 1000 μM) (**B**). (**C**,**D**) Protective effect of post-fermented GBE on AF64A-induced damage in F3 cells (**C**) and F3.ChAT cells. Donepezil was used as a reference control. LDH, lactate dehydrogenase. Data are presented as mean ± SD in triplicates. * $p < 0.05$, significantly different from normal control (NC); # $p < 0.05$, significantly different from vehicle.

3.4. Post-Fermented GBE's Effects on Cholinergic Pathway in AF64A-Damaged F3 and F3.ChAT Cells

To investigate the neuroprotective effects of post-fermented GBE, the genes related to the cholinergic pathway in F3 (Figure 5) and F3.ChAT (Figure 6) cells were analyzed by real-time PCR. As expected, AF64A significantly reduced the gene expression related to acetylcholine synthesis, including CHT, ChAT, and VAChT, as well as the cholinergic receptors nAChR α5, nAChR β2, and m1AChR, and the growth factors NGF and BDNF. However, treatment with post-fermented GBE significantly increased the expression of these genes in a concentration-dependent manner. Coincidently, Western blot analysis showed that AF64A treatment (100 μM) decreased the expression of BDNF, NGF, ChAT, and VAChT, while treatment with post-fermented GBE increased their expression (Figure 7). Treatment with donepezil (1 μM) also increased the expression of these genes and proteins; however, the effect of post-fermented GBE was overall better than that of donepezil.

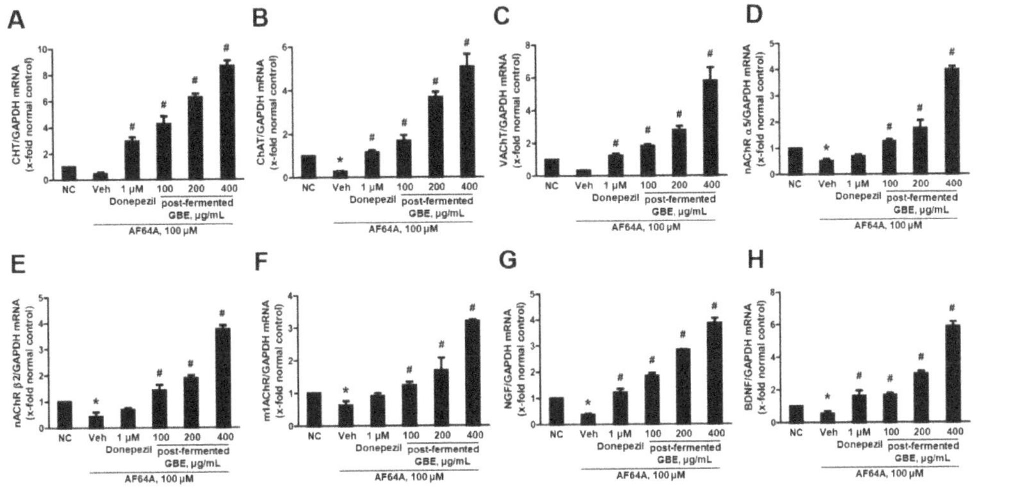

Figure 5. Effects of post-fermented GBE on the cholinergic pathway in AF64A-induced damage in human neural stem cells (F3 cells). (**A**) Choline transporter (CHT), (**B**) choline acetyltransferase (ChAT), (**C**) vesicular acetylcholine transporter (VAChT), (**D**) nicotinic acetylcholine receptors (nAChR) α5, (**E**) nAChR β2, (**F**) muscarinic 1 acetylcholine receptor (m1AChR), (**G**) nerve growth factor (NGF), and (**H**) brain-derived neurotrophic factor (BDNF) gene expression were analyzed by real-time PCR and normalized to GAPDH. Data are presented as mean ± SD in triplicates. * $p < 0.05$, significantly different from normal control (NC); # $p < 0.05$, significantly different from vehicle.

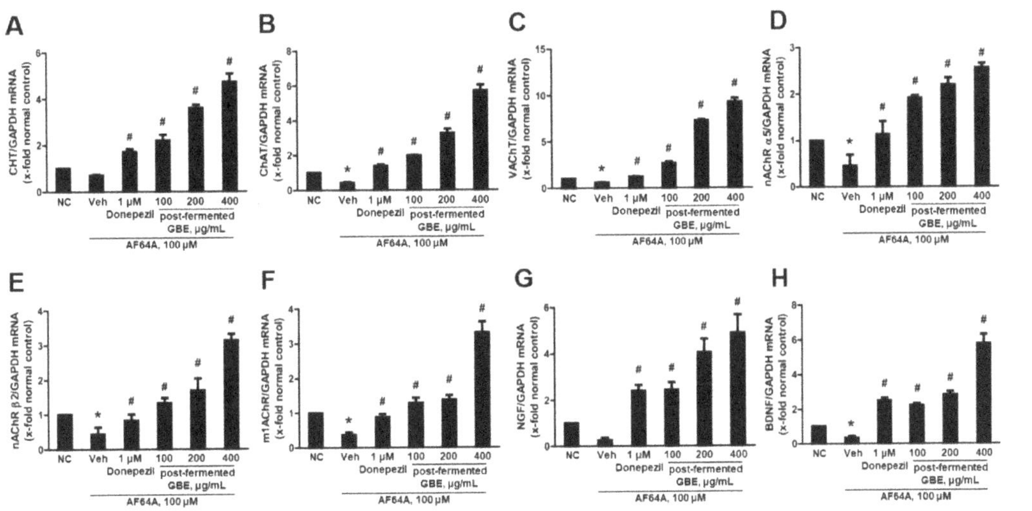

Figure 6. Effects of post-fermented GBE on the cholinergic pathway in AF64A-induced damage in ChAT overexpressing human neural stem cells (F3.ChAT cells). (**A**) CHT, (**B**) ChAT, (**C**) VAChT, (**D**) nAChR α5, (**E**) nAChR β2, (**F**) m1AChR, (**G**) NGF, and (**H**) BDNF gene expression were analyzed by real-time PCR and normalized to GAPDH. Data are presented as mean ± SD in triplicates. * $p < 0.05$, significantly different from normal control (NC); # $p < 0.05$, significantly different from vehicle.

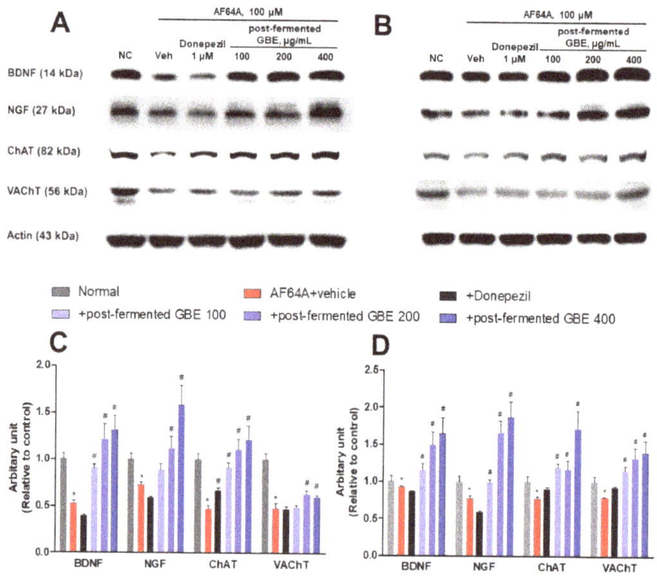

Figure 7. Effects of post-fermented GBE on protein expression in AF64A-induced damage in F3 (**A**,**C**) and F3.ChAT cells (**B**,**D**). (**A**,**B**) Representative bands of F3 (**A**) and F3.ChAT (**B**) cells. Protein expression was analyzed by Western blotting. (**C**,**D**) The band densities of F3 (**C**) and F3.ChAT (**D**) cells were quantified in arbitrary units and normalized to actin. Data are presented in triplicates as mean ± SD. * $p < 0.05$, significantly different from normal control (NC); # $p < 0.05$, significantly different from vehicle.

3.5. Restoration of Cognitive Function in AF64A-Induced Memory Deficit Animals

Two weeks after AF64A injection, memory deficit was confirmed in some animals using passive avoidance and Morris water maze performances. The mice were then orally administered with post-fermented GBE (0, 100, 200, and 400 mg/kg) and donepezil (2 mg/kg) for 6 weeks, during which no adverse effects such as weight loss were observed (Supplementary Figure S1). If no significant changes in body weight were observed, we proceeded with the next phase of cognitive testing. After 6 weeks, learning and memory function in mice were analyzed by passive avoidance and Morris water maze performances (Figure 8). In the passive avoidance performance, the retention time of animals in the normal group increased from the 3rd trial, reaching a maximum from the 5th trial. The retention time of animals in the AF64A + vehicle group did not increase. However, the retention time of animals in the AF64A + post-fermented GBE group increased, especially at 400 mg/kg, with the time increasing from the 4th trial and reaching a maximum from the 5th trial, similar to the normal group. Similarly, in the Morris water maze performance, the escape time of animals in the normal group decreased as the number of trials increased; however, the AF64A + vehicle group did not decrease. However, animals in the AF64A + post-fermented GBE group had a reduced escape time as in the normal group.

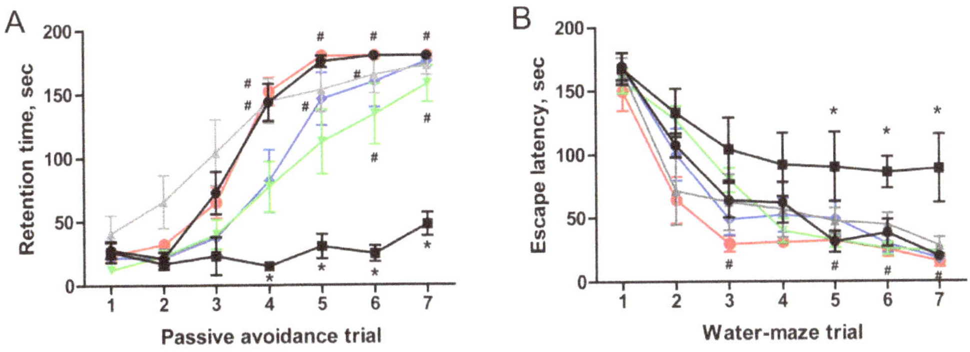

Figure 8. Recovery of cognitive function in AF64A-induced memory deficit animals (n = 7 in each group): (**A**) passive avoidance performance and (**B**) Morris water maze performance. The endpoint was set at 180 s if the animals stayed in the light chamber in the passive avoidance test or failed to find the platform in the Morris water maze test. ●, Normal; ■, AF64A (3 nmol) + vehicle; ▲, AF64A (3 nmol) + Donepezil (2 mg/kg); ▼, AF64A (3 nmol) + post-fermented GBE (100 mg/kg); ♦, AF64A (3 nmol) + post-fermented GBE (200 mg/kg); ●, AF64A (3 nmol) + post-fermented GBE (400 mg/kg). Data are presented as mean ± SD in triplicates. * $p < 0.05$, significantly different from normal control (NC); # $p < 0.05$, significantly different from vehicle.

3.6. Cholinergic Pathway Modulation by Post-Fermented GBE in AF64A-Induced Brain Damage in Mice

The effect on the cholinergic pathway was analyzed by real-time RT-PCR in cells (Figure 9). In the AF64A + vehicle group, there was a significant reduction in the gene expression of CHT, ChAT, VAChT, nAChR α5, nAChR β2, m1AChR, NGF, and BDNF. However, animals treated with post-fermented GBE in the AF64A + group showed a dose-dependent increase in the expression of these genes.

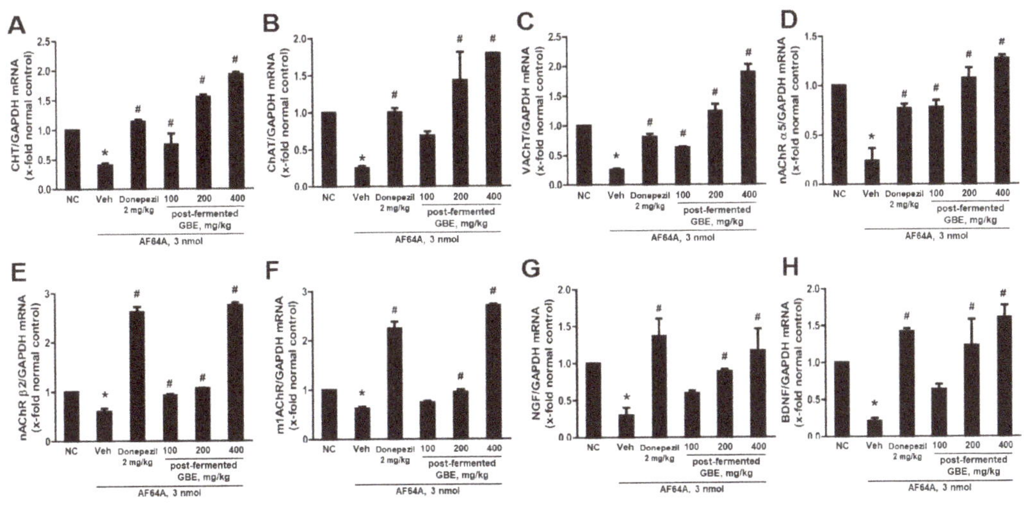

Figure 9. Effects of post-fermented GBE on the cholinergic pathway in AF64A-induced brain damage in mice (n = 5 in each group). (**A**) CHT, (**B**) ChAT, (**C**) VAChT, (**D**) nAChR α5, (**E**) nAChR β2, (**F**) m1AChR, (**G**) NGF, and (**H**) BDNF gene expression were analyzed by real-time PCR and normalized to GAPDH. Data are presented as mean ± SD in triplicates. * $p < 0.05$, significantly different from normal control (NC); # $p < 0.05$, significantly different from vehicle.

In the Western blotting (Figure 10), the expression of CHT, ChAT, VAChT, BDNF, and NGF was significantly decreased by AF64A injection. However, their expression was increased by the administration of post-fermented GBE. Also, the expression of GFAP and amyloid beta (Aβ) was significantly increased by AF64A injection. However, their expression was significantly decreased by the administration of post-fermented GBE.

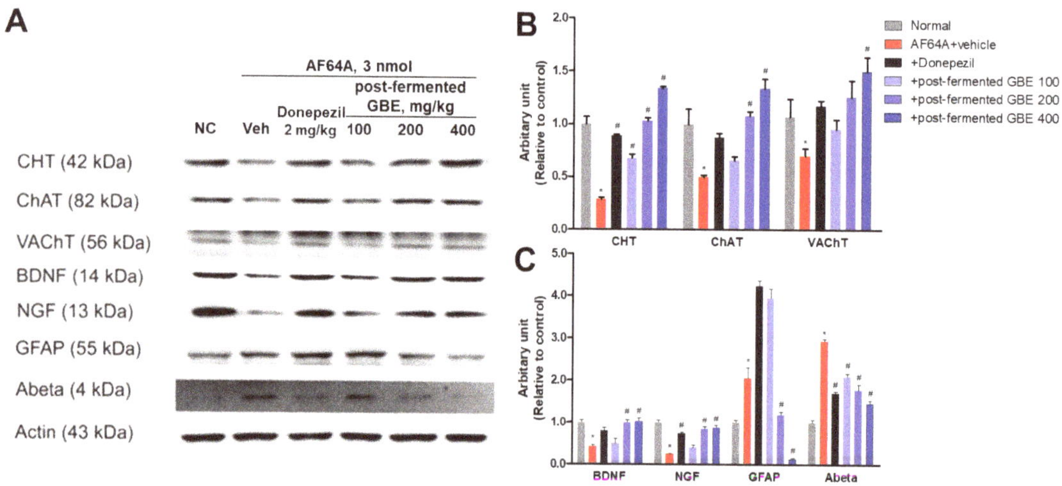

Figure 10. Effects of post-fermented GBE on protein expression in AF64A-induced brain damage in mice (n = 5 in each group). (**A**) Representative bands of brain tissues in mice. Protein expression was analyzed by Western blotting. (**B**,**C**) The band densities of brain tissues in mice were quantified in arbitrary units and normalized to actin. Data are presented as mean ± SD in triplicates. * $p < 0.05$, significantly different from normal control (NC); # $p < 0.05$, significantly different from vehicle.

3.7. GFAP Inactivation by Post-Fermented GBE in the Context of AF64A-Induced Brain Damage in Mice

Inflammation-activated central nervous system astrocytes are characterized by hypertrophy and proliferation, along with an upregulation of their cytoskeletal protein, GFAP. As shown in Figure 11, intensive GFAP-immunoreactivities (red-colored) were observed in activated astrocytes in the subventricular zone of AF64A-injected mice. However, astrocytic activation was significantly inhibited by the administration of post-fermented GBE (100–400 mg/kg) to normal levels in the subventricular zone.

3.8. ACh Concentration Improvement in AF64A-Induced Brain Damage through Post-Fermented GBE Administration

Our study revealed a significant increase in the number of activated astrocytes in the vehicle group following AF64A injection. However, the administration of post-fermented GBE reduced the number of these activated astrocytes in a dose-dependent manner, as shown in Figure 12A, where the count of activated astrocytes was measured using ImageJ software. Additionally, in the vehicle group, we observed a significant reduction in ACh levels after the AF64A injection, as depicted in Figure 12B. Intriguingly, post-fermented GBE administration led to a dose-dependent recovery of ACh concentration. Notably, we observed a direct correlation between the increase in ACh levels and the dosage of post-fermented GBE administered.

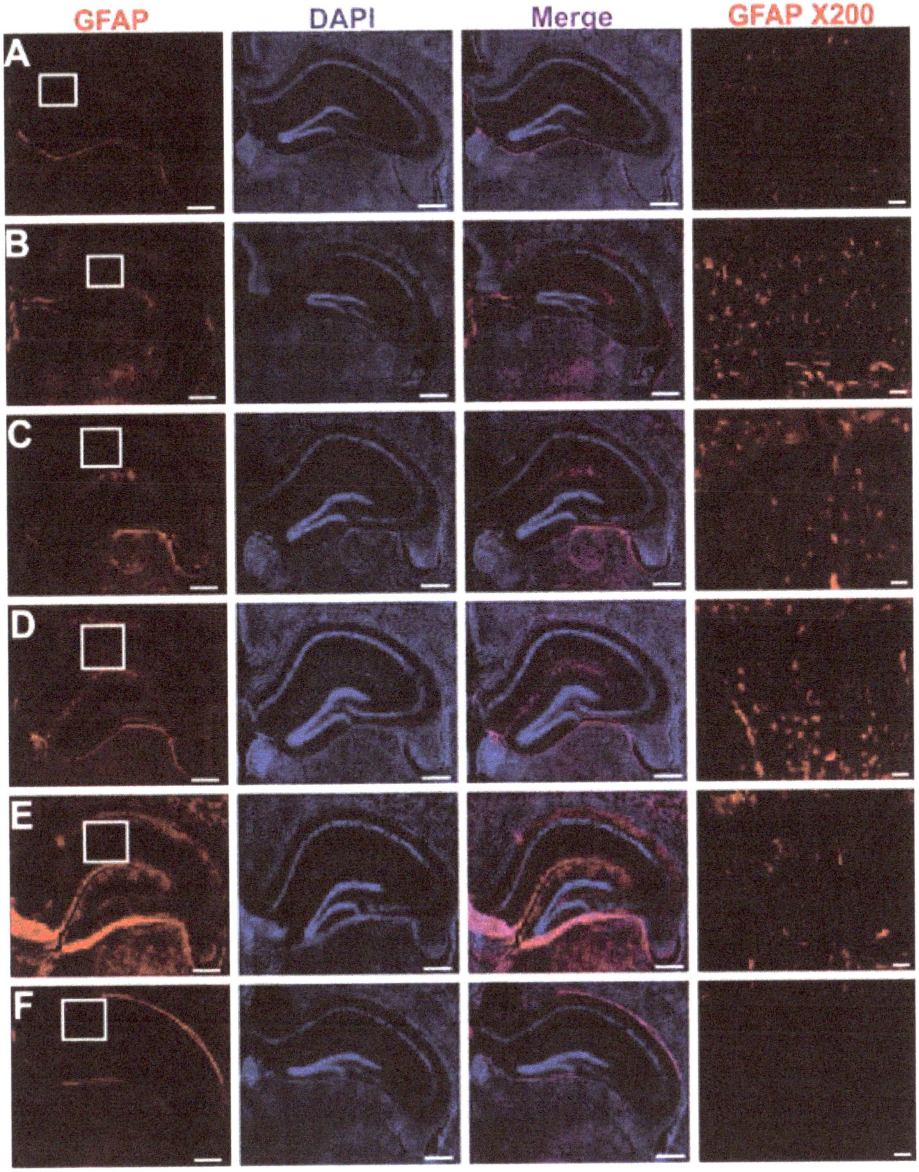

Figure 11. Inactivation of Glial Fibrillary Acidic Protein (GFAP) by post-fermented GBE in AF64A-induced brain damage in mice (n = 2 in each group). (**A–F**) These panels present representative microscopic images of activated (GFAP-positive) astrocytes, colored in red, scale bar = 500 μm. DAPI was used as a counterstain. The white square in the GFAPx200 image shows an enlarged photograph of GFAP, scale bar = 50 μm. (**A**) Normal, (**B**) AF64A (3 nmol) + vehicle, (**C**) AF64A (3 nmol) + Donepezil (2 mg/kg), (**D**) AF64A (3 nmol) + post-fermented GBE (100 mg/kg), (**E**) AF64A (3 nmol) + post-fermented GBE (200 mg/kg), and (**F**) AF64A (3 nmol) + post-fermented GBE (400 mg/kg).

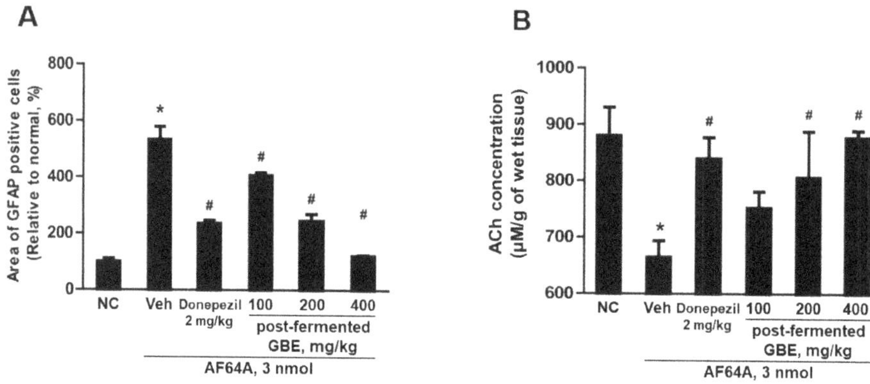

Figure 12. Illustration of the effects of post-fermented GBE on activated astrocytes count and acetylcholine (ACh) concentration following AF64A-induced brain damage. (**A**) Quantification of activated astrocytes (GFAP-positive) was performed using ImageJ software (n = 2 in each group). (**B**) The concentration of ACh in brain tissue was evaluated using an acetylcholine/acetylcholinesterase assay kit, following the protocol outlined in the Materials and Methods section (n = 5 in each group). Data are presented as mean ± SD in triplicates. * $p < 0.05$, significantly different from normal control (NC); # $p < 0.05$, significantly different from vehicle.

4. Discussion and Conclusions

The present study investigated the potential cognitive benefits of fermented GBE in a rodent model of AF64A-induced memory deficits. In this study, the active ingredients of GBE were found to be enhanced after fermentation, as evidenced by a chromatographic analysis comparing pre- and post-fermented GBE. Furthermore, the treatment with fermented GBE restored the cholinergic nervous system in human neural stem cells and animals damaged by AF64A. Thus, these findings suggest that fermented GBE could hold the potential for treating memory deficits in clinical applications. Ginseng has long been utilized in traditional oriental medicine due to its therapeutic effects, which are primarily attributed to its bioactive components, ginsenosides, that are extensively studied in ginseng roots [43]. Recently, ginseng berries have been considered a potential alternative source of bioactive compounds, as they contain a relatively high concentration of ginsenosides, primarily Re and Rd [23]. Additionally, the bioactivity of ginseng can be enhanced through processing methods, such as red ginseng preparation, which can result in higher levels of ginsenosides [44,45]. Our previous studies demonstrated that fermenting ginseng berries using *L. plantarum* can alter the composition of ginsenosides and increase their pharmacological activities [35,46]. Similarly, in this study, we confirmed that the content of Rg3, total polyphenols, and flavonoids increased after fermentation with *L. plantarum*.

The change in ginsenoside composition led to altered physiological activity, resulting in increased antioxidant and anti-inflammatory effects, as confirmed by the DPPH assay, hydroxyl radiated oxidation assay, and MDA assay. Additionally, the AChE activity test showed an inhibitory effect on AChE activity in both pre- and post-fermented GBE. The key ginsenosides of pre-fermented GBE, Re and Rc, are known to regulate the cholinergic nervous system [47,48], while Rg3, Rg5, and Rk1 in post-fermented GBE are reported to inhibit AChE activity [48,49]. In vitro and in vivo tests were conducted to investigate the effects of post-fermented GBE on the cholinergic nervous system. AF64A, a cholinergic toxin, is widely used in screening drugs for the development of dementia treatments [41,50]. In this study, AF64A induced overall inhibition of the cholinergic nervous system in human neural stem cells, reduced the concentration of acetylcholine in brain tissue, and increased the expression of GFAP, an indicator of inflammation and brain damage in animal tests [12,42,51,52]. However, treatment with post-fermented GBE counteracted the effect of

AF64A, enhancing the activity of the cholinergic nervous system. This increase in activity was attributed to increased expression of NGF and BDNF, which prevent nerve cell death and promote their proliferation, as well as increased activity of the cholinergic nervous system [12,53–55]. Thus, an increase in ginsenosides, such as Rg3, Rg5, and Rk1, in post-fermented GBE seems to inhibit inflammation caused by AF64A and increase antioxidant effects to protect cells [56,57], as well as increase BDNF and NGF to regulate the expression of the cholinergic nervous system [58–60]. Interestingly, the administration of AF64A led to an increase in amyloid-beta, which is thought to be due to the change of the amyloidogenic pathway by increased inflammation [41]. Additionally, the administration of GBE reduced the level of Aβ. Although this study demonstrated that the cholinergic nervous system was restored by increasing the levels of BDNF and NGF through the administration of GBE, further research is needed to investigate the reduction of Aβ through the administration of post-fermented GBE. These findings strongly suggest that the robust antioxidant properties of fermented GBE could aid in protecting against oxidative stress, known to contribute to cognitive decline. Furthermore, it may modulate neurotransmitter systems, such as the cholinergic system, as well as Aβ levels, which play crucial roles in memory, learning, and neuropathogenesis.

Although our study provides valuable insights into the effects of pre- and post-fermented GBE and AF64A on cholinergic neurons, it is important to recognize the limitations of our experimental model. Despite these, the findings from this research carry significant clinical implications for the development of new treatments for Alzheimer's disease and other cognitive disorders. Future studies employing more complex and comprehensive models of AD could provide further insights into the effects of these treatments on AD pathogenesis.

In summary, this study demonstrates that GBE fermented by *L. plantarum* leads to an increase in bioactive compounds, such as Rg3, Rg5, Rk1, total polyphenols, and flavonoids, compared to pre-fermented GBE. This results in enhanced pharmacological activities, including antioxidant and anti-inflammatory effects. Notably, post-fermented GBE also seems to upregulate the expression of NGF and BDNF while reducing AChE activity. These effects may help protect against brain damage and restore memory in AF64A-induced memory-deficient animals. Overall, these findings suggest that fermented GBE holds potential as a therapeutic agent for AD and other neurodegenerative disorders. However, further research is needed to elucidate the underlying mechanisms of the observed effects and to determine the optimal dosage and treatment duration for maximum efficacy. Additionally, future studies should employ more comprehensive and accurate models of AD that better represent the disease's pathological features to assess the therapeutic potential of fermented GBE more reliably. This would aid in determining the feasibility of fermented GBE as a treatment for AD and related neurodegenerative disorders. Moreover, clinical trials involving human subjects are necessary to evaluate the safety, tolerability, and efficacy of fermented GBE in real-world settings. By conducting these future studies, researchers can build upon the current findings and potentially develop novel treatment options for patients suffering from Alzheimer's disease and other neurodegenerative conditions.

AD is a progressive neurodegenerative disorder that currently has no known curative treatment. However, there are several therapeutic and preventive treatments available that can help to manage symptoms and slow disease progression. These treatments include medications like AChE inhibitors (donepezil, rivastigmine, and galantamine) and memantine, as well as non-pharmacological interventions like cognitive stimulation therapy and physical exercise. While these treatments can provide some relief to patients, there is still a need for more effective treatments and preventative measures due to an incomplete understanding of the pathophysiology of AD. Therefore, there is a growing interest in the application of natural extracts as potential therapeutic agents for AD. Our study provides valuable insights into the potential cognitive benefits of fermented GBE, underscoring the need for continued research to fully comprehend its clinical applications. The findings suggest that fermented GBE, rich in the major active ginsenosides verified in this study, holds promise as a candidate for developing new therapeutic interventions for memory deficits and cognitive disorders. However, it is important to note that the current study was conducted in animal models, and further research is needed to determine the safety, tolerability, and efficacy of fermented GBE in human populations. Future clinical trials involving human subjects will be necessary to evaluate the potential therapeutic benefits of fermented GBE in real-world settings. By conducting these future studies, researchers can build upon the current findings and potentially develop novel treatment options for patients suffering from Alzheimer's disease and other neurodegenerative conditions.

In conclusion, our study sheds light on the potential cognitive benefits of fermented GBE, thus emphasizing the necessity for further research to fully unravel its clinical implications. The results imply that fermented GBE, enriched with the primary active ginsenosides confirmed in our study, presents itself as a promising avenue for the creation of novel therapeutic interventions to address memory impairments and cognitive dysfunctions. Nevertheless, it is crucial to recognize that our study relied on animal models, warranting subsequent studies to validate the safety, tolerability, and effectiveness of fermented GBE in human subjects. Future clinical trials involving human participants will be indispensable for gauging the potential therapeutic advantages of fermented GBE in practical scenarios. By executing these prospective investigations, scientists can expand on our current knowledge and potentially formulate innovative treatment strategies for patients afflicted with Alzheimer's disease and other neurodegenerative disorders.

Supplementary Materials: The following supporting information can be downloaded at https://www.mdpi.com/article/10.3390/nu15153389/s1, Table S1: Primer sequences used for PCR analysis in this study; Table S2: List of antibodies used in the current study; Table S3: Contents of ginsenoside in pre- and post-fermented GBE (mg/g). Figure S1: The body weights during the experimental period.

Author Contributions: Conceptualization, S.-S.J. and D.P.; methodology, H.-S.K.; software, Y.C.; validation, E.-J.Y., J.J. and J.-W.A.; formal analysis, E.-J.Y. and J.-W.A.; investigation, S.-S.J. and D.P.; data curation, E.-J.Y. and D.P.; writing—original draft preparation, E.-J.Y. and J.-W.A. writing—review and editing, S.-S.J. and D.P.; visualization, E.-J.Y. and J.-W.A.; supervision, S.-S.J. and D.P.; project administration, S.-S.J. and D.P.; funding acquisition, S.-S.J. and D.P. All authors have read and agreed to the published version of the manuscript.

Funding: This research was supported by the Republic of Korea Health Technology R&D Project through the Republic of Korea Health Industry Development Institute (KHIDI) and Republic of Korea Dementia Research Center (KDRC), funded by the Ministry of Health and Welfare and Ministry of Science and ICT, Republic of Korea (grant number: HU21C0332).

Institutional Review Board Statement: The animal study protocol was approved by the Institutional Animal Care and Use Committee of Chungbuk National University, Republic of Korea ((#CBNUA-1398-20-01).

Informed Consent Statement: Not applicable.

Data Availability Statement: All data generated from this study are contained within the article.

Conflicts of Interest: The authors declare no conflict of interest.

References

1. Pardo-Moreno, T.; Gonzalez-Acedo, A.; Rivas-Dominguez, A.; Garcia-Morales, V.; Garcia-Cozar, F.J.; Ramos-Rodriguez, J.J.; Melguizo-Rodriguez, L. Therapeutic approach to Alzheimer's disease: Current treatments and new perspectives. *Pharmaceutics* **2022**, *14*, 1117. [CrossRef] [PubMed]
2. Alzheimer, A.; Stelzmann, R.A.; Schnitzlein, H.N.; Murtagh, F.R. An english translation of Alzheimer's 1907 paper, "Uber eine eigenartige Erkankung der Hirnrinde". *Clin. Anat.* **1995**, *8*, 429–431. [PubMed]
3. DeTure, M.A.; Dickson, D.W. The neuropathological diagnosis of Alzheimer's disease. *Mol. Neurodegener.* **2019**, *14*, 32. [CrossRef]
4. Ashrafian, H.; Zadeh, E.H.; Khan, R.H. Review on Alzheimer's disease: Inhibition of amyloid beta and tau tangle formation. *Int. J. Biol. Macromol.* **2021**, *167*, 382–394. [CrossRef]
5. Gao, Y.; Tan, L.; Yu, J.T.; Tan, L. Tau in Alzheimer's disease: Mechanisms and therapeutic strategies. *Curr. Alzheimer Res.* **2018**, *15*, 283–300. [CrossRef]

6. Pinheiro, L.; Faustino, C. Therapeutic strategies targeting amyloid-beta in Alzheimer's disease. *Curr. Alzheimer Res.* **2019**, *16*, 418–452. [CrossRef]
7. Arvanitakis, Z.; Shah, R.C.; Bennett, D.A. Diagnosis and management of dementia: Review. *JAMA* **2019**, *322*, 1589–1599. [CrossRef] [PubMed]
8. Cummings, J.; Lee, G.; Zhong, K.; Fonseca, J.; Taghva, K. Alzheimer's disease drug development pipeline: 2021. *Alzheimers Dement.* **2021**, *7*, e12179. [CrossRef] [PubMed]
9. Huang, L.K.; Chao, S.P.; Hu, C.J. Clinical trials of new drugs for Alzheimer disease. *J. Biomed. Sci.* **2020**, *27*, 18. [CrossRef] [PubMed]
10. Garcia-Morales, V.; Gonzalez-Acedo, A.; Melguizo-Rodriguez, L.; Pardo-Moreno, T.; Costela-Ruiz, V.J.; Montiel-Troya, M.; Ramos-Rodriguez, J.J. Current understanding of the physiopathology, diagnosis and therapeutic approach to Alzheimer's disease. *Biomedicines* **2021**, *9*, 1910. [CrossRef]
11. Dou, K.X.; Tan, M.S.; Tan, C.C.; Cao, X.P.; Hou, X.H.; Guo, Q.H.; Tan, L.; Mok, V.; Yu, J.T. Comparative safety and effectiveness of cholinesterase inhibitors and memantine for Alzheimer's disease: A network meta-analysis of 41 randomized controlled trials. *Alzheimers Res. Ther.* **2018**, *10*, 126. [CrossRef] [PubMed]
12. Park, D.; Choi, E.K.; Cho, T.H.; Joo, S.S.; Kim, Y.B. Human neural stem cells encoding ChAT gene restore cognitive function via acetylcholine synthesis, Aβ elimination, and neuroregeneration in APPswe/PS1dE9 Mice. *Int. J. Mol. Sci.* **2020**, *21*, 3958. [CrossRef] [PubMed]
13. Vaz, M.; Silva, V.; Monteiro, C.; Silvestre, S. Role of Aducanumab in the treatment of Alzheimer's disease: Challenges and opportunities. *Clin. Interv. Aging* **2022**, *17*, 797–810. [CrossRef]
14. Thapa, A.; Carroll, N.J. Dietary modulation of oxidative stress in Alzheimer's disease. *Int. J. Mol. Sci.* **2017**, *18*, 1583. [CrossRef]
15. Carregosa, D.; Carecho, R.; Figueira, I.; Claudia, N.S. Low-molecular-weight metabolites from polyphenols as effectors for attenuating neuroinflammation. *J. Agric. Food Chem.* **2020**, *68*, 1790–1807. [CrossRef]
16. Phan, H.T.T.; Samarat, K.; Takamura, Y.; Azo-Oussou, A.F.; Nakazono, Y.; Vestergaard, M.C. Polyphenols modulate Alzheimer's amyloid beta aggregation in a structure-dependent manner. *Nutrients* **2019**, *11*, 756. [CrossRef]
17. Congdon, E.E.; Sigurdsson, E.M. Tau-targeting therapies for Alzheimer disease. *Nat. Rev. Neurol.* **2018**, *14*, 399–415. [CrossRef]
18. Cha, Y.; Lee, S.H.; Jang, S.K.; Guo, H.; Ban, Y.H.; Park, D.; Jang, G.Y.; Yeon, S.; Lee, J.Y.; Choi, E.K.; et al. A silk peptide fraction restores cognitive function in AF64A-induced Alzheimer disease model rats by increasing expression of choline acetyltransferase gene. *Toxicol. Appl. Pharmacol.* **2017**, *314*, 48–54. [CrossRef]
19. Verkhratsky, A.; Parpura, V.; Rodriguez-Arellano, J.J.; Zorec, R. Astroglia in Alzheimer's disease. *Adv. Exp. Med. Biol.* **2019**, *1175*, 273–324. [PubMed]
20. Fan, Q.I.; Hanin, I. Effects of AF64A on gene expression of choline acetyltransferase (ChAT) in the septo-hippocampal pathway and striatum in vivo. *Neurochem. Res.* **1999**, *24*, 15–24. [CrossRef] [PubMed]
21. Rapaka, D.; Adiukwu, P.C.; Bitra, V.R. Experimentally induced animal models for cognitive dysfunction and Alzheimer's disease. *MethodsX* **2022**, *9*, 101933. [CrossRef] [PubMed]
22. More, S.V.; Kumar, H.; Cho, D.Y.; Yun, Y.S.; Choi, D.K. Toxin-induced experimental models of learning and memory impairment. *Int. J. Mol. Sci.* **2016**, *17*, 1447. [CrossRef] [PubMed]
23. Han, S.Y.; Bae, M.G.; Choi, Y.H. Stereoselective and simultaneous analysis of ginsenosides from ginseng berry extract in rat plasma by UPLC-MS/MS: Application to a pharmacokinetic study of ginseng berry extract. *Molecules* **2018**, *23*, 1835. [CrossRef] [PubMed]
24. Xue, Q.; He, N.; Wang, Z.; Fu, X.; Aung, L.H.H.; Liu, Y.; Li, M.; Cho, J.Y.; Yang, Y.; Yu, T. Functional roles and mechanisms of ginsenosides from *Panax ginseng* in atherosclerosis. *J. Ginseng Res.* **2021**, *45*, 22–31. [CrossRef]
25. Bai, L.; Gao, J.; Wei, F.; Zhao, J.; Wang, D.; Wei, J. Therapeutic potential of ginsenosides as an adjuvant treatment for diabetes. *Front. Pharmacol.* **2018**, *9*, 423. [CrossRef]
26. Kim, J.; Cho, S.Y.; Kim, S.H.; Cho, D.; Kim, S.; Park, C.W.; Shimizu, T.; Cho, J.Y.; Seo, D.B.; Shin, S.S. Effects of Korean ginseng berry on skin antipigmentation and antiaging via FoxO3a activation. *J. Ginseng Res.* **2017**, *41*, 277–283. [CrossRef]
27. Hu, J.R.; Chun, Y.S.; Kim, J.K.; Cho, I.J.; Ku, S.K. Ginseng berry aqueous extract prevents scopolamine-induced memory impairment in mice. *Exp. Ther. Med.* **2019**, *18*, 4388–4396. [CrossRef] [PubMed]
28. Lee, D.Y.; Park, C.W.; Lee, S.J.; Park, H.R.; Kim, S.H.; Son, S.U.; Park, J.; Shin, K.S. Anti-cancer effects of *Panax ginseng* berry polysaccharides via activation of immune-related cells. *Front. Pharmacol.* **2019**, *10*, 1411. [CrossRef] [PubMed]
29. Sanlier, N.; Gokcen, B.B.; Sezgin, A.C. Health benefits of fermented foods. *Crit. Rev. Food Sci. Nutr.* **2019**, *59*, 506–527. [CrossRef] [PubMed]
30. Juraskova, D.; Ribeiro, S.C.; Silva, C.C.G. Exopolysaccharides produced by lactic acid bacteria: From biosynthesis to health-promoting properties. *Foods* **2022**, *11*, 156. [CrossRef] [PubMed]
31. Melini, F.; Melini, V.; Luziatelli, F.; Ficca, A.G.; Ruzzi, M. Health-promoting components in fermented foods: An up-to-date systematic review. *Nutrients* **2019**, *11*, 1189. [CrossRef] [PubMed]
32. Akbarian, M.; Khani, A.; Eghbalpour, S.; Uversky, V.N. Bioactive peptides: Synthesis, sources, applications, and proposed mechanisms of action. *Int. J. Mol. Sci.* **2022**, *23*, 1445. [CrossRef]

33. Jang, S.K.; Ahn, J.W.; Jo, B.R.; Kim, H.S.; Kim, S.J.; Sung, E.A.; Lee, D.I.; Park, H.Y.; Jin, D.H.; Joo, S.S. Double-processed ginseng berry extracts enhance learning and memory in an Aβ42-induced Alzheimer's mouse model. *Korean J. Food Sci. Technol.* **2019**, *51*, 160–168.
34. Lee, D.I.; Kim, S.T.; Lee, D.H.; Yu, J.M.; Jang, S.K.; Joo, S.S. Ginsenoside-free molecules from steam-dried ginseng berry promote ethanol metabolism: An alternative choice for an alcohol hangover. *J. Food Sci.* **2014**, *79*, C1323–C1330. [CrossRef] [PubMed]
35. Kim, S.T.; Kim, H.B.; Lee, K.H.; Choi, Y.R.; Kim, H.J.; Shin, I.S.; Gyoung, Y.S.; Joo, S.S. Steam-dried ginseng berry fermented with *Lactobacillus plantarum* controls the increase of blood glucose and body weight in type 2 obese diabetic db/db mice. *J. Agric. Food Chem.* **2012**, *60*, 5438–5445. [CrossRef] [PubMed]
36. Ahn, J.W.; Jang, S.K.; Jo, B.R.; Kim, H.S.; Park, J.Y.; Park, H.Y.; Yoo, Y.M.; Joo, S.S. A therapeutic intervention for Alzheimer's disease using ginsenoside Rg3: Its role in M2 microglial activation and non-amyloidogenesis. *J. Physiol. Pharmacol.* **2021**, *72*, 185–193.
37. Choi, J.K.; Lee, Y.B.; Lee, K.H.; Im, H.C.; Kim, Y.B.; Choi, E.K.; Joo, S.S.; Jang, S.K.; Han, N.S.; Kim, C.H. Extraction conditions for phenolic compounds with antioxidant activities from white rose petals. *J. Appl. Biol. Chem.* **2015**, *58*, 117–124. [CrossRef]
38. Aryal, S.; Baniya, M.K.; Danekhu, K.; Kunwar, P.; Gurung, R.; Koirala, N. Total phenolic content, flavonoid content and antioxidant potential of wild vegetables from Western Nepal. *Plants* **2019**, *8*, 96. [CrossRef]
39. Yoon, E.J.; Lee, M.Y.; Choi, B.I.; Lim, K.J.; Hong, S.Y.; Park, D. Pharmaceutical advantages of genotx-407, a combination of extracts from *Scutellaria baicalensis* root and *Magnolia officinalis* bark. *Antioxidants* **2020**, *9*, 1111. [CrossRef]
40. Park, D.; Jeon, J.H.; Kwon, S.C.; Shin, S.; Jang, J.Y.; Jeong, H.S.; Lee, D.I.; Kim, Y.B.; Joo, S.S. Antioxidative activities of white rose flower extract and pharmaceutical advantages of its hexane fraction via free radical scavenging effects. *Biochem.Cell Biol.* **2009**, *87*, 943–952. [CrossRef]
41. Yoon, E.J.; Choi, Y.; Park, D. Effects of AF64A induction on the cholinergic and amyloidogenic pathways in human neural stem cells and rat brain for Alzheimer's disease models. *Brain Digit. Learn.* **2022**, *12*, 607–620.
42. Yon, J.M.; Kim, Y.B.; Park, D. The ethanol fraction of white rose petal extract abrogates excitotoxicity-induced neuronal damage in vivo and in vitro through inhibition of oxidative stress and proinflammation. *Nutrients* **2018**, *10*, 1375. [CrossRef] [PubMed]
43. Ratan, Z.A.; Haidere, M.F.; Hong, Y.H.; Park, S.H.; Lee, J.O.; Lee, J.; Cho, J.Y. Pharmacological potential of ginseng and its major component ginsenosides. *J. Ginseng Res.* **2021**, *45*, 199–210. [CrossRef]
44. Shin, J.H.; Park, Y.J.; Kim, W.; Kim, D.O.; Kim, B.Y.; Lee, H.; Baik, M.Y. Change of ginsenoside profiles in processed ginseng by drying, steaming, and puffing. *J. Microbiol. Biotechnol.* **2019**, *28*, 222–229. [CrossRef]
45. Hyun, S.H.; Bhilare, K.D.; In, G.; Park, C.K.; Kim, J.H. Effects of *Panax ginseng* and ginsenosides on oxidative stress and cardiovascular diseases: Pharmacological and therapeutic roles. *J. Ginseng Res.* **2022**, *46*, 33–38. [CrossRef] [PubMed]
46. Kim, S.T.; Kim, H.J.; Jang, S.K.; Lee, D.I.; Joo, S.S. Establishment of optimal fermentation conditions for steam-dried ginseng berry via friendly bacteria and its antioxidant activities. *Korean J. Food Sci. Technol.* **2013**, *45*, 77–83. [CrossRef]
47. Kim, M.S.; Yu, J.M.; Kim, H.J.; Kim, H.B.; Kim, S.T.; Jang, S.K.; Choi, Y.W.; Lee, D.I.; Joo, S.S. Ginsenoside Re and Rd enhance the expression of cholinergic markers and neuronal differentiation in Neuro-2a cells. *Biol. Pharm. Bull.* **2014**, *37*, 826–833. [CrossRef]
48. Zheng, M.; Xin, Y.; Li, Y.; Xu, F.; Xi, X.; Guo, H.; Cui, X.; Cao, H.; Zhang, X.; Han, C. Ginsenosides: A potential neuroprotective agent. *Biomed. Res. Int.* **2018**, 8174345. [CrossRef] [PubMed]
49. An, K.S.; Choi, Y.O.; Lee, S.M.; Ryu, H.Y.; Kang, S.J.; Yeon, Y.; Kim, Y.R.; Lee, J.G.; Kim, C.J.; Lee, Y.J. Ginsenosides Rg5 and Rk1 enriched cultured wild ginseng root extract bioconversion of *Pediococcus pentosaceus* HLJG0702: Effect on scopolamine-induced memory dysfunction in mice. *Nutrients* **2019**, *11*, 1120. [CrossRef]
50. Park, D.; Lee, H.J.; Joo, S.S.; Bae, D.K.; Yang, G.; Yang, Y.H.; Lim, I.; Matsuo, A.; Tooyama, I.; Kim, Y.B.; et al. Human neural stem cells over-expressing choline acetyltransferase restore cognition in rat model of cognitive dysfunction. *Exp. Neurol.* **2012**, *234*, 521–526. [CrossRef]
51. Amalia, L. Glial fibrillary acidic protein (GFAP): Neuroinflammation biomarker in acute ischemic stroke. *J. Inflamm. Res.* **2021**, *14*, 7501. [CrossRef] [PubMed]
52. Zwirner, J.; Lier, J.; Franke, H.; Hammer, N.; Matschke, J.; Trautz, F.; Tse, R.; Ondruschka, B. GFAP positivity in neurons following traumatic brain injuries. *Int. J. Legal Med.* **2021**, *135*, 2323–2333. [CrossRef] [PubMed]
53. Amadoro, G.; Latina, V.; Balzamino, B.O.; Squitti, R.; Varano, M.; Calissano, P.; Micera, A. Nerve growth factor-based therapy in Alzheimer's disease and age-related macular degeneration. *Front. Neurosci.* **2021**, *15*, 735928. [CrossRef] [PubMed]
54. Miranda, M.; Morici, J.F.; Zanoni, M.B.; Bekinschtein, P. Brain-derived neurotrophic factor: A key molecule for memory in the healthy and the pathological brain. *Front. Cell. Neurosci.* **2019**, *13*, 363. [CrossRef]
55. Yoon, E.J.; Choi, Y.; Park, D. Improvement of cognitive function in ovariectomized rats by human neural stem cells overexpressing choline acetyltransferase via secretion of NGF and BDNF. *Int. J. Mol. Sci.* **2022**, *23*, 5560. [CrossRef]
56. Kim, H.J.; Oh, T.K.; Kim, Y.H.; Lee, J.; Moon, J.M.; Park, Y.S.; Sung, C.M. Pharmacokinetics of ginsenoside Rb1, Rg3, Rk1, Rg5, F2, and Compound K from red ginseng extract in healthy Korean volunteers. *Evid. Based Complement. Alternat. Med.* **2022**, *2022*, 8427519. [CrossRef]
57. Xiong, J.; Yang, J.; Yan, K.; Guo, J. Ginsenoside Rk1 protects human melanocytes from H_2O_2-induced oxidative injury via regulation of the PI3K/AKT/Nrf2/HO-1 pathway. *Mol. Med. Rep.* **2021**, *24*, 821. [CrossRef]
58. Xu, D.; Wang, C.; Zhao, W.; Gao, S.; Cui, Z. Antidepressant-like effects of ginsenoside Rg5 in mice: Involving of hippocampus BDNF signaling pathway. *Neurosci. Lett.* **2017**, *645*, 97–105. [CrossRef]

59. You, Z.; Yao, Q.; Shen, J.; Gu, Z.; Xu, H.; Wu, Z.; Chen, C.; Li, L. Antidepressant-like effects of ginsenoside Rg3 in mice via activation of the hippocampal BDNF signaling cascade. *J. Nat. Med.* **2017**, *71*, 367–379. [CrossRef] [PubMed]
60. Kim, M.; Mok, H.; Yeo, W.S.; Ahn, J.H.; Choi, Y.K. Role of ginseng in the neurovascular unit of neuroinflammatory diseases focused on the blood-brain barrier. *J. Ginseng Res.* **2021**, *45*, 599–609. [CrossRef]

nutrients

MDPI

Article

Chebulic Acid Prevents Hypoxia Insult via Nrf2/ARE Pathway in Ischemic Stroke

Rong Zhou [1,†], Kuan Lin [1,2,†], Changlong Leng [1,2], Mei Zhou [1], Jing Zhang [1], Youwei Li [1], Yujing Liu [1], Xiansheng Ye [1,2], Xiaoli Xu [1], Binlian Sun [1], Xiji Shu [1] and Wei Liu [1,2,*]

1 Wuhan Institutes of Biomedical Sciences, School of Medicine, Jianghan University, Wuhan 430056, China
2 Institute of Cerebrovascular Disease, Jianghan University, Wuhan 430056, China
* Correspondence: liuwei@jhun.edu.cn
† These authors contributed equally to this work.

Abstract: Excessive reactive oxygen species (ROS) production contributes to brain ischemia/reperfusion (I/R) injury through many mechanisms including inflammation, apoptosis, and cellular necrosis. Chebulic acid (CA) isolated from *Terminalia chebula* has been found to have various biological effects, such as antioxidants. In this study, we investigated the mechanism of the anti-hypoxic neuroprotective effect of CA in vitro and in vivo. The results showed that CA could protect against oxygen-glucose deprivation/reoxygenation (OGD/R) induced neurotoxicity in SH-SY5Y cells, as evidenced by the enhancement of cell viability and improvement of total superoxide dismutase (T-SOD) in SH-SY5Y cells. CA also attenuated OGD/R-induced elevations of malondialdehyde (MDA) and ROS in SH-SY5Y cells. Nuclear factor-E2-related factor 2 (Nrf2) is one of the key regulators of endogenous antioxidant defense. CA acted as antioxidants indirectly by upregulating antioxidant-responsive-element (ARE) and Nrf2 nuclear translocation to relieve OGD/R-induced oxidative damage. Furthermore, the results showed that CA treatment resulted in a significant decrease in ischemic infarct volume and improved performance in the motor ability of mice 24 h after stroke. This study provides a new niche targeting drug to oppose ischemic stroke and reveals the promising potential of CA for the control of ischemic stroke in humans.

Keywords: ischemic stroke; Chebulic acid; Nrf2; neuroprotection; antioxidants

1. Introduction

Stroke is one of the leading causes of death and disability in the global population, placing a heavy burden on families and society. Ischemic stroke accounts for 60~70% of stroke cases and is caused by a narrowing or occlusion of the arteries, resulting in insufficient blood and oxygen supply to the brain. Currently, the primary treatments for ischemic stroke are surgery and drug therapy, and the pathological intervention of ischemic injury is focused on improving cerebral blood circulation and neuroprotection [1]. Although significant progress has been made in the treatment of stroke, there are still many deficiencies in the treatment methods and effects [2]. For example, intravenous recombinant tissue plasminogen activator (R-TPA) is currently approved for the clinical treatment of ischemic stroke [3]; however, most patients do not have access to thrombolytic therapy because of the three-hour treatment window. Therefore, it is of great importance to find new drugs that can prevent stroke and reduce its poor prognosis.

Currently, drug discovery based on a single target is unsatisfactory, and research and development of new drugs from the perspective of multiple targets are increasingly recognized by researchers in the field of medicine worldwide [4,5]. Traditional Chinese medicines (TCMs) have been used to treat human diseases for thousands of years. The unique advantage of TCMs is that they are characterized by multiple active components that can act on multiple targets in the treatment of diseases. Thus, it is an effective approach to research drugs utilized in traditional Chinese medicine for the treatment of ischemic stroke.

Numerous studies have shown that oxidative stress plays a key role in ischemic brain injury [6]. When cerebral ischemia and reperfusion occur, a harmful cycle of inflammation, oxidative stress, and apoptosis occur, ultimately leading to neuronal cell death. Under normal circumstances, the production and clearance of oxygen-free radicals in the body are balanced. During cerebral ischemia, especially during reperfusion, the production of free radicals exceeds the scavenging capacity to activate a series of inflammatory markers in ischemic areas, which can directly damage cells and induce cell necrosis and apoptosis, a process known as oxidative stress injury [7–9]. Nrf2 is an important regulatory factor in endogenous antioxidant defense [10], which can promote the transcription of a variety of antioxidant genes to reduce oxidative stress damage [11,12].

Terminalia chebula, a traditional medicine widely used in Asia to treat various diseases, is the dried ripe fruit of *Terminalia chebula* Retz. tomentella Kurt. It contains a variety of bioactive components such as tannins, organic acids, triterpenes, and CA, which have been reported to have strong antioxidant and anticancer effects [13].

Although CA has various biological effects, the specific neuroprotective effects and mechanisms of CA in ischemic stroke have not been reported. Therefore, in this study, we investigated the neuroprotective effects of CA on ischemic stroke both in vitro and in vivo and examine its related mechanisms.

2. Materials and Methods

2.1. Cell Culture

SH-SY5Y cells were obtained from Procell Life Science and Technology (Wuhan, China). Cells were cultured in Dulbecco's modified Eagle's medium (DMEM)/F12 (1:1) (Gibco) supplemented with 10% fetal bovine serum. For OGD/R model, the glucose-containing medium was first removed and the cells were cleaned with PBS, followed by the addition of glucose-free DMEM to the cells. The cells were then exposed to hypoxia (37 °C, 94% N_2, 5% CO_2, 1% O_2) for 5 h. After that, Oxygen-glucose deprivation was then terminated and cells were cultured under normal conditions (37 °C, 95% air, 5% CO_2) for 2 h.

2.2. CA Preparation and Treatment

CA (Biopurify, Chengdu, China) was first dissolved in DMSO (Sigma, St. Louis, MO, USA) to a stock solution at a concentration of 60 μg/μL. It was further diluted with DMEM or glucose-free DMEM and sterile filtered using a 0.22 μm filter before being added to the SH-SY5Y cells. As mentioned above, the OGD/R model was constructed, and the cells were divided into different groups according to the experimental requirements. The final concentration of DMSO was 0.05% (*v*/*v*).

2.3. CCK8 Assay

The CCK8 assay (Beyotime, Shanghai, China) was used to evaluate cell viability. For the CA toxicity test, cells were inoculated into 96-well plates (10^4/mL) with CA (10–300 μg/mL), and cells without CA were used as the positive control. For the detection of CA protection, cells were divided into the following groups: (1) normal control groups, (2) OGD/R groups, and (3) OGD/R+ CA (10–100 μg/mL) groups. After 24 h, 10 μL of CCK8 was added to each well and then incubated for 1 h. Absorbance at 450 nm was measured with a microplate reader.

2.4. CA Antioxidant Activity

SH-SY5Y cells were grouped as follows: (1) normal control, (2) OGD/R, (3) 10 μg/mL CA + OGD/R, (4) 20 μg/mL CA + OGD/R, and (5) 40 μg/mL CA + OGD/R. Total superoxide dismutase (T-SOD) activity and lipid peroxidation levels were determined with a WST-8 and MDA assay kit (Beyotime, Shanghai, China).

2.5. Immunofluorescence of the ROS

A 2′,7′-dichlorofluorescein diacetate (DCFH-DA) was prepared in a serum-free medium using a ROS detection kit (Beyotime, Shanghai, China). Cells in each group were collected and suspended in DCFH-DA solution for 20 min. DAPI was dropped, sealed, and observed under a forward microscope (DP72, Olympus, Tokyo, Japan).

2.6. Detection of the ROS and Apoptosis Rate by Flow Cytometry

DCFH-DA was diluted with serum-free medium at 1:1000. After modeling, the medium was removed, and 500 μL of diluted DCFH-DA was added. After incubating for 20 min in the cell culture box at 37 °C, ROS content was determined using flow cytometry.

Cell apoptosis rate was detected with a Cell Apoptosis Kit (Beyotime, Shanghai, China). Cells were first digested with trypsin, and then obtained cell precipitates. The cell precipitates were resuspended in a mixture of binding buffer and FITC-labeled annexin V, and then incubated at room temperature for 10 min. After 10 μL propidium iodide was added and incubated on ice for 10 min, apoptotic cells were measured by FACS analysis.

2.7. Immunofluorescence of Nrf2 Nuclear Translocation

Cells were seeded in a cell slide (JinAn Biological, Shanghai, China). After modeling, 300 μL 4% pre-cooled paraformaldehyde was added to each well and fixed for 20 min. The cells were then sealed with 5% BSA. They rested for 40 min, then cleaned with PBS. Nrf2 antibody (1:500) was used to incubate at 4 °C overnight. After adding fluorescent secondary antibody (1:200), incubated at 37 °C for 1 h. TBST was cleaned three times for 5 min, the cell culture slide was removed, DAPI was dropped, and observed under a forward microscope.

2.8. Animals and Middle Cerebral Artery Occlusion (MCAO) Model Establishment

C57BL/6 mice were obtained from the Laboratory Animal Center of Yangzhou University (Yangzhou, China; certificate number SCXK, 2017–0007). The MCAO model was established, and the mice were first anesthetized. After the skin was disinfected, it was incised; the carotid arteries were separated by blunt dissection. A silk suture was advanced from the external carotid artery to the internal carotid artery. Only mice with a ≥60% reduction in cerebral blood flow were included in this study. For mice in the sham group, only external carotid artery was separated, and no suture was placed.

2.9. Animal Experiments Drug Administration

The mice were randomly divided into six groups: (1) sham (control group); (2) MCAO group; (3) 10 mg/kg CA + MCAO group; (4) 20 mg/kg CA + MCAO group; (5) 40 mg/kg CA + MCAO group; (6) 80 mg/kg CA + MCAO group. Each group received intraperitoneal injection of different concentrations of the CA or vehicle (PBS), and CA was first dissolved in DMSO to a stock at a concentration of 60 μg/mL, and was further diluted with PBS and sterile filtered using a 0.22 μm filter before intraperitoneal injection. The final concentration of DMSO was 2% (*v/v*). Vehicle or CA was administered once daily from three days before modeling, and then given again 1.5 h after modeling on the fourth day. The intraperitoneal injection concentration was 0.1 mL/10 mg. All experiments began 24 h after the MCAO.

2.10. Behavioral Tests

The rotarod test was used to evaluate balance and motor coordination in mice. Before surgery, all mice received three days of pre-training. The time taken for each mouse to walk on the rotarod was recorded and repeated three times for each mouse. Finally, the average time value was taken.

The modified neurological severity score (mNSS) was used to evaluate the level of neurological deficits in mice, including motion, sensation, beam balance, and reflection/abnormal motion. With higher scores indicating greater damage. The score for all mice was obtained 24 h after ischemia treatment.

2.10.1. 2,3,5-Triphenyl-tetrazolium Chloride (TTC) Staining

The mice were decapitated 24 h after MCAO, anesthetized with 10% chloral hydrate, and the volume of cerebral infarction was determined. Immediately after the brain tissue was removed, it was placed in a freezer at −20 °C for 20 min, cut into 2 mm thick slices, and incubated in 2% TTC (Sigma, USA) 37 °C solution for 15–30 min. The infarct volume was then calculated.

2.11. TUNEL Staining

Brain tissue was embedded in paraffin, then cut into 5 μm slices and baked for 2 h. After brain tissue was dewaxed and hydrated, 20 μg/mL DNase-free protease K (Beyotime, Shanghai, China) was added for 15 min, and 50 μL TUNEL assay solution was added for 60 min, washed with PBS three times. The red signal of the apoptotic cells was observed using a fluorescence microscope.

2.12. Western Blot Experiment

Cell particles were lysed with RIPA lysate. Proteins were normalized to 30 μg per lane, resolved on 10% polyacrylamide gels, and subsequently blotted onto PVDF membranes. The membrane was placed in 5% (*w/v*) skim milk for 1 h, it was then incubated at 4 °C overnight with primary antibodies (all at 1:1000), followed by 1 h at room temperature with secondary antibodies. The bands were visualized using enhanced chemiluminescence and quantified using densitometry. All blots presented are representative of at least three independent experiments.

2.13. Statistical Analysis

All results were expressed as mean ± SD. One-way analysis of variance (ANOVA) was used for statistical analysis. All experiments were repeated at least three times, and $p < 0.05$ was considered statistically significant.

3. Results

3.1. Cytotoxicity of CA and Its Protective Effects on OGD/R-Induced SH-SY5Y Cells

The cytotoxic potential of CA (Figure 1A) in SH-SY5Y cells was evaluated using a CCK8 assay (Figure 1B). CA showed no cytotoxicity at the concentrations of 10–100 μg/mL (Figure 1B). Meanwhile, CA distinctly increased the survival rate of SH-SY5Y cells treated with OGD/R in a dose-dependent manner compared to the model group (Figure 1C). These results indicate that CA has a wide safe concentration range and has a protective effect on OGD/R-induced cells. We found that the optimal concentration of CA administered to the cells for subsequent experiments was 10–40 μg/mL. Superoxide dismutase (SOD) is an important antioxidant enzyme that catalyzes the disproportionation of superoxide anions to produce hydrogen peroxide and oxygen (O_2). In our results, enzymatic antioxidant (T-SOD) activity increased 1.3 times in the 40 μg/mL CA group compared with the control group (Figure 1D). Malondialdehyde (MDA) is a natural product of lipid oxidation that is markedly increased in animal or plant cells suffering from oxidative stress. The lipid peroxidation level significantly decreased when the SH-SY5Y cells was CA-treated at a concentration of 20 μg/mL (Figure 1E).

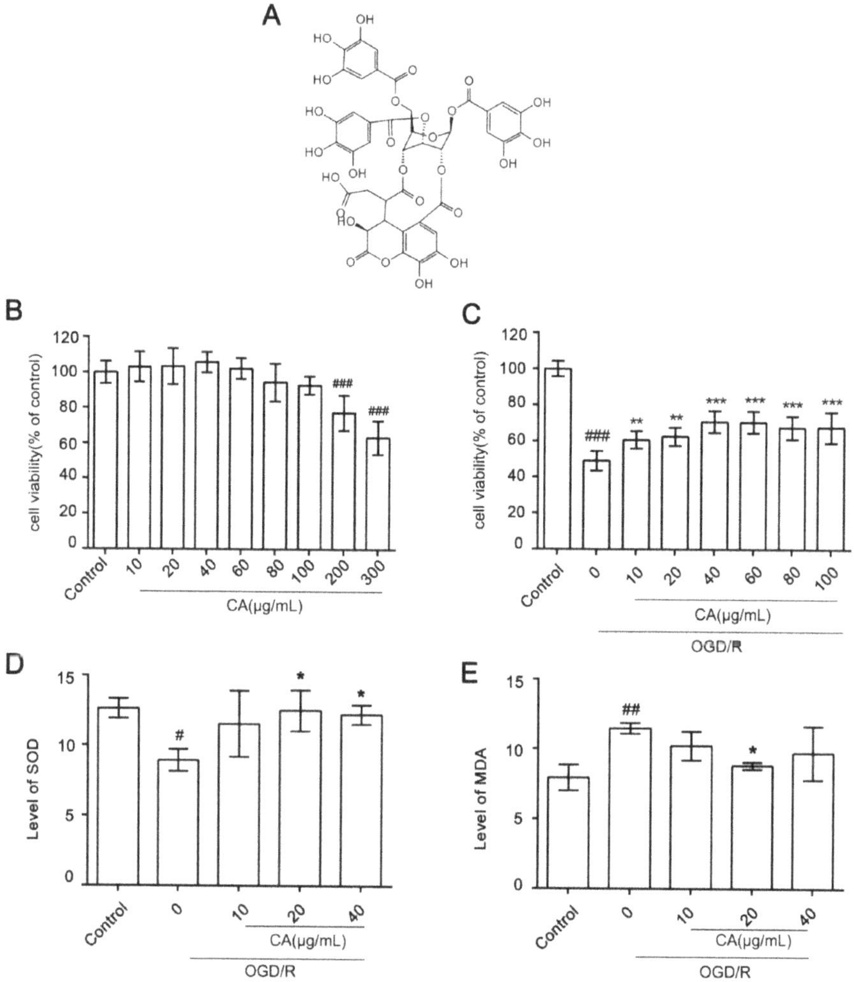

Figure 1. Chebulic acid attenuates OGD/R induced cell death in SH-SY5Y cells. (**A**) Chemical structure of chebulinic acid (CA). (**B**) SH-SY5Y cells were incubated for 24 h with various concentrations of CA (10–300 μg/mL). Cell viability was determined using CCK8 assay; bars represent the percentage of cell viability. (**C**) SH-SY5Y cells were inoculated with different concentrations of CA (10–100 μg /mL) and exposed to OGD/R. (**D**) T-SOD levels in cells. (**E**) MDA levels in cells. Results are expressed as mean ± SD. # $p < 0.05$, ## $p < 0.01$, and ### $p < 0.001$ compared with the control. * $p < 0.05$, ** $p < 0.01$, and *** $p < 0.001$ versus OGD/R group.

3.2. CA Reduced OGD/R-Induced ROS Production and Apoptosis in SH-SY5Y Cells

To investigate the effect of CA on oxidative stress, immunofluorescence assays, and flow cytometry was used to detect the content of ROS in different groups of SH-SY5Y cells. Immunofluorescence assays showed that the production of ROS in SH-SY5Y cells was inhibited in a dose-dependent manner in the CA group compared with that in the OGD/R group (Figure 2A,B). The same trend was observed using flow cytometry (Figure 2C,D).

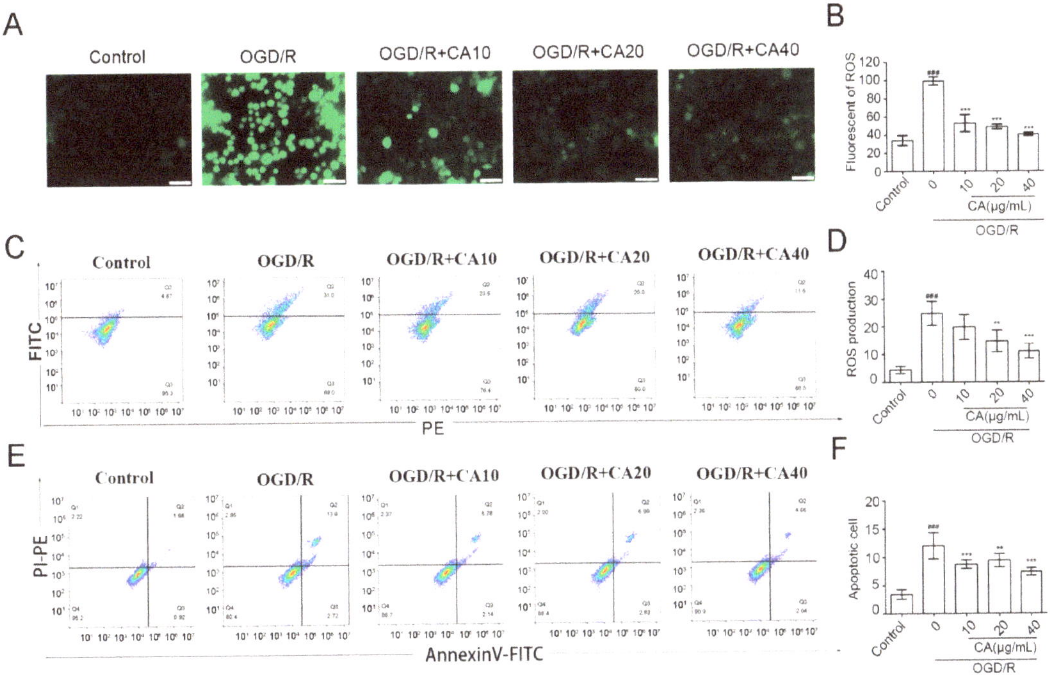

Figure 2. Effect of CA on ROS levels. (**A**,**B**) Representative images of ROS with magnification at 20×. (**C**,**D**) ROS production was detected in each condition. (**E**,**F**) The apoptosis rate was measured using flow cytometry. Results are expressed as mean ± SD. ### $p < 0.001$ compared with the control. ** $p < 0.01$, and *** $p < 0.001$ versus OGD/R group.

A series of injuries after ischemia-reperfusion eventually lead to cell apoptosis; therefore, the apoptotic cells in each group of cells were detected by flow cytometry using Annexin V labeled with FITC. The number of apoptotic cells increased 3.4-fold after OGD/R treatment compared to the control group, while CA treatment reduced OGD/R-induced apoptosis in all treatment groups. The number of apoptotic cells decreased to 61.7% in the model group when treated with CA at the concentration of 40 μg/mL (Figure 2E,F).

3.3. CA Promotes Nuclear Translocation of Nrf2 in SH-SY5Y Cells Induced by OGD/R

Nrf2 is an important regulatory factor in antioxidant defense. Increasing evidence has confirmed that Nrf2 plays an important role in protecting brain cells from ischemic injury. Nrf2 is a promising therapeutic target for stroke prevention [14]. Therefore, we investigated whether CA induced Nrf2 translocation into the nucleus of SH-SY5Y cells. Immunofluorescence microscopy showed that CA promoted Nrf2 transfer into the nucleus of SH-SY5Y cells after OGD/R induction (Figure 3A,B). Similar results were also reflected in the western blot analysis, which showed that the expression levels of total Nrf2 and Nrf2 in the nucleus in the CA-treated groups were increased compared to the OGD/R group (Figure 3B–D). These results suggest that the antioxidant effects of CA may be related to the activation of proteins in the Nrf2 pathway. It has been shown that the Keap1- Nrf2-ARE signaling pathway is involved in the protective effect of stroke on brain tissue [15]. Nrf2 is released from Kelch-like ech-associated protein 1 (Keap1), and then translocated to the nucleus, where it binds to AREs in the nucleus and regulates the transcription of downstream targets to promote the expression of a variety of antioxidant genes [16], such as heme oxygenase-1 (HO-1) and SODs. During a stroke, excessive nitric oxide produced by inducible nitric oxide synthase (iNOS) contributes to a cascade of inflammation and neuronal death and further worsens primary brain injury [17]. Figure 3E–H shows that CA promoted the expression of the antioxidant factor HO-1 and decreased the expression of iNOS after OGD/R.

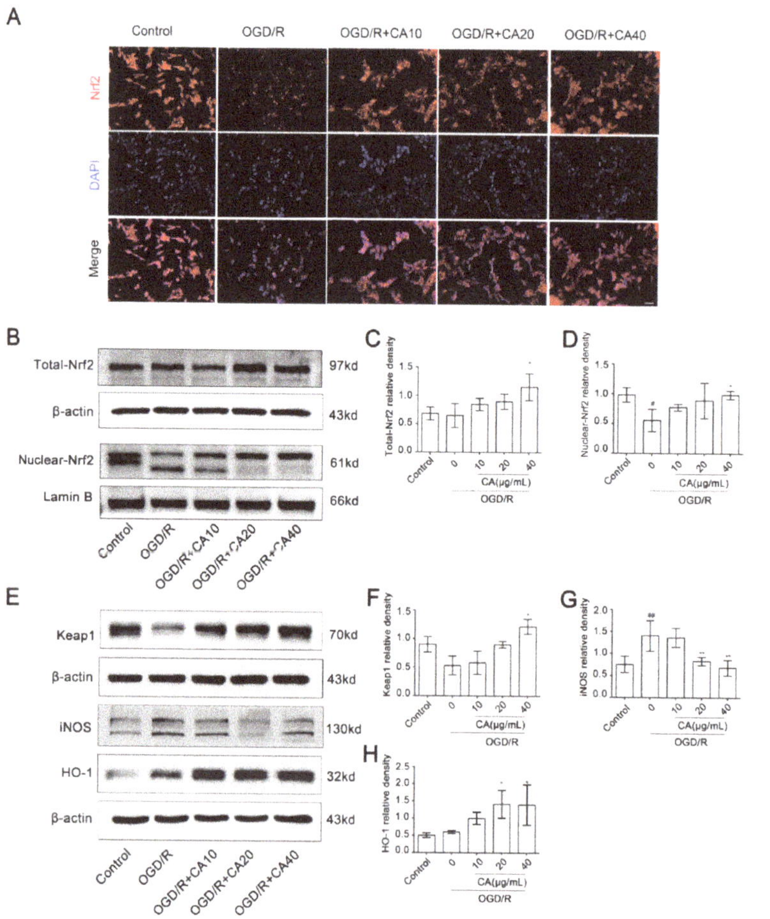

Figure 3. Nrf2 nuclear translocation was enhanced by CA in OGD/R-insulted SH-SY5Y cells. (**A**) SH-SY5Y cells in different groups were first stained with anti- Nrf2 antibody (red) and then counterstained with DAPI (blue) (40×). (**B–D**) The expression of nuclear Nrf2 and total Nrf2 were determined by western blot. (**E–H**) Chebulinic acid promoted the activation of Nrf2-ARE pathways. Western blot analysis was carried out with specific antibodies for detecting the activation of Keap1, iNOS, HO-1. Results are expressed as mean ± SD. # $p < 0.05$, and ## $p < 0.01$ compared with the control. * $p < 0.05$, and ** $p < 0.01$ versus OGD/R group.

3.4. CA Decreased Cerebral Damage and Apoptosis Following Ischemia-Reperfusion In Vivo

To investigate whether CA has the same protective effect in vivo, C57 mice were randomly divided into Sham, MCAO, and MCAO + CA groups. Reperfusion was performed for 24 h according to the surgical methods mentioned above (see Figure 4A for schematic diagram). First, neurological deficit score (mNSS) and infarct volume were measured. The results showed that the neurological deficit score in the CA groups was significantly lower than that in the MCAO group (Figure 4B,C). The effect of CA on the apoptosis of brain cells was measured by TUNEL staining. As shown in Figure 4D,E, the number of TUNEL-positive neurons in the MCAO group significantly increased after ischemia-reperfusion injury, whereas CA administration effectively reduced the apoptosis of nerve cells in vivo.

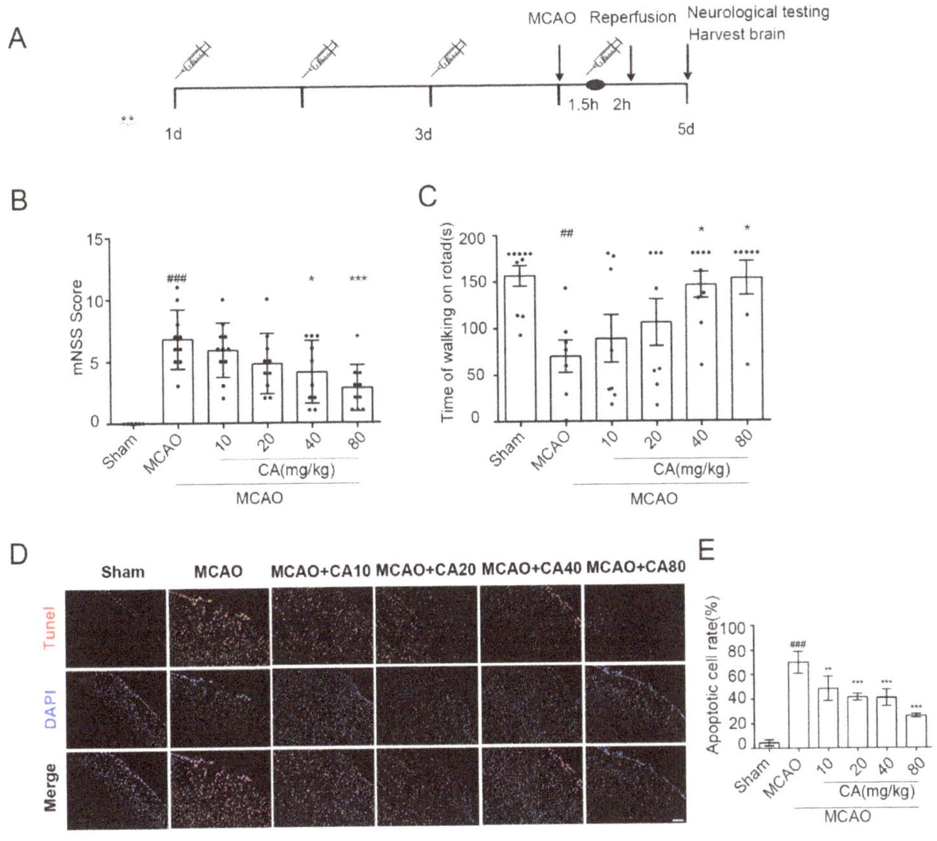

Figure 4. CA decreased cerebral damage and apoptosis following ischemia-reperfusion in vivo. (**A**) The timeline of CA administration in the OGD/R model. (**B**,**C**) Mouse behavioral performance in the mNSS score test and rotarod test with different treatments. (**D**,**E**) Effect of CA on apoptosis on the affected side of mice (TUNEL staining). Three animals were randomly selected from each group, and five fields of view were randomly selected from each section. ## $p < 0.01$, and ### $p < 0.001$ compared with the sham group. * $p < 0.05$, ** $p < 0.01$, and *** $p < 0.001$ versus MCAO group.

3.5. CA Reduced Infarct Volume after Ischemia-Reperfusion In Vivo

TTC staining was used to quantify infarct volume (Figure 5A,B). Normal brain tissue appears scarlet, whereas infarcts appear white in color. After MCAO, the cerebral infarction volume increased significantly, while the cerebral infarction volume in the treatment groups decreased in a quantitative dependence. At a dose of 80 mg/kg, the infarct volume was reduced to 5.9 times that in the MCAO group. The expression of Nrf2, Keap1, HO−1, and iNOS in brain tissue was also observed. Similarly, the expression of antioxidant stress-related proteins was upregulated after CA compared with that in the MCAO group, while iNOS was downregulated (Figure 5C–G).

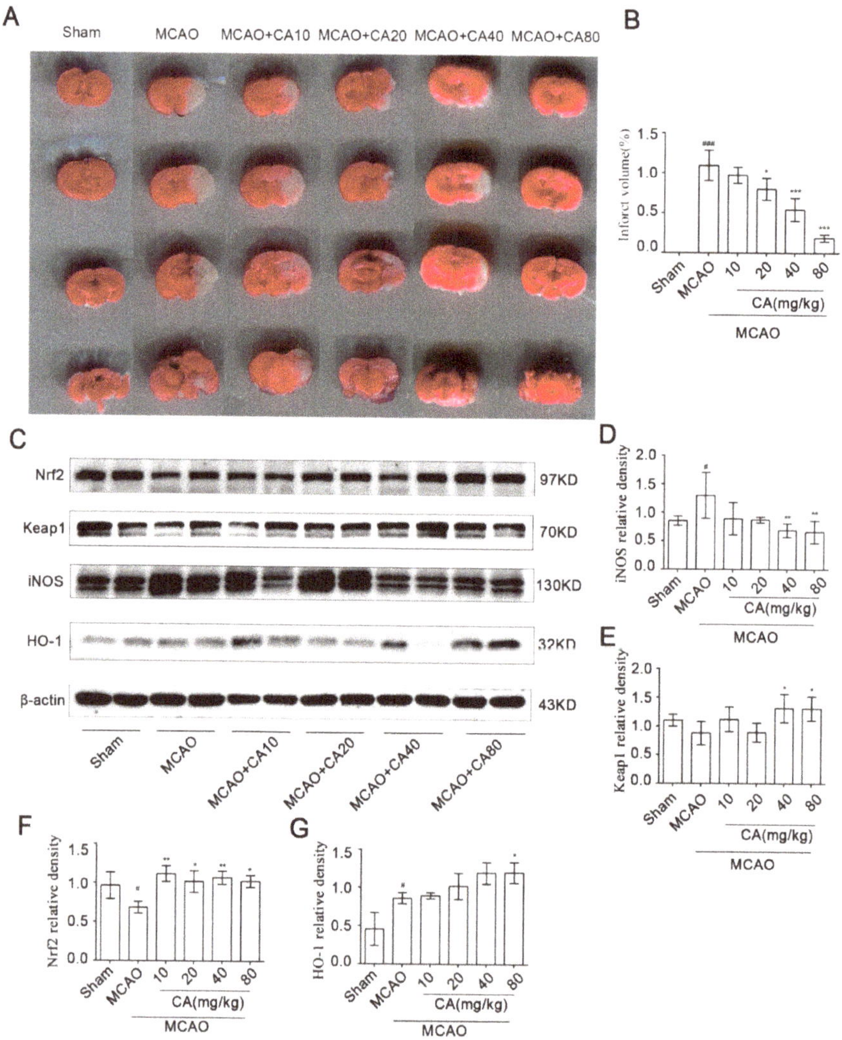

Figure 5. CA reduced infarct volume after ischemia-reperfusion in vivo. (**A**,**B**) Cerebral infarct volumes of rats in different treatment groups. Red staining represents normal tissues, and white staining represents the infarct region. (**C**–**G**) Chebulic acid increases activation of the Nrf2-ARE pathway in vivo. Western blot analysis was performed with specific antibodies to detect the activation of Nrf2, Keap1, iNOS, and HO−1 in the ischemic hemisphere (representative images from three independent experiments are shown). The results are expressed as mean ± SD. # $p < 0.05$ and ### $p < 0.001$ compared with the sham group. * $p < 0.05$, ** $p < 0.01$, and *** $p < 0.001$ versus MCAO group.

4. Discussion

Stroke is one of the most important diseases that threaten human life and health worldwide [18]. Stroke includes hemorrhagic stroke and ischemic stroke, of which ischemic stroke accounts for 60~70% of all stroke cases [19]. Many studies have shown that the rapid increase of ROS after the occurrence of acute ischemic stroke can cause an imbalance in the body's antioxidant response, leading to a series of pathophysiological events, including inflammatory response, apoptosis, and autophagy, ultimately leading to neurodegeneration and nerve cell death [20,21].

Ischemic stroke occurs when an artery in the brain is blocked, resulting in insufficient oxygen and glucose supply to the damaged area to maintain normal cellular activity. This in turn leads to changes in the electrochemical and metabolic levels of cells and increases the release of toxic substances [22], one of which is the increased production of ROS [23,24]. Although reperfusion therapy is currently the widely accepted treatment for ischemic stroke, reperfusion also has a significant negative impact on brain cells, including a significant increase in ROS levels [25]. At this point, the body's antioxidant mechanism cannot cope with the damage caused by oxidative substances, such as reactive oxygen species, which eventually leads to apoptosis and necrosis of nerve cells.

Studies have shown that CA can reduce cellular damage by reducing the level of ROS and the content of oxidized glutathione [26,27]. Some studies have also shown that CA participates in the antioxidant process by regulating Nrf2 expression in glomerular mesangial cells and hepatocytes [28–30]. However, whether CA can also regulate Nrf2 expression in neurocytes to resist oxidative stress injury has rarely been studied.

Many studies have proved that Nrf2 plays a vital role in protecting brain cells from ischemic injury. As our study showed, in vitro, nuclear translocation of Nrf2 in SH-SY5Y cells was not obvious after cerebral ischemia-reperfusion simulation using the OGD/R model. However, the nuclear translocation of Nrf2 increased significantly after treatment with different concentrations of CA, and the same trend was verified by western blot analysis. These findings indicate that CA effectively activates the Nrf2-ARE regulatory element and protects the collective from oxidative stress in an OGD/R mouse model. Similarly, ROS expression in SH-SY5Y cells increased significantly after OGD/R, whereas it decreased in the CA treatment groups.

Inflammatory factors also play critical roles in cerebral I/R injury. In the early stages of cerebral ischemia, a large number of pro-inflammatory factors are produced in the tissues [31]. Meanwhile, the interaction between oxidative stress and neuroinflammation in ischemic stroke has been extensively studied [32,33]. Nerve cell death, damage to the integrity of the blood-brain barrier (BBB), and enlarged cerebral infarction are related to a variety of inflammatory factors triggered by ROS [34]. Our study showed that the brain tissue of mice in the MCAO group expressed more inflammatory factors, which significantly decreased after treatment with CA. However, the exact molecular mechanisms need to be further explored.

The pathological processes after cerebral ischemia-reperfusion mainly include oxidative stress, excitatory toxicity, intracellular calcium overload, inflammation, and apoptosis, which ultimately determine the size of the infarction [35]. Although the antioxidant effects of CA have been demonstrated, its neuroprotective effects after ischemia-reperfusion have rarely been studied. Our study found that neurological and motor impairment occurred in mice 24 h after MCAO; however, compared with the model group, both impairments were improved in the CA-treated groups, and the high-dose groups showed more significant improvement than the low-dose groups. Similarly, neuronal apoptosis and the size of cerebral infarction after MCAO were improved in mice treated with CA.

In conclusion, in our study, we found that CA promoted the migration of antioxidant regulator Nrf2 from the cytoplasm to the nucleus and that Nrf2 into the nucleus promotes the increased expression of antioxidant proteins such as HO-1and SOD, these antioxidant proteins can resist the damage of cells and brain tissue caused by excessive reactive oxygen species and inflammatory factors such as iNOS produced during ischemia. Our results found that CA has excellent neuroprotective effects and can be used as a promising new drug for the treatment of acute ischemic stroke; however, its mechanism of action needs to be further elucidated.

Author Contributions: Conceptualization, W.L.; methodology, R.Z., K.L. and W.L.; data curation, resources, writing-original draft, R.Z. and K.L.; writing—review and editing, C.L., M.Z., X.Y., B.S. and X.X.; validation, J.Z., X.S., Y.L. (Youwei Li) and Y.L. (Yujing Liu). All authors have read and agreed to the published version of the manuscript.

Funding: This work was supported by grants from the Scientific Research Projects of Jianghan University (2021, No.140) to Mei Zhou.

Institutional Review Board Statement: This study was approved by the Institutional Review Board of Jianghan University.

Informed Consent Statement: Not applicable.

Data Availability Statement: Not applicable.

Acknowledgments: This work was supported by the Wuhan Institutes of Biomedical Sciences of Jianghan University.

Conflicts of Interest: The authors declare no conflict of interest.

References

1. Meng, W.T.; Li, D.X.; Tong, L. Progress in research of the treatment of ischemic stroke. *Chin. J. New Drugs* **2016**, *25*, 1114–1120.
2. Stapf, C.; Mohr, J.P. Ischemic stroke therapy. *Annu. Rev. Med.* **2002**, *53*, 453–475. [CrossRef] [PubMed]
3. Donnan, G.A.; Fisher, M.; Macleod, M.M. Stroke. *Lancet* **2008**, *371*, 1612–1623. [PubMed]
4. Ahmad, M.; Dar, N.J.; Bhat, Z.S.; Hussain, A.; Shah, A.; Liu, H.; Graham, S.H. Inflammation in ischemic stroke: Mechanisms, consequences and possible drug targets. *CNS Neurol. Disord. Drug Targets* **2014**, *13*, 1378–1396. [CrossRef] [PubMed]
5. Zhu, J.B.; Wang, Y.H.; Hu, Z.D.; Li, H. Research progress on pathogenesis of ischemic stroke and traditional Chinese medicine commonly used for treatment of ischemic stroke. *China J. Chin. Mater. Med.* **2019**, *44*, 422–432.
6. Cai, M.; Yu, Z.; Wang, L.; Song, X.; Zhang, J.; Zhang, Z.; Zhang, W.; Li, W.; Xiang, J.; Cai, D. Tongxinluo reduces brain edema and inhibits post-ischemic inflammation after middle cerebral artery occlusion in rats. *J. Ethnopharmacol.* **2016**, *181*, 136–145. [CrossRef] [PubMed]
7. Chan, P.H. Reactive oxygen radicals in signaling and damage in the ischemic brain. *J. Cereb. Blood Flow Metab.* **2001**, *21*, 2–14. [CrossRef]
8. Manzanero, S.; Santro, T.; Arumugam, T.V. Neuronal oxidative stress in acute ischemic stroke: Sources and contribution to cell injury. *Neurochem. Int.* **2013**, *62*, 712–718.
9. Rodrigo, R.; Fernández, G.R.; Gutiérrez, R.; Matamala, J.M.; Carrasco, R.; Miranda, M.A.; Feuerhake, W. Oxidative stress and pathophysiology of ischemic stroke: Novel therapeutic opportunities. *CNS Neurol. Disord. Drug Targets* **2013**, *12*, 698–714. [CrossRef]
10. Kaur, J.; Arora, S.; Singh, B.; Thakur, L.C.; Gambhir, J.; Prabhu, K.M. Role of oxidative stress in pathophysiology of transient ischemic attack and stroke. *Int. J. Biol. Med. Res.* **2011**, *3*, 94–98.
11. Shah, Z.A.; Li, R.C.; Thimmulappa, R.K.; Kensler, T.W.; Yamamoto, M.; Biswal, S.; Doré, S. Role of reactive oxygen species in modulation of Nrf2 following ischemic reperfusion injury. *Neuroscience* **2007**, *47*, 53–59. [CrossRef] [PubMed]
12. Shih, A.Y.; Li, P.; Murphy, T.H. A small-molecule-inducible Nrf2-mediated antioxidant response provides effective prophylaxis against cerebral ischemia in vivo. *J. Neurosci.* **2005**, *25*, 10321–10335. [CrossRef] [PubMed]
13. Pfundstein, B.; El Desouky, S.K.; Hull, W.E.; Haubner, R.; Erben, G.; Owen, R.W. Polyphenolic compounds in the fruits of Egyptian medicinal plants (*Terminalia bellerica*, *Terminalia chebula* and *Terminalia horrida*): Characterization, quantitation and determination of antioxidant capacities. *Phytochemistry* **2010**, *71*, 1132–1148. [CrossRef]
14. Wu, S.; Yue, Y.; Peng, A.; Zhang, L.; Xiang, J.; Cao, X.; Ding, H.; Yin, S. Myricetin ameliorates brain injury and neurological deficits via Nrf2 activation after experimental stroke in middle-aged rats. *Food Funct.* **2016**, *15*, 2624–2634. [CrossRef] [PubMed]
15. Zhang, R.; Xu, M.; Wang, Y.; Xie, F.; Zhang, G.; Qin, X. Nrf2-a Promising therapeutic target for defensing against oxidative stress in stroke. *Mol. Neurobiol.* **2017**, *54*, 6006–6017. [CrossRef] [PubMed]
16. Xu, X.; Zhang, L.; Ye, X.; Hao, Q.; Zhang, T.; Cui, G.; Yu, M. Nrf2/ARE pathway inhibits ROS-induced NLRP3 inflammasome activation in BV2 cells after cerebral ischemia reperfusion. *Inflamm. Res.* **2018**, *67*, 57–65. [CrossRef] [PubMed]
17. Liu, H.T.; Mu, D.Z. Inducible nitric oxide synthase and brain hypoxic-ischemic brain damage. *Chin. J. Contemp. Pediatr.* **2014**, *16*, 962–967.
18. Rajsic, S.; Gothe, H.; Borba, H.H.; Sroczynski, G.; Vujicic, J.; Toell, T.; Siebert, U. Economic burden of stroke: A systematic review on post-stroke care. *Eur. J. Health Econ.* **2019**, *20*, 107–134. [CrossRef]
19. Liu, X.; Rao, S.; Wang, J. Intravenous thrombolysis in combination with mild hypothermia therapy in the treatment of acute cerebral infarction. *Pak. J. Med. Sci.* **2019**, *35*, 1161–1166. [CrossRef]
20. Chen, H.; Yoshioka, H.; Kim, G.S.; Jung, J.E.; Okami, N.; Sakata, H.; Maier, C.M.; Narasimhan, P.; Goeders, C.E.; Chan, P.H. Oxidative stress in ischemic brain damage: Mechanisms of cell death and potential molecular targets for neuroprotection. *Antioxid. Redox Signal.* **2011**, *14*, 1505–1517. [CrossRef]

21. Shirley, R.; Ord, E.N.; Work, L.M. Oxidative Stress and the Use of Antioxidants in Stroke. *Antioxidants* **2014**, *3*, 472–501. [CrossRef] [PubMed]
22. Woodruff, T.M.; Thundyil, J.; Tang, S.C.; Sobey, C.G.; Taylor, S.M.; Arumugam, T.V. Pathophysiology, treatment, and animal and cellular models of human ischemic stroke. *Mol. Neurodegener.* **2011**, *6*, 11. [CrossRef] [PubMed]
23. Yang, Z.J.; Xie, Y.; Bosco, G.M.; Chen, C.; Camporesi, E.M. Hyperbaric oxygenation alleviates MCAO-induced brain injury and reduces hydroxyl radical formation and glutamate release. *Eur. J. Appl. Physiol.* **2010**, *108*, 513–522. [CrossRef] [PubMed]
24. Olmez, I.; Ozyurt, H. Reactive oxygen species and ischemic cerebrovascular disease. *Neurochem. Int.* **2012**, *60*, 208–212. [CrossRef] [PubMed]
25. Yamato, M.; Egashira, T.; Utsumi, H. Application of in vivo ESR spectroscopy to measurement of cerebrovascular ROS generation in stroke. *Free Radic. Biol. Med.* **2003**, *35*, 1619–1631. [CrossRef] [PubMed]
26. Lee, H.S.; Jung, S.H.; Yun, B.S.; Lee, K.W. Isolation of chebulic acid from *Terminalia chebula* Retz. and its antioxidant effect in isolated rat hepatocytes. *Arch. Toxicol.* **2007**, *81*, 211–218. [CrossRef]
27. Nam, M.H.; Son, W.R.; Yang, S.Y.; Lee, Y.S.; Lee, K.W. Chebulic acid inhibits advanced glycation end products-mediated vascular dysfunction by suppressing ros via the erk/nrf2 pathway. *J. Funct. Foods* **2017**, *36*, 150–161. [CrossRef]
28. Koo, Y.C.; Pyo, M.C.; Nam, M.H.; Hong, C.O.; Yang, S.Y.; Lee, K.W. Chebulic acid prevents hepatic fibrosis induced by advanced glycation end-products in LX-2 cell by modulating Nrf2 translocation via ERK pathway. *Toxicol. In Vitro* **2016**, *34*, 8–15. [CrossRef]
29. Jung, H.L.; Yang, S.Y.; Pyo, M.C.; Hong, C.O.; Nam, M.H.; Lee, J.W.; Lee, K.W. Protective effects of chebulic acid from *Terminalia chebula* Retz. against t-BHP-induced oxidative stress by modulations of Nrf2 and its related enzymes in HepG2 cells. *Food. Sci. Biotechnol.* **2018**, *28*, 555–562. [CrossRef]
30. Huang, K.; Huang, J.; Xie, X.; Wang, S.; Chen, C.; Shen, X.; Liu, P.; Huang, H. Sirt1 resists advanced glycation end products-induced expressions of fibronectin and TGF-β1 by activating the Nrf2/ARE pathway in glomerular mesangial cells. *Free Radic. Biol. Med.* **2013**, *65*, 528–540. [CrossRef]
31. Jayaraj, R.L.; Azimullah, S.; Beiram, R.; Jalal, F.Y.; Rosenberg, G.A. Neuroinflammation: Friend and foe for ischemic stroke. *J. Neuroinflamm.* **2019**, *16*, 142. [CrossRef] [PubMed]
32. Chehaibi, K.; Trabelsi, I.; Mahdouani, K.; Slimane, M.N. Correlation of Oxidative Stress Parameters and Inflammatory Markers in Ischemic Stroke Patients. *J. Stroke Cerebrovasc. Dis.* **2016**, *25*, 2585–2593. [CrossRef] [PubMed]
33. Yang, Q.; Huang, Q.; Hu, Z.; Tang, X. Potential Neuroprotective Treatment of Stroke: Targeting Excitotoxicity, Oxidative Stress, and Inflammation. *Front. Neurosci.* **2019**, *13*, 1036. [CrossRef] [PubMed]
34. Crack, P.J.; Taylor, J.M. Reactive oxygen species and the modulation of stroke. *Free Radic. Biol. Med.* **2005**, *38*, 1433–1444. [CrossRef] [PubMed]
35. Kaushal, V.; Schlichter, L.C. Mechanisms of microglia-mediated neurotoxicity in a new model of the stroke penumbra. *J. Neurosci.* **2008**, *28*, 2221–2230. [CrossRef] [PubMed]

nutrients

MDPI

Article

Extra Virgin Olive Oil and Cardiovascular Protection in Chronic Kidney Disease

Giulia Marrone [1], Silvia Urciuoli [2], Manuela Di Lauro [1], Jessica Ruzzolini [3], Francesca Ieri [2], Pamela Vignolini [2], Francesca Di Daniele [4,5], Cristina Guerriero [1], Chiara Nediani [3], Nicola Di Daniele [1] and Annalisa Noce [1,*]

[1] UOC of Internal Medicine—Center of Hypertension and Nephrology Unit, Department of Systems Medicine, University of Rome Tor Vergata, 00133 Rome, Italy
[2] PHYTOLAB (Pharmaceutical, Cosmetic, Food Supplement, Technology and Analysis)—DiSIA, University of Florence, 50019 Florence, Italy
[3] Department of Experimental and Clinical Biomedical Sciences "Mario Serio", University of Florence, 50121 Florence, Italy
[4] School of Applied Medical, Surgical Sciences, University of Rome Tor Vergata, 00133 Rome, Italy
[5] Department of Systems Medicine, UOSD of Dermatology, University of Rome Tor Vergata, 00133 Rome, Italy
* Correspondence: annalisa.noce@uniroma2.it; Tel.: +39-062-090-2194

Abstract: The high mortality related to chronic kidney disease (CKD) is not only due to the disease itself; in fact, CKD also represents an important risk factor for cardiovascular (CV) morbidity and mortality. Among the functional foods that seems to have cardioprotective action, extra virgin olive oil (EVOO) plays a pivotal health-promoting role. The aim of this study was to evaluate the possible cardioprotective effects of an EVOO containing a very high content (>900 ppm) of minor phenolic compounds (MPCs). The selected EVOO was analyzed by HPLC-DAD-MS to establish the MPC content. The Olea extract obtained from the selected EVOO was tested against the RAW 264.7 cell line in order to investigate its anti-inflammatory activity. We enrolled 40 CKD patients under conservative therapy for in vivo clinical testing. All CKD patients consumed 40 mL/day of raw EVOO for 9 weeks (T1). At baseline (T0) and at T1, we monitored the patients' blood and urinary parameters. The patients' body composition was assessed using bioelectrical impedance analysis and the carotid intima-media thickness (CIMT) using ultrasound imaging. At T1, we observed a decrease in inflammatory parameters, CIMT, and oxidative stress biomarkers. We also noticed improvements in lipid and purine metabolism, atherogenic indices, and body composition. Thus, this study highlighted the cardioprotective action of EVOO in nephropathic patients.

Keywords: cardiovascular protection; extra virgin olive oil; chronic kidney disease; inflammatory state; oxidative stress; minor phenolic compounds; atherogenic indices; carotid intima-media thickness

1. Introduction

The incidence of chronic kidney disease (CKD) has increased significantly in the last three decades due to the explosive spread of related risk factors such as arterial hypertension, diabetes mellitus, metabolic syndrome, etc. In 2016, CKD reached 13th place in the leading causes of death in the world, and it has been hypothesized that by 2040, it will be the 5th leading cause of death in the world [1]. The high mortality related to CKD cannot be explained only by the disease itself; rather, CKD also represents an important risk factor for cardiovascular (CV) mortality and morbidity [2,3]. In fact, the presence of CKD has been observed to be associate with the onset of a series of comorbidities that are risk factors for CV diseases. Among these comorbidities, special mention is due to alterations of calcium–phosphorus metabolism [4,5], hyperhomocysteinemia [6,7], the increase of asymmetric dimethylarginine (ADMA), malnutrition, uremic sarcopenia [8,9], the accumulation of toxic substances, including those derived from the gut microbiota [10,11], a low-grade chronic inflammatory state, and dyslipidaemia and metabolic acidosis [12–15].

All these factors contribute to the development of accelerated atherosclerosis in which the primum movens is represented by endothelial dysfunction (ED) [16,17]. Physiologically, the endothelium can be considered a "pervasive" organ that performs numerous functions, among which is the maintenance of vascular tone. In fact, it regulates vascular permeability, the immune response, and angiogenesis [17]. During CKD, ED is amplified and all the previously mentioned CV risk factors contribute to its genesis. As a matter of fact, an increase in ED prevalence was previously observed in relation to CKD stage [18]. Moreover, several studies have demonstrated a worsening of ED directly related to the reduction of the glomerular filtration rate (GFR) in CKD patients [17]. Low-grade chronic inflammatory states are due to an increased production of pro-inflammatory cytokines (interleukin-IL-6, tumor necrosis factor-TNF-α, IL-1β) in association with an enhanced formation of reactive oxygen species (ROS), with consequent induction of oxidative stress (OS). Both inflammatory states and OS cause a reduction in the bioavailability of nitric oxide (NO), a compound with antithrombotic, anti-inflammatory, and vasorelaxation action [18,19]. In particular, a NO reduction induced by the accumulation of NO synthetase endogenous inhibitors through the nuclear factor kappa-light-chain-enhancer of activated B cells (NF-kB) pathway was observed in CKD patients [20]. Furthermore, increased OS provokes the glycation of proteins, carbohydrates, and lipids and leads to the formation of advanced glycation end products (AGEs), which appear to have a direct toxic effect on the myocardium [21]. AGEs also increase the ED phenomenon by inhibiting the enzyme dimethylarginine dimethylaminohydrolase (DDAH), which degrades the ADMA, an endogenous inhibitor of NO production via reduction of the activity of endothelial NO synthetase [22–24].

Extra virgin olive oil (EVOO) plays a pivotal role among the functional foods that seem to reduce the risk of CV morbidity and mortality. In fact, the European Prospective Investigation (EPIC)-Spain study [25], the PREvención con DIeta MEDditerránea (PREDIMED) study [26], and the EUROLIVE study [27] have all highlighted the important cardioprotective action of EVOO. This beneficial effect seems to be related to the presence of minor phenolic compounds (MPCs), such as oleocanthal, oleacin, tyrosol and hydroxytyrosol (HT), and monounsaturated fatty acids (MUFAs), in which EVOO is rich [28–30]. In fact, these compounds exert an anti-inflammatory, antioxidant, and antiatherogenic effect, reducing the global CV risk.

To date, we have tested two EVOOs other than the one selected for this clinical study. In particular, we previously administered two EVOOs to CKD patients—the first was characterized by a medium (>400 ppm) MPC content and the second one was characterized by a high (>700 ppm) MPC content—in order to assess EVOO's potential beneficial effects on quality of life and on CKD-related comorbidities [31,32]. Moreover, in the study conducted by Nocc et al. [32], we assessed whether the beneficial effects were maintained over time, namely after a two-month washout period. At this regard, we demonstrated that only the consumption of EVOO with a high MPC content resulted in the positive effects being maintained over time.

In the light of our previous results, in this study, we evaluated the possible cardioprotective action of an EVOO with a very high (>900 ppm) MPC content in CKD patients under conservative therapy. This EVOO has never been tested before in in vivo study. Furthermore, in this study, we examined several parameters that were not investigated in our previous studies, namely atherogenic indices, carotid intima-media thickness (CIMT), and some inflammatory biomarkers (namely TNF-α, platelet-to-lymphocyte ratio (PLR), neutrophil-to-lymphocyte ratio (NLR), and lymphocyte-to-monocyte ratio (LMR)). In addition, in this study, we conducted a preliminary in vitro test on an extract, rich in oleocanthal, obtained from the selected EVOO in order to evaluate the effective anti-inflammatory activity of our EVOO.

2. Materials and Methods

2.1. Selection and Characterization of the Organic EVOO

For this study, we selected an organic EVOO from Ophena (Abruzzo), a town in central Italy, with a very high content of active MPCs [31]. This EVOO is produced from a mix of two cultivars of *Olea europaea* L., namely Leccino and Intosso, which are widespread in the Abruzzo region.

This EVOO was produced using a biphasic and controlled pressing technology in order to preserve and maintain the very high content of active MPCs. The selected EVOO was analyzed using high-performance liquid chromatography coupled with diode array detector mass spectrometry (HPLC-DAD-MS) (Agilent Technologies, Palo Alto, CA, USA) to evaluate the contents of single active molecules such as HT, tyrosol, elenolic acid and its derivatives, oleacin, oleocanthal, oleuropein aglycone, secoiridoid derivatives, and lignans. The analyses were performed according to the protocol described by Romani et al. [31].

EVOO product analysis was carried out using the Oxitester system (CDR srl Florence, Italy) for parameters such as acidity (expressed as % of oleic acid), peroxides (expressed as meq O_2/kg), and total polyphenols (expressed in mg of tyrosol) [31].

2.1.1. Olea Extract

The used EVOO for the extraction had a total MPC content of 1145.95 mg/kg. The extract tested in this study was obtained using a liquid/liquid multiple extraction method starting with 10 L of EVOO. The selected EVOO blend was extracted with a 70% EtOH-H_2O solution adjusted to pH 3.2 with formic acid in the dark for 30 min at room temperature in a mechanical orbital shaker. The solution was transferred to a separating funnel to remove the lipid portion with hexane. The liquid extract was dried under vacuum (Laborota 4000, Heidolph, Schwabach, Germany) and dissolved in 50 mL of 70% EtOH-H_2O solution adjusted to pH 3.2 with formic acid. The obtained extract was mixed and dried again and then dissolved in 50 mL of H_2O. The final redissolved extract was then degreased twice with hexane directly in the test tube and subjected to HPLC-DAD-MS analysis for qualitative and quantitative characterization.

2.1.2. HPLC-DAD-MS Analysis of Olea Extract

The analyses for the qualitative and quantitative characterization of bioactive compounds of the Olea extract were achieved using an HP-1260 liquid chromatograph equipped with a DAD (Agilent-Technologies, Palo Alto, CA, USA). The HPLC system was interfaced with an Agilent MS system equipped with an ESI source (Agilent Corp, Santa Clara, CA, USA). The analyses were acquired in full-scan mode and the mass range was set to m/z 100–1500 in negative mode. The analytical columns and chromatographic methods used were described in a previous study of ours [31]. Polyphenols found in the extract were identified by comparing retention times and UV/Vis spectra with those of the authentic standards. Each compound was quantified at the selected wavelength (240, 280, 330, 350 nm) using a five-point regression curve and applying the correction of the molecular weights [31].

2.2. In Vitro Study

Murine macrophage RAW 264.7 cell line was purchased from the American Type Culture Collection (ATCC, Manassas, VA, USA). Cells were cultured in Dulbecco's modified Eagle's medium/high glucose (DMEM 4500, EuroClone, Milan, Italy) supplemented with 10% fetal bovine serum (FBS, EuroClone) and maintained at 37 °C in a humidified atmosphere containing 90% air and 10% CO_2. Cells were harvested from subconfluent cultures via incubation with a trypsin-EDTA solution (EuroClone) and propagated every three days. Viability of the cells was determined by trypan blue exclusion test. Cultures were periodically monitored for Mycoplasma contamination using Chen's fluorochrome test, as described in a previous study of ours [33].

2.2.1. MTT Assay

Cell viability was assessed using a 3-(4,5-Dimethylthiazol-2-yl)-2,5-diphenyltetrazolium bromide (MTT) assay (Sigma Aldrich, Milan, Italy). Cells were placed into 96-well plates in complete medium in the absence and in the presence of different concentrations of oleocanthal standard (oleo std) or Olea extract that was rich in oleocanthal fraction (oleo fr) for 72 h. Next, MTT reagent was added to the medium and incubated at 37 °C. After 2 h, the blue MTT–formazan product was solubilized with dimethyl sulfoxide (DMSO, Sigma Aldrich) and its absorbance was read at 595 nm using a microplate reader (Bio-Rad, Milan, Italy), as previously described [34].

2.2.2. Nitrite Assay

NO metabolite concentration was measured in the culture medium of RAW cells, using the Griess reaction, which is specific for nitrite dosage. First, 100 μL of cell culture medium from RAW264.7 cells was mixed with an equal volume of Griess reagent (1% sulfanilamide, 0.1% N-1-naphthalenediamine dihydrochloride, and 2.5% H_3PO_4) and transferred to 96-well plates. Plates were incubated at room temperature for 10 min. The absorbance was then measured at 540 nm in a microplate reader (BioTek, Winooski, VT, USA). The amount of nitrite in the media was calculated from the sodium nitrite ($NaNO_2$) standard curve. Results were normalized to protein concentration. For RAW264.7 cells, nitrite production was expressed with reference to lipopolysaccharide (LPS; Sigma) as 100% [33].

2.2.3. Western Blotting Analysis

Cells were lysed and separated using electrophoresis as previously described in the literature [35]. The primary antibodies were as follows: rabbit anti-inducible NO syntethase (iNOS) (1:1000, Cell Signaling Technology, Danvers, MA, USA) and rabbit anti-cyclooxigenase (COX)-2 (1:1000, Cell Signaling Technology, Danvers, MA, USA). The membrane was washed in T-PBS buffer, incubated for 1 h at room temperature with goat anti-rabbit IgG Alexa Fluor 750 antibody or with goat anti-mouse IgG Alexa Fluor 680 antibody (Invitrogen, Monza, Italy), and then visualized using an Odyssey Infrared Imaging System (LI-COR® Bioscience, Lincoln, NE, USA). Mouse anti-alpha tubulin monoclonal antibody (1:1000, Cell Signaling Technology) was used to confirm that equal amounts of protein were loaded into each lane.

2.3. In Vivo Study

The aim of in vivo study was to evaluate the potential beneficial effects of an organic EVOO with a very high content of MPCs (>900 ppm) in CKD patients under conservative therapy.

2.3.1. Sample Size

In this study, we enrolled 40 CKD patients under conservative therapy distributed according to a Gauss curve of known mean and unknown variance. Therefore, the aforementioned sample size of 40 patients derived from the following probabilistic considerations:

A. The null hypothesis was rejected if the mean of the population from which the sample was extracted differed from the sample mean by an amount, expressed in absolute value, equal to or greater than 46.2% of the standard deviation;
B. For the hypotheses' (null and alternative) verification, the one-tailed Gauss z test with $\alpha = 0.05$ (first type error) and $\beta = 0.10$ (second type error) was adopted in order to give a test power equal to 90%.

2.3.2. Enrolled Patients

Consequently, 40 CKD patients under conservative therapy, stage I-IV (according to kidney disease: improving global outcomes—KDIGO guidelines [36]) were enrolled at the Hypertension and Nephrology Unit of Policlinico Tor Vergata (PTV), Rome (Italy). The inclusion criteria of study population were as follows: acceptance and signature of informed consent, age between 18 and 80 years, both sexes, and CKD stage I-IV. The exclusion criteria were as follows: the presence of either solid or hematological malignancies in the active phase, or of inflammatory and/or infectious pathologies.

At the time of enrolment, all patients were instructed to consume 40 mL/day of the EVOO selected for clinical experimentation. The EVOO was to be consumed raw in the patients' culinary preparations [37]. The study lasted 9 weeks. At baseline (T0) and after 9 weeks (T1), all the enrolled patients underwent blood and urinary analysis, body composition assessment via bioelectrical impedance analysis (BIA), Doppler ultrasound imaging of epiaortic vessels, monitoring of systolic and diastolic blood pressure, and evaluation of style and quality of life through specific questionnaires described below. The study protocol was declared to be compliant with the Helsinki Declaration by the PTV Independent Ethics Committee (protocol number 36/20). The flowchart of the study is represented in Figure 1.

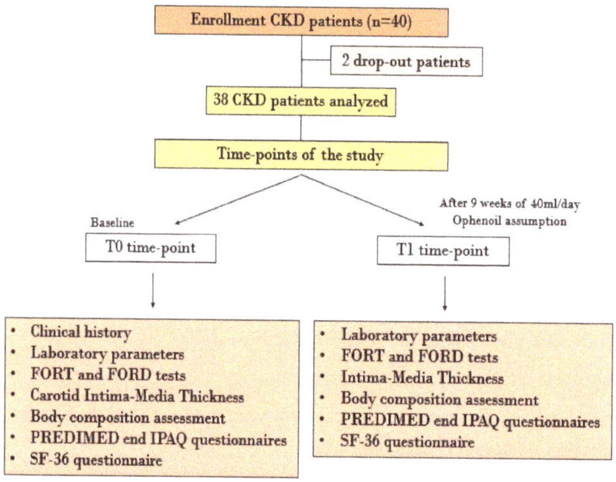

Figure 1. Flowchart of in vivo study. Abbreviations: CKD, chronic kidney disease; FORD, Free Oxygen Radical Defense; FORT, Free Oxygen Radical Test; IPAQ, International Physical Activity Questionnaires; PREDIMED, Preventiòn con dieta Mediterrànea; SF-36, Short Form Health Survey-36.

2.3.3. Blood and Urinary Analysis

At baseline (T0) and after 9 weeks (T1), all patients were assessed via blood and urinary analysis. In particular, glycemia, uricemia, intact parathyroid hormone, serum albumin, renal function parameters (like creatininemia, azotemia, albuminuria), electrolytes (like potassium, calcium, phosphorus, sodium), and lipid profile (like total cholesterol (TC), low-density lipoprotein cholesterol (LDL-C), high-density lipoprotein cholesterol (HDL-C), and triglycerides) were detected. Moreover, the patients underwent evaluation of inflammatory status via C-reactive protein (CRP), erythrocyte sedimentation rate (ESR), IL-6, TNF-α, PLR, NLR, and LMR and evaluation of OS biomarkers (like free oxygen radical defense (FORD) and free oxygen radical test (FORT)). In particular, the last ones allowed us to evaluate the antioxidant defenses and OS of the patients by means of capillary sampling, with a CR4000 instrument used for analysis [38].

2.3.4. Atherogenic Indices

At both time-points of the study, we calculated the atherogenic indices. In particular, we calculated TC/HDL-C, LDL-C/HDL-C, and log(triglycerides/HDL-C) indices. These indices can provide additional information regarding CV risk, as they are closely related to the patient lipid profile [39].

2.3.5. Body Composition Assessment

At T0 and T1, all patients underwent an anthropometric parameter assessment. Body weight was measured to the nearest 0.01 Kg using a balance (Seca 711, Hamburg, Germany), and height was measured using a stadiometer to the nearest 0.1 cm (Seca 220, Hamburg, Germany). Subsequently, the body mass index (BMI) was calculated as weight divided by the height squared.

Moreover, the study population underwent BIA to evaluate the body composition at T0 and at T1. The BIA parameters were determined at 50 KHz frequency, using a BIA 101 S instrument (Akern/RIL System, Florence, Italy). In particular, resistance, reactance, phase angle, fat mass (FM), fat-free mass (FFM), intracell water (ICW), extracell water (ECW), total body water (TBW), body cellular mass (BCM), body cellular mass index (BCMI), and basal metabolic rate (BMR) were evaluated [40].

2.3.6. Doppler Ultrasound of Epiaortic Vessels

All nephropathic patients underwent Doppler ultrasound to estimate CIMT. This examination was done using a MyLab70 VXG ultrasound device (Esaote, Genova, Italy) with a linear LA523 probe, at a 2–9 MHz frequency range. All examinations were conducted by the same operator (A.N.) to rule out operator-dependent bias. The CIMT was measured through a B-mode ultrasound examination at the level of the right common carotid artery. A longitudinal section of the right common carotid artery was obtained; three different CIMT measurements were performed, about 1 cm below the bifurcation, in the plaque-free area on the distal wall of the right common carotid artery, using a semiautomatic application. The CIMT was calculated as the average value of the three different measurements. This procedure was executed in accordance with the Mannheim protocol [41].

2.3.7. Questionnaires

Three questionnaires were administered to all enrolled patients, evaluating both their lifestyle (PREDIMED and International Physical Activity Questionnaires-IPAQ) and their quality of life (Short Form 36 Health Survey-SF-36), at T0 and at T1.

The lifestyle questionnaires were administered in order to exclude any bias due to lifestyle changes during the study period. In particular, the PREDIMED questionnaire monitors eating habits and adherence to the Mediterranean diet, while the IPAQ monitors the degree of physical activity of the patient [26,42].

The SF-36 questionnaire evaluates the quality of life as perceived by the patient through 36 questions regarding nine areas: general health, health change, physical functioning, pain, social functioning, emotional well-being, energy/fatigue, role limitation due to physical health, and role limitation due to emotional problems.

2.3.8. Statistical Analysis

All data were entered into an Excel spreadsheet (Microsoft, Redmond, Washington, DC, USA) and the analyses were done using the Windows Social Science Statistics Package, version 25.0 (IBM_SPSS, Chicago, IL, USA).

The descriptive analysis results are represented as mean ± standard deviation (SD) for the parameters with normal distributions (after confirmation with the histograms and the Kolgomorov–Smirnov test), while for the non-normal variables, the median and the interval (minimum:maximum) are used.

The comparisons between the normal variables were done with one-way ANOVA, while the comparisons between the two time-points of the study (T0 versus T1) were performed using paired T-tests for normal variables, while Mann–Whitney tests were used for non-normal variables. Regarding occurrences (percentages), the chi-square test, possibly corrected by Fisher's exact test, was applied. A p value < 0.05 was considered statistically significant.

3. Results

3.1. Qualitative and Quantitative Characterization of the Organic EVOO

The HPLC-DAD-MS characterization of the EVOO selected for this study showed a very high content of MPCs, equal to 1145.98 mg/L. By evaluating the single molecules, we confirmed that the EVOO met the criteria required in order to claim CV protection according to the European Food Safety Authority (EFSA), as reported in Commission Regulation n. 432/2012 [43,44]. This regulation establishes that a daily intake of 20 g EVOO containing 5 mg of HT and its derivatives protects against blood lipid oxidation. In particular, in the EVOO selected for this study, the content of HT and its derivatives reached 778.43 mg/L. Moreover, in the EVOO administered in this study, we detected the contents of oleacin (315.46 mg/L) and oleocanthal (197.84 mg/L), molecules characterized by important anti-inflammatory activities [45,46].

Table 1 shows the chemical characterization of the single compounds identified in the EVOO sample.

Table 1. HPLC-DA-MS analysis of Ophena EVOO.

Compounds	EVOO mg/L
Hydroxytyrosol	3.10 ± 0.09
Tyrosol	1.02 ± 0.03
Elenolic Acid Derivatives	9.31 ± 0.28
Elenolic acid	150.06 ± 4.50
Oleacin (10-hydroxy-oleocanthal)	315.46 ± 9.46
Oleocanthal	197.84 ± 5.04
Secoiridoid derivatives	96.43 ± 2.89
Lignans	208.17 ± 6.25
Oleuropein aglycone	164.58 ± 4.94
Total MPCs	1145.97 ± 34.38
MPCs excluding elenolic acid and derivatives	986.60 ± 29.60

Abbreviation: MPCs, minor phenolic compounds.

Analyses relating to qualitative parameters of EVOO were carried out using the Oxitester system. We obtained low peroxide values (4.98 meqO_2/kg) and acidity equal to 0.17%, indicating a high quality of the selected product (Table 2).

Table 2. Acidity, peroxides, and polyphenols of EVOO.

EVOO	
Acidity (% acid oleic)	0.17
Peroxides (meqO_2/kg)	4.98
Polyphenols (mg tyrosol/kg)	890

All results are expressed as average of three determinations. The standard error was <3% for acidity, <5% for peroxides, and <10% for polyphenols.

Oleocanthal Fraction Characterization

The HPLC-DAD-MS characterization analyses of the Olea extract showed high contents of oleacin (411.73 mg/g) and oleocanthal (331.73 mg/g) (Table 3). As we previously reported, for the analyzed EVOO sample, the high presence of these molecules permitted us to hypothesize a possible anti-inflammatory action of this extract. In fact, this action is added to the massive antioxidant properties already ascribed to these molecules and to HT, tyrosol, elenolic acid, oleuropein aglycone, ligstriside, and secoiridoidic derivatives [28,47,48].

3.2. In Vitro Study

To evaluate whether the oleo fr extracted from EVOO was more effective in terms of anti-inflammatory properties than the oleocanthal standard (oleo std), we compared their potential toxicities. In this way, equimolar doses of both oleo std and fr were administered to RAW 264.7 cells for 72 h and cell viability was determined via MTT assay.

Table 3. HPLC-DAD-MS characterization of Olea extract.

Olea Extract	mg/g
Hydroxytyrosol	7.93 ± 0.24
Tyrosol	7.12 ± 0.22
Elenolic acid	89.19 ± 2.68
Oleacin (10-hydroxy-oleocanthal)	411.73 ± 12.35
Oleocanthal	331.73 ± 9.95
Oleuropein aglycone	75.87 ± 2.27
Ligstroside	4.93 ± 0.15
Secoiridoid derivatives	59.03 ± 1.77
Total	987.53 ± 29.63

Figure 2A shows that oleo fr was nontoxic up to a 15 μM dose, whereas oleo std did not affect cell viability even at high doses. To assess the anti-inflammatory property of oleo fr, we measured NO metabolite (specifically nitrite) production induced by 1 μg/mL of LPS (a marker of inflammation) in the same RAW 264.7culture medium, in either the presence or the absence of oleo fr. Oleo fr showed a higher capability to reduce NO production (Figure 2C) compared to oleo std (Figure 2B) and also compared to LPS, which was used as the positive control for nitrite production. In fact, it was already effective at a dose of 7.5 μM, compared to 30 μM of the oleo std. To study the anti-inflammatory capability of oleo fr in more depth, we also analyzed the expression levels of two enzymes directly implicated in the inflammatory response: iNOS and COX-2. Western blotting and densitometric analysis showed significant decreases of both iNOS and COX-2 expression, starting from a concentration of 15 μM (Figure 3).

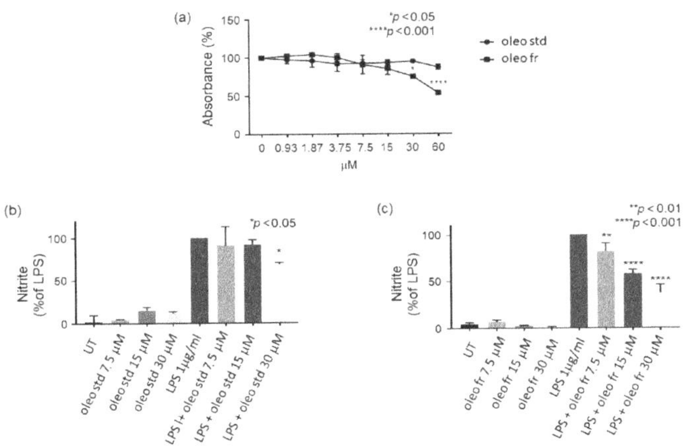

Figure 2. Cell viability assessed by MTT assay. (**a**) Cell viability assessed by MTT assay after 72 h of exposure to different doses of oleocanthal fraction (oleo fr) or oleocanthal standard (oleo std). Significance is indicated with * and relates to the untreated control (UT). Statistics were determined using two-way ANOVA and Sidak's multiple-comparisons test; (**b**) Nitrite production by RAW 264.7 treated for 24 h with 1 μg/mL LPS and oleo std at different doses. Significance is indicated with * and relates to LPS as 100% of nitrite production. Statistics were determined using ordinary one-way ANOVA and Dunnett's multiple-comparisons test; (**c**) Nitrite production by RAW 264.7 treated for 24 h with 1 μg/mL LPS and oleol fr at different doses. Significance is indicated with * and relates to LPS as 100% of nitrite production. Statistics were determined using ordinary one-way ANOVA and Dunnett's multiple-comparisons test.

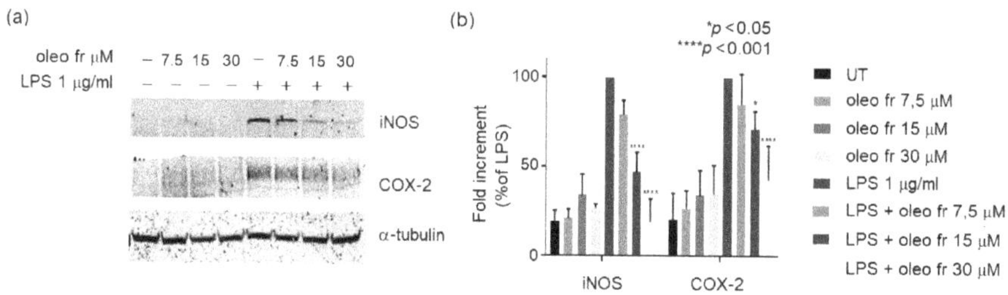

Figure 3. (**a**) Representative western blot panels of iNOS and COX-2 protein levels. Each band in the western blot was quantified via densitometric analysis and (**b**) the corresponding histogram was constructed by normalizing the density of each band to that of α-tubulin. The significance is indicated with * and relates to LPS. Statistical analyses were conducted using two-way ANOVA and Dunnett's multiple-comparisons test.

These results suggest a greater effectiveness of the fraction compared to the standard, probably due to the synergistic effect induced by all components present in the fraction.

3.3. *In Vivo Study*

The main epidemiological features of the study population (40 CKD patients under conservative therapy) are shown in Table 4. In particular, the mean age of the study population was 70.7 ± 10.6 years (CI: 49.5–80). The values of systolic and diastolic blood pressure monitored in the different time-points did not demonstrate any statistical significance.

Table 4. Epidemiological features of study population.

N°	**40**
Age (years)	70.7 ± 10.6
Sex (M/F)	24/16
BMI (kg/m^2)	27.6 ± 5.2

Data are expressed as mean ± standard deviation. Abbreviation: BMI, body mass index.

Only 38 patients completed the clinical trial. We recorded two drop-outs, for reasons not related to the experiment.

Table 5 shows the results of the laboratory and urinary parameters assessed at T0 and at T1. At the end of the study (T1), we observed an improvement of renal function parameters, with a significant reduction of serum level of creatinine ($p = 0.013$), azotemia ($p = 0.017$), and albuminuria ($p = 0.027$). Moreover, we noticed an amelioration of lipid and purine metabolism, with a significant increase of HDL-C and a significant decrease of triglycerides ($p = 0.002$) and uric acid serum levels ($p = 0.039$). The results also showed an improvement in the nutritional status of the patients after EVOO consumption, with a significant increase in serum albumin levels ($p = 0.001$).

As for the OS and the inflammation parameters, after 9 weeks of EVOO consumption, we observed significant reductions of FORT level ($p = 0.013$) and of CRP ($p = 0.046$), ESR (0.0006), TNF-α ($p = 0.0001$), and IL-6 ($p = 0.019$) serum levels, as reported in Table 6. In contrast, the patients' antioxidant defenses seemed to remain stable.

Table 7 expresses the data regarding atherogenic indices. At the end of the study, we observed significant reductions of TC/HDL-C ($p = 0.0171$), LDL-C/HDL-C ($p = 0.0098$), and log(triglycerides/HDL-C) ($p = 0.0067$).

After 9 weeks of EVOO consumption, we also observed an amelioration in the other inflammatory parameters, namely the PLR ($p = 0.0003$) and LMR ($p = 0.0406$), and in the absolute number of lymphocytes ($p = 0.0007$), as reported in Table 8.

Table 5. Laboratory and urinary parameters assessed at baseline and after 9 weeks of study.

	T0	T1	*p*-Value
Creatinine (mg/dL)	2.17 ± 0.17	2.08 ± 0.16	0.013
e-GFR (mL/min/1.73 m^2)	33.73 ± 2.81	35.35 ± 2.96	0.040
Albuminuria (mg/dL)	223.43 ± 60.95	120.88 ± 32.35	0.027
Albumin (g/dL)	4.22 ± 0.26	4.38 ± 0.31	0.001
Azotaemia (mg/dL)	79.03 ± 5.86	69.82 ± 4.69	0.017
Sodium (mEq/L)	141.24 ± 2.24	136.62 ± 2.34	n.s.
Potassium (mEq/L)	4.59 ± 0.64	4.69 ± 0.37	n.s.
Calcium (mg/dL)	9.51 ± 0.53	9.46 ± 0.50	n.s.
Phosphorus (mg/dL)	3.66 ± 0.63	3.67 ± 0.61	n.s.
TC (mg/dL)	176.20 ± 40.51	175.91 ± 38.64	n.s.
HDL-C (mg/dL)	45.26 ± 1.81	49.02 ± 2.29	0.004
LDL-C (mg/dL)	105.74 ± 37.22	103.71 ± 32.33	n.s.
Triglycerides (mg/dL)	124.45 ± 9.71	111.03 ± 8.27	0.002
PTHI (mg/dL)	90.15 ± 28.80	75.63 ± 11.77	n.s.
Glycaemia (mg/dL)	95.39 ± 27.01	100.97 ± 30.17	n.s.
Uric acid (mg/dL)	6.34 ± 0.31	5.68 ± 0.29	0.039

Data are expressed as mean ± standard deviation; Abbreviations: E-GFR, Estimated Glomerular Filtration Rate; TC, Total Cholesterol; HDL-C, High-Density Lipoprotein Cholesterol; LDL-C, Low-Density Lipoprotein Cholesterol; n.s., Not Significant; PTHI, Parathyroid Hormone Intact.

Table 6. Oxidative stress and inflammatory parameters assessed at baseline and after 9 weeks of study.

	T0	T1	*p*-Value
FORT (U)	397.60 ± 27.74	303.17 ± 25.65	0.013
FORD (mmol/L Trolox)	1.37 ± 0.49	1.51 ± 0.50	n.s.
CRP (mg/L)	5.39 ± 1.22	3.13 ± 0.82	0.046
ESR (mm/h)	46.43 ± 4.70	39.22 ± 3.96	0.0006
TNF-α (pg/mL)	89.70 ± 66.53	36.65 ± 32.83	0.0001
IL-6 (pg/mL)	71.22 ± 23.81	10.13 ± 2.50	0.019

Data are expressed as mean ± standard deviation. *t*-test was applied for paired data. Values of $p \leq 0.05$ are considered statistically significant. Abbreviations: CRP, C-Reactive Protein; ESR, Erythrocyte Sedimentation Rate; FORD, Free Oxygen Radical Defense; FORT, Free Oxygen Radical Test; IL, Interleukin; n.s., Not Significant; TNF, Tumor Necrosis Factor.

Table 7. Atherogenic indices.

	T0	T1	*p*-Value
TC/HDL-C	3.90 (2.62–6.58)	3.42 (2.31–6.57)	0.0171
LDL-C/HDL-C	2.27 (1.20–5.47)	1.91 (1.20–4.15)	0.0098
log(triglycerides/HDL-C)	0.05 (0.03–0.11)	0.04 (0.02–0.09)	0.0067

Data are expressed as a median and the minimum-maximum range; Abbreviations: TC, Total Cholesterol; HDL-C, High-Density Lipoprotein Cholesterol; LDL-C, Low-Density Lipoprotein Cholesterol; n.s., Not Significant.

Table 8. Other inflammatory parameters.

	T0	T1	*p*-Value
Platelet-to-lymphocyte ratio	135.09 (51.08–337.84) [a]	116.01 (55.08–227.00) [a]	0.0003
Neutrophil-to-lymphocyte ratio	2.22 (0.75–7.00) [a]	2.14 (0.86–7.45) [a]	n.s.
Lymphocyte-to-monocyte ratio	3.75 (0.27–7.74) [a]	3.50 (0.15–8.21) [a]	0.0406
Lymphocytes (n/mm^3)	2.03 ± 0.70 [b]	1.78 ± 0.65 [b]	0.0007

[a] Data are expressed as a median and the minimum-maximum range; [b] Data are expressed as mean ± standard deviation. Abbreviation: n.s., Not Significant.

The Doppler ultrasound imaging showed a significant reduction of CIMT ($p = 0.017$), as summarized in Table 9.

Table 9. CIMT values assessed at baseline and after 9 weeks of study.

	T0	T1	*p*-Value
Carotid Intima-Media Thickness (mm)	1.10 ± 0.44	1.02 ± 0.35	0.017

Data are expressed as mean ± standard deviation.

Finally, the body composition assessment by BIA highlighted a significant increase of reactance (0.007) and of BCM % (p = 0.025), as reported in Table 10.

Table 10. Body composition parameters assessed at baseline and after 9 weeks of study.

	T0	T1	*p*-Value
Weight (kg)	74.1 ± 13.8	73.7 ± 13.7	n.s.
BMI (kg/m^2)	27.76 ± 5.27	28.62 ± 4.50	n.s.
Resistance (ohm)	496.0 ± 80.3	493.6 ± 104.8	n.s.
Reactance (ohm)	40.78 ± 1.71	43.63 ± 1.80	0.007
Phase angle (°)	4.80 ± 0.86	4.90 ± 1.01	n.s.
TBW (%)	52.6 ± 9.1	72.4 ± 10.6	n.s.
ICW (%)	47.2 ± 5.3	49.1 ± 8.5	n.s.
ECW (%)	52.8 ± 5.3	50.9 ± 8.5	n.s.
FM (%)	28.6 ± 9.7	29.4 ± 10.6	n.s.
FFM (%)	69.6 ± 11.6	70.7 ± 9.4	n.s.
BCM (%)	44.6 ± 9.2	47.0 ± 6.4	0.025
BCMI	9.0 ± 1.7	9.1 ± 1.8	n.s.
BMR (Kcal)	1452.3 ± 154.7	1453.3 ± 157–5	n.s.

Data are expressed as mean ± standard deviation. Abbreviations: BCM, Body Cellular Mass; BCMI, Body Cellular Mass Index; BMI, Body Mass Index, BMR, Basal Metabolic Rate; ECW, Extra Cell Water, FM, Fat Mass; FFM, Fat Free Mass; ICW, Intra Cell Water; n.s., Not Significant; TBW, Total Body Water.

The lifestyle questionnaires PREDIMED and IPAQ did not show statistically significant differences between the two observation time-points, highlighting that the results obtained may be attributable to EVOO consumption. Moreover, at baseline (T0) and after 9 weeks (T1) of in vivo study, the SF-36 questionnaire was administered to assess patients' perception of their quality of life. At T1, we observed an improvement in the general health and emotional well-being spheres (Figure 4).

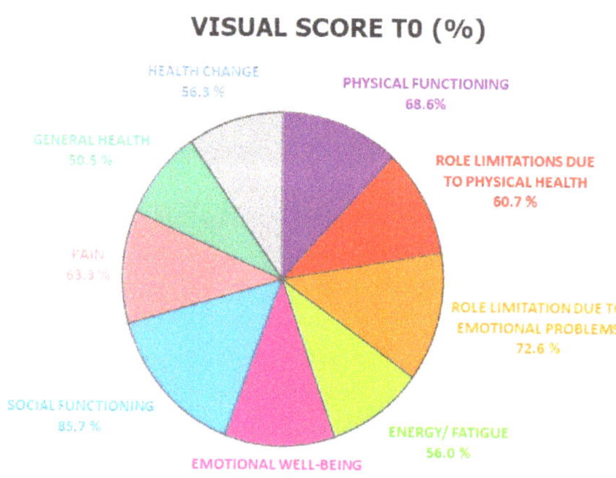

Figure 4. *Cont.*

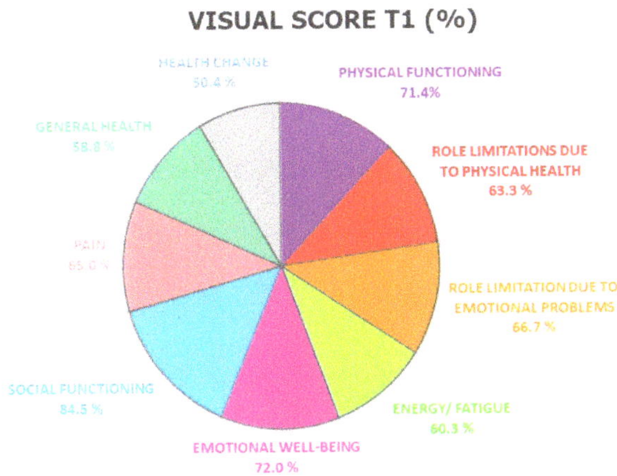

Figure 4. Visual scores, expressed in % for each sphere, of the SF-36 questionnaire administered at baseline and after 9 weeks of study.

4. Discussion

In our study population, we observed a significant improvement of lipid metabolism after 9 weeks of treatment with an EVOO with a very high MPC content. In particular, we observed a significant increase of HDL-C and a reduction of triglycerides. These results could be partly related to the high content of HT. In fact, in a previous animal study, Jemai et al. [49] demonstrated a lipid-lowering action of HT and its derivatives, related to their antioxidant effects which counteract the lipid peroxidation. Moreover, Cao and co-authors [50] showed that HT supplementation, at a dose of 50 mg/kg/day for 17 weeks in obese mice, induced a decrease of sterol regulatory element-binding protein 1 (SREBP-1c) levels, which is a cholesterol-sensitive transcription factor that stimulates the activity of hydroxy-methyl-glutaryl-coenzyme A (HMG-CoA) reductase. In subsequent human studies, conducted on metabolic syndrome patients treated with oral food supplements with a high HT content [51,52], the hypolipemic effect of HT was confirmed.

Interestingly, in our study population, we also observed an amelioration of atherogenic indices. In detail, we detected significant decreases of TC/HDL-C, LDL-C/HDL-C, and log (triglycerides/HDL-C). These data are in accordance with the results obtained in the EUROLIVE Study [27], which reported an amelioration of fatty acid profile in LDL-C, probably correlated to a decrease in lipid oxidative injury. The observed reduction of TC/HDL-C is very important as it highlights the possible cardioprotective action of EVOO with a very high MPC content in nephropathic patients. In fact, this ratio represents a milestone biomarker in lipid atherogenesis, because it is linked to the balance between the passage of cholesterol in and out of the arterial intima [53]. Moreover, the Framingham Offspring Study showed that TC/HDL-C and LDL-C/HDL-C are the most important biomarkers for CV events, among all lipid parameters [54].

In the light of the CV protection induced by the EVOO administered to our study population, it was of utmost importance to observe not only an amelioration of lipid profile, but also a reduction of the chronic inflammatory state typical of CKD patients. In fact, atherosclerotic CV disease cannot be considered only a pathological condition related to the cholesterol accumulation, but is characterized by a more complex pathogenic mechanism and is frequently triggered by a chronic inflammatory status [55]. Inflammatory cell infiltrates have been isolated in atherosclerotic plaque [56], corroborating this hypothesis. Moreover, in the Physicians' Health Study [57] and Women's Health Study [58], a direct association was shown between pro-inflammatory cytokine (such as IL-6 and IL-1β) levels and atherosclerotic CV disease. In our study, we highlighted significant reductions of CRP, ESR, TNF-α, and IL-6 after 9 weeks of EVOO administration, confirming the cardioprotective action of EVOO with a very high MPC content in CKD patients. This anti-inflammatory effect was related to the high content of oleocanthal in the EVOO selected. In fact, several studies have pointed out the anti-inflammatory action induced by oleocanthal, as it is an unselective inhibitor of COX-1 and -2 [46,59]. This anti-inflammatory action is also supported by our in vitro data, as discussed above.

In addition, the inflammatory status improvement seemed to positively influence the degree of ED related to CKD. In fact, in the initial stages of atherosclerotic disease, pro-inflammatory cytokines (like IL-6 and TNF-α, which are significantly reduced at T1 in our study) play a key role. These molecules, on one hand, induce the migration of leukocytes into the subendothelial space and, on the other hand, alter the gene expression of the adhesion molecules. The latter, in turn, favor the adhesion, chemotaxis, and subendothelial migration of the same leukocytes [60]. In detail, the physiopathological process that induces atherosclerotic plaque formation is mediated by the accumulation of monocytes in the subendothelial space [61]. We consider the reduction of CIMT observed at the end of our study to support this hypothesis. In detail, upon analyzing the data obtained from the ultrasound examination of the epiaortic vessels, we detected a CIMT improvement in patients presenting a slight increase of CIMT, but not in those who had already developed a carotid atherosclerotic plaque. In this regard, in the carotid atherosclerosis progression study (CAPS), the authors observed a direct correlation between serum CRP levels and an increase in CIMT [62]; at the T1 time-point, we registered a significant decrease of CRP levels, as previously described. In addition to traditional inflammatory biomarkers such as ESR and CRP, we also calculated, the following ratios in order to monitor the inflammatory state: NLR, PLR, and LMR. The latter parameters, which are easy and quite cheap to monitor, were significantly decreased at the end of the study. Furthermore, they are associated with the inflammatory state of the subject and they seem to be correlated to the CV risk. In particular, NLR appears to be a reliable predictor of cardiac arrhythmia and it represents a short- and long-term biomarker of CV disease [63]. On the other hand, PLR seems to be an integrated parameter able to monitor both thrombotic and inflammatory pathways [64]. Historically, it has been used as inflammatory biomarker in cancer patients [65,66], and a possible role has only recently identified as a predictor for CV events [67]. Finally, in a human study conducted on 199 patients that underwent coronary angiography, LMR was associated directly and independently with the severity of coronary atherosclerosis [68]. Therefore, the reduction of these three ratios observed in our study allows further speculation regarding the strong CV protection induced by EVOO with a very high MPC content. A further possible explanation of the CIMT improvement relies on the reduction of LDL-C/HDL-C observed. In fact, a meta-analysis demonstrated that this ratio is related to CIMT. Moreover, low HDL-C concentrations seem to be inversely related to CIMT [69].

In this paper, we confirmed the positive impact of EVOO on slowing CKD progression, as already demonstrated in our previous studies [16,32]. In fact, we observed at T1 a significant reduction of creatinine and uric acid, and an increase of estimated-GFR. Moreover, at the end of the study, we noticed a reduction of microalbuminuria, which on one hand represents a biomarker of renal dysfunction and CKD progression [29,31,70], and on the other hand is related to the CV risk [71]. Therefore, its significant reduction confirms both the cardioprotective and nephroprotective action of EVOO.

We also obtained an additional result, namely a reduction of OS as monitored by FORT. This interesting observation supports the cardioprotective action induced by EVOO and it is probably related to its high content of oleocanthal. This molecule also exerts an antioxidant action, reducing the activity of nicotamide adenine dinucleotide phosphate oxidase and, at the same time, ROS production [72].

Finally, we showed an improvement of the nutritional status of patients, related to the significant enhancement of albuminemia observed at the end of the study. In fact, hypoalbuminemia is frequently present in CKD patients under conservative therapy, and it is correlated with both a low caloric intake and a chronic inflammatory status. In this regard, EVOO consumption at a dose of 40 mL/day is able to counteract the inflammation and, at the same time, provide the correct caloric intake [73].

Moreover, regarding body composition assessment, we observed a significant increase of BCM% after our intervention. This parameter is not only directly related to albumin, as previous demonstrated in the literature, but it is a useful tool to evaluate inflammation in CKD and elderly patients [74].

As for the SF-36 questionnaire, this test allowed us to underline an enhancement of quality of life as perceived by patients, likely related to their enhanced health status.

5. Conclusions

We would like to stress that this study highlighted the cardioprotective action of EVOO in nephropathic patients for the first time. This positive health effect could be due to the reduction of the chronic inflammatory state produced by the oleocanthal and to the improvement of lipid metabolism induced by HT and oleuropein.

Previous clinical trials (such as PREDIMED [26], EPIC [25], and EUROLIVE [27]) have shown this beneficial effect only in other CV high-risk populations, but not in CKD patients.

In order to reduce CV mortality in CKD, the traditional nutritional treatment, planned according to CKD stage, should be combined with functional foods. Among these, according also to EFSA's health claim [43,44], EVOO with a high content of MPCs seems to be one of the most important functional foods exerting cardioprotective action.

Author Contributions: Conceptualization, A.N.; methodology, S.U., J.R., F.I., P.V. and C.N.; investigation, G.M., M.D.L. and C.G.; data curation, G.M.; writing—original draft preparation, G.M., M.D.L. and A.N.; writing—review and editing, N.D.D. and A.N.; visualization, M.D.L., J.R. and F.D.D.; supervision, N.D.D. and A.N. All authors have read and agreed to the published version of the manuscript.

Funding: This research received no external funding.

Institutional Review Board Statement: The study was conducted in accordance with the Declaration of Helsinki, and approved by the Independent Ethics Committee of Policlinico Tor Vergata (protocol code 36, approved in 2020).

Informed Consent Statement: Informed consent was obtained from all subjects involved in the study.

Data Availability Statement: Data supporting reported results can be found upon request to the corresponding author.

Acknowledgments: This article is dedicated to the memory of our beloved and esteemed full professor Annalisa Romani, who recently passed away. We would like to thank Gabriella Venafro for the English language revision. We would like to thank Lazio Region and ARSIAL (Regional Agency for Development and Innovation of Lazio Agriculture)—Research project "Food culture well-being and natural cuisine" and Tuscany Region (BIOSYNOL PSGO 52 2017). We would like to thank Goldmed Suisse for the extra-virgin olive oil supply for free.

Conflicts of Interest: The authors declare no conflict of interest.

Abbreviation

ADMA	Asymmetric Dimethylarginine
AGEs	Advanced Glycation End Products
BCM	Body Cellular Mass
BCMI	Body Cellular Mass Index
BIA	Bioelectrical Impedance Analysis
BMI	Body Mass Index
BMR	Basal Metabolic Rate
CAPS	Carotid Atherosclerosis Progression Study
CIMT	Carotid Intima-Media Thickness
CKD	Chronic Kidney Disease
COX	Cyclooxygenase Enzymes

CRP	C-Reactive Protein
CV	Cardiovascular
DDAH	Enzyme Dimethylarginine Di-Methylaminohydrolase
ECW	Extra Cell Water
ED	Endothelial Dysfunction
EFSA	European Food Safety Authority
EPIC	European Prospective Investigation
ESR	Erythrocyte Sedimentation Rate
EVOO	Extra Virgin Olive Oil
FFM	Fat Free Mass
FM	Fat Mass
FORD	Free Oxygen Radical Defense
FORT	Free Oxygen Radical Test
SF-36	Short Form 36 Health Survey
GFR	Glomerular Filtration Rate
HDL-C	High-Density Lipoprotein Cholesterol
HMG-CoA	Hydroxy-methyl-glutaryl-coenzyme A
HPLC-DAD-MS	High-Performance Liquid Chromatography Coupled with Diode Array Detector-Mass Spectrometry
HT	Hydroxytyrosol
ICW	Intra Cell Water
IL	Interleukin
IPAQ	International Physical Activity Questionnaires
KDIGO	Kidney Disease: Improving Global Outcomes
LDL-C	Low-Density Lipoprotein Cholesterol
LMR	Lymphocyte-To-Monocyte Ratio
LPS	Lipopolysaccharide
MPCs	Minor Phenolic Compounds
MTT	3-(4,5-Dimethylthiazol-2-yl)-2,5-diphenyltetrazolium bromide
MUFAs	Monounsaturated Fatty Acids
NF-kB	Nuclear Factor Kappa-Light-Chain-Enhancer of Activated B Cells
NLR	Neutrophil-To-Lymphocyte Ratio
NO	Nitric Oxide
Oleo fr	Oleocanthal fraction
Oleo std	Oleocanthal standard
OS	Oxidative Stress
PLR	Platelet-To-Lymphocyte Ratio
PREDIMED	Prevención Con Dieta Mediterránea
PTV	Policlinico Tor Vergata
ROS	Reactive Oxygen Species
SD	Standard Deviation
TBW	Total Body Water
TC	Total Cholesterol
TNF	Tumor Necrosis Factor

References

1. Foreman, K.J.; Marquez, N.; Dolgert, A.; Fukutaki, K.; Fullman, N.; McGaughey, M.; Pletcher, M.A.; Smith, A.E.; Tang, K.; Yuan, C.W.; et al. Forecasting life expectancy, years of life lost, and all-cause and cause-specific mortality for 250 causes of death: Reference and alternative scenarios for 2016-40 for 195 countries and territories. *Lancet* **2018**, *392*, 2052–2090. [CrossRef]
2. Weiner, D.E.; Tighiouart, H.; Elsayed, E.F.; Griffith, J.L.; Salem, D.N.; Levey, A.S.; Sarnak, M.J. The Framingham predictive instrument in chronic kidney disease. *J. Am. Coll. Cardiol.* **2007**, *50*, 217–224. [CrossRef]
3. Reichel, H.; Zee, J.; Tu, C.; Young, E.; Pisoni, R.L.; Stengel, B.; Duttlinger, J.; Lonnemann, G.; Robinson, B.M.; Pecoits-Filho, R.; et al. Chronic kidney disease progression and mortality risk profiles in Germany: Results from the Chronic Kidney Disease Outcomes and Practice Patterns Study. *Nephrol. Dial. Transplant.* **2020**, *35*, 803–810. [CrossRef] [PubMed]
4. Noce, A.; Canale, M.P.; Capria, A.; Rovella, V.; Tesauro, M.; Splendiani, G.; Annicchiarico-Petruzzelli, M.; Manzuoli, M.; Simonetti, G.; Di Daniele, N. Coronary artery calcifications predict long term cardiovascular events in non diabetic Caucasian hemodialysis patients. *Aging* **2015**, *7*, 269–279. [CrossRef] [PubMed]

5. Pires, A.; Sobrinho, L.; Ferreira, H.G. The Calcium/Phosphorus Homeostasis in Chronic Kidney Disease: From Clinical Epidemiology to Pathophysiology. *Acta Med. Port.* **2017**, *30*, 485–492. [CrossRef]
6. Pastore, A.; Noce, A.; Di Giovamberardino, G.; De Stefano, A.; Calla, C.; Zenobi, R.; Dessi, M.; Di Daniele, N. Homocysteine, cysteine, folate and vitamin B(1)(2) status in type 2 diabetic patients with chronic kidney disease. *J. Nephrol.* **2015**, *28*, 571–576. [CrossRef]
7. Cianciolo, G.; De Pascalis, A.; Di Lullo, L.; Ronco, C.; Zannini, C.; La Manna, G. Folic Acid and Homocysteine in Chronic Kidney Disease and Cardiovascular Disease Progression: Which Comes First? *Cardiorenal. Med.* **2017**, *7*, 255–266. [CrossRef]
8. Pereira, R.A.; Cordeiro, A.C.; Avesani, C.M.; Carrero, J.J.; Lindholm, B.; Amparo, F.C.; Amodeo, C.; Cuppari, L.; Kamimura, M.A. Sarcopenia in chronic kidney disease on conservative therapy: Prevalence and association with mortality. *Nephrol. Dial. Transplant.* **2015**, *30*, 1718–1725. [CrossRef]
9. Noce, A.; Marrone, G.; Ottaviani, E.; Guerriero, C.; Di Daniele, F.; Pietroboni Zaitseva, A.; Di Daniele, N. Uremic Sarcopenia and Its Possible Nutritional Approach. *Nutrients* **2021**, *13*, 147. [CrossRef]
10. Noce, A.; Marchetti, M.; Marrone, G.; Di Renzo, L.; Di Lauro, M.; Di Daniele, F.; Albanese, M.; Di Daniele, N.; De Lorenzo, A. Link between gut microbiota dysbiosis and chronic kidney disease. *Eur. Rev. Med. Pharmacol. Sci.* **2022**, *26*, 2057–2074. [CrossRef] [PubMed]
11. Noce, A.; Marrone, G.; Di Daniele, F.; Ottaviani, E.; Wilson Jones, G.; Bernini, R.; Romani, A.; Rovella, V. Impact of Gut Microbiota Composition on Onset and Progression of Chronic Non-Communicable Diseases. *Nutrients* **2019**, *11*, 1073. [CrossRef]
12. Noce, A.; Marrone, G.; Di Lauro, M.; Urciuoli, S.; Pietroboni Zaitseva, A.; Wilson Jones, G.; Di Daniele, N.; Romani, A. Cardiovascular Protection of Nephropathic Male Patients by Oral Food Supplements. *Cardiovasc. Ther.* **2020**, *2020*, 1807941. [CrossRef]
13. Noce, A.; Marrone, G.; Wilson Jones, G.; Di Lauro, M.; Pietroboni Zaitseva, A.; Ramadori, L.; Celotto, R.; Mitterhofer, A.P.; Di Daniele, N. Nutritional Approaches for the Management of Metabolic Acidosis in Chronic Kidney Disease. *Nutrients* **2021**, *13*, 2534. [CrossRef]
14. Mihai, S.; Codrici, E.; Popescu, I.D.; Enciu, A.M.; Albulescu, L.; Necula, L.G.; Mambet, C.; Anton, G.; Tanase, C. Inflammation-Related Mechanisms in Chronic Kidney Disease Prediction, Progression, and Outcome. *J. Immunol. Res.* **2018**, *2018*, 2180373. [CrossRef]
15. Noce, A.; Di Lauro, M.; Di Daniele, F.; Pietroboni Zaitseva, A.; Marrone, G.; Borboni, P.; Di Daniele, N. Natural Bioactive Compounds Useful in Clinical Management of Metabolic Syndrome. *Nutrients* **2021**, *13*, 630. [CrossRef]
16. Grazioli, E.; Romani, A.; Marrone, G.; Di Lauro, M.; Cerulli, C.; Urciuoli, S.; Murri, A.; Guerriero, C.; Tranchita, E.; Tesauro, M.; et al. Impact of Physical Activity and Natural Bioactive Compounds on Endothelial Dysfunction in Chronic Kidney Disease. *Life* **2021**, *11*, 841. [CrossRef]
17. Roumeliotis, S.; Mallamaci, F.; Zoccali, C. Endothelial Dysfunction in Chronic Kidney Disease, from Biology to Clinical Outcomes: A 2020 Update. *J. Clin. Med.* **2020**, *9*, 2359. [CrossRef]
18. Vanhoutte, P.M.; Zhao, Y.; Xu, A.; Leung, S.W. Thirty Years of Saying NO: Sources, Fate, Actions, and Misfortunes of the Endothelium-Derived Vasodilator Mediator. *Circ. Res.* **2016**, *119*, 375–396. [CrossRef]
19. Bocedi, A.; Fabrini, R.; Lai, O.; Alfieri, L.; Roncoroni, C.; Noce, A.; Pedersen, J.Z.; Ricci, G. Erythrocyte glutathione transferase: A general probe for chemical contaminations in mammals. *Cell Death Discov.* **2016**, *2*, 16029. [CrossRef]
20. Vila Cuenca, M.; van Bezu, J.; Beelen, R.H.J.; Vervloet, M.G.; Hordijk, P.L. Stabilization of cell-cell junctions by active vitamin D ameliorates uraemia-induced loss of human endothelial barrier function. *Nephrol. Dial. Transplant.* **2019**, *34*, 252–264. [CrossRef]
21. Noce, A.; Rovella, V.; Marrone, G.; Cattani, G.; Zingaretti, V.; Limongi, D.; D'Agostini, C.; Sorge, R.; Casasco, M.; Di Daniele, N.; et al. Hemodialysis biomarkers: Total advanced glycation end products (AGEs) against oxidized human serum albumin (HSAox). *Acta Diabetol.* **2019**, *56*, 1323–1331. [CrossRef] [PubMed]
22. Yilmaz, M.I.; Saglam, M.; Caglar, K.; Cakir, E.; Sonmez, A.; Ozgurtas, T.; Aydin, A.; Eyileten, T.; Ozcan, O.; Acikel, C.; et al. The determinants of endothelial dysfunction in CKD: Oxidative stress and asymmetric dimethylarginine. *Am. J. Kidney Dis.* **2006**, *47*, 42–50. [CrossRef]
23. Ando, R.; Ueda, S.; Yamagishi, S.; Miyazaki, H.; Kaida, Y.; Kaifu, K.; Yokoro, M.; Nakayama, Y.; Obara, N.; Fukami, K.; et al. Involvement of advanced glycation end product-induced asymmetric dimethylarginine generation in endothelial dysfunction. *Diab. Vasc. Dis. Res.* **2013**, *10*, 436–441. [CrossRef]
24. Goligorsky, M.S. Pathogenesis of endothelial cell dysfunction in chronic kidney disease: A retrospective and what the future may hold. *Kidney Res. Clin. Pract.* **2015**, *34*, 76–82. [CrossRef]
25. Buckland, G.; Mayen, A.L.; Agudo, A.; Travier, N.; Navarro, C.; Huerta, J.M.; Chirlaque, M.D.; Barricarte, A.; Ardanaz, E.; Moreno-Iribas, C.; et al. Olive oil intake and mortality within the Spanish population (EPIC-Spain). *Am. J. Clin. Nutr.* **2012**, *96*, 142–149. [CrossRef]
26. Estruch, R.; Ros, E.; Salas-Salvado, J.; Covas, M.I.; Corella, D.; Aros, F.; Gomez-Gracia, E.; Ruiz-Gutierrez, V.; Fiol, M.; Lapetra, J.; et al. Primary Prevention of Cardiovascular Disease with a Mediterranean Diet Supplemented with Extra-Virgin Olive Oil or Nuts. *N. Engl. J. Med.* **2018**, *378*, e34. [CrossRef]
27. Cicero, A.F.; Nascetti, S.; Lopez-Sabater, M.C.; Elosua, R.; Salonen, J.T.; Nyyssonen, K.; Poulsen, H.E.; Zunft, H.J.; Kiesewetter, H.; de la Torre, K.; et al. Changes in LDL fatty acid composition as a response to olive oil treatment are inversely related to lipid oxidative damage: The EUROLIVE study. *J. Am. Coll. Nutr.* **2008**, *27*, 314–320. [CrossRef]

28. Romani, A.; Ieri, F.; Urciuoli, S.; Noce, A.; Marrone, G.; Nediani, C.; Bernini, R. Health Effects of Phenolic Compounds Found in Extra-Virgin Olive Oil, By-Products, and Leaf of *Olea europaea* L. *Nutrients* **2019**, *11*, 1776. [CrossRef]
29. Romani, A.; Campo, M.; Urciuoli, S.; Marrone, G.; Noce, A.; Bernini, R. An Industrial and Sustainable Platform for the Production of Bioactive Micronized Powders and Extracts Enriched in Polyphenols from *Olea europaea* L. and *Vitis vinifera* L. Wastes. *Front Nutr.* **2020**, *7*, 120. [CrossRef]
30. Senesi, R.; Andreani, C.; Baglioni, P.; Batista de Carvalho, L.A.E.; Licoccia, S.; Marques, M.P.M.; Moretti, G.; Noce, A.; Paolesse, R. Parker, S.F.; et al. Looking for Minor Phenolic Compounds in Extra Virgin Olive Oils Using Neutron and Raman Spectroscopies. *Antioxidants* **2021**, *10*, 643. [CrossRef]
31. Romani, A.; Bernini, R.; Noce, A.; Urciuoli, S.; Di Lauro, M.; Pietroboni Zaitseva, A.; Marrone, G.; Di Daniele, N. Potential Beneficial Effects of Extra Virgin Olive Oils Characterized by High Content in Minor Polar Compounds in Nephropathic Patients A Pilot Study. *Molecules* **2020**, *25*, 4757. [CrossRef] [PubMed]
32. Noce, A.; Marrone, G.; Urciuoli, S.; Di Daniele, F.; Di Lauro, M.; Pietroboni Zaitseva, A.; Di Daniele, N.; Romani, A. Usefulness of Extra Virgin Olive Oil Minor Polar Compounds in the Management of Chronic Kidney Disease Patients. *Nutrients* **2021**, *13*, 581 [CrossRef] [PubMed]
33. Ruzzolini, J.; Chioccioli, S.; Monaco, N.; Peppicelli, S.; Andreucci, E.; Urciuoli, S.; Romani, A.; Luceri, C.; Tortora, K. Calorini, L.; et al. Oleuropein-Rich Leaf Extract as a Broad Inhibitor of Tumour and Macrophage iNOS in an Apc Mutant Rat Model. *Antioxidants* **2021**, *10*, 1577. [CrossRef] [PubMed]
34. Ruzzolini, J.; Peppicelli, S.; Bianchini, F.; Andreucci, E.; Urciuoli, S.; Romani, A.; Tortora, K.; Caderni, G.; Nediani, C.; Calorini, L Cancer Glycolytic Dependence as a New Target of Olive Leaf Extract. *Cancers* **2020**, *12*, 317. [CrossRef]
35. Ruzzolini, J.; Peppicelli, S.; Andreucci, E.; Bianchini, F.; Scardigli, A.; Romani, A.; la Marca, G.; Nediani, C.; Calorini, L. Oleuropein, the Main Polyphenol of *Olea. europaea* Leaf Extract, Has an Anti-Cancer Effect on Human BRAF Melanoma Cells and Potentiates the Cytotoxicity of Current Chemotherapies. *Nutrients* **2018**, *10*, 1950. [CrossRef]
36. Holden, R.M.; Mustafa, R.A.; Alexander, R.T.; Battistella, M.; Bevilacqua, M.U.; Knoll, G.; Mac-Way, F.; Reslerova, M.; Wald, R.; Acott, P.D.; et al. KDIGO 2017 Clinical Practice Guideline Update for the Diagnosis, Evaluation, Prevention, and Treatment of Chronic Kidney Disease-Mineral and Bone Disorder (CKD-MBD). *Kidney Int. Suppl.* **2017**, *7*, 1–59. [CrossRef]
37. Ramirez-Anaya, J.D.P.; Castaneda-Saucedo, M.C.; Olalla-Herrera, M.; Villalon-Mir, M.; Serrana, H.L.; Samaniego Sanchez, C. Changes in the Antioxidant Properties of Extra Virgin Olive Oil after Cooking Typical Mediterranean Vegetables. *Antioxidants* **2019**, *8*, 246. [CrossRef]
38. Gaman, M.A.; Epingeac, M.E.; Diaconu, C.C.; Gaman, A.M. Evaluation of oxidative stress levels in obesity and diabetes by the free oxygen radical test and free oxygen radical defence assays and correlations with anthropometric and laboratory parameters. *World. J. Diabetes* **2020**, *11*, 193–201. [CrossRef]
39. Millan, J.; Pinto, X.; Munoz, A.; Zuniga, M.; Rubies-Prat, J.; Pallardo, L.F.; Masana, L.; Mangas, A.; Hernandez-Mijares, A.; Gonzalez-Santos, P.; et al. Lipoprotein ratios: Physiological significance and clinical usefulness in cardiovascular prevention. *Vasc. Health Risk Manag.* **2009**, *5*, 757–765.
40. Bellizzi, V.; Scalfi, L.; Terracciano, V.; De Nicola, L.; Minutolo, R.; Marra, M.; Guida, B.; Cianciaruso, B.; Conte, G.; Di Iorio, B.R. Early changes in bioelectrical estimates of body composition in chronic kidney disease. *J. Am. Soc. Nephrol.* **2006**, *17*, 1481–1487. [CrossRef]
41. Touboul, P.J.; Hennerici, M.G.; Meairs, S.; Adams, H.; Amarenco, P.; Bornstein, N.; Csiba, L.; Desvarieux, M.; Ebrahim, S.; Hernandez Hernandez, R.; et al. Mannheim carotid intima-media thickness and plaque consensus (2004-2006-2011). An update on behalf of the advisory board of the 3rd, 4th and 5th watching the risk symposia, at the 13th, 15th and 20th European Stroke Conferences, Mannheim, Germany, 2004, Brussels, Belgium, 2006, and Hamburg, Germany, 2011. *Cerebrovasc. Dis.* **2012**, *34*, 290–296. [CrossRef]
42. Wanner, M.; Probst-Hensch, N.; Kriemler, S.; Meier, F.; Autenrieth, C.; Martin, B.W. Validation of the long international physical activity questionnaire: Influence of age and language region. *Prev. Med. Rep.* **2016**, *3*, 250–256. [CrossRef]
43. EFSA. Scientific Opinion on the Substantiation of Health Claims Related to Polyphenols in Olive and Protection of LDL Particles from Oxidative Damage (ID 1333, 1638, 1639, 1696, 2865), Maintenance of Normal Blood HDL Cholesterol Concentrations (ID 1639), Maintenance of Normal Blood Pressure (ID 3781), "Anti-Inflammatory Properties" (ID 1882), "Contributes to the Upper Respiratory Tract Health" (ID 3468), "Can Help to Maintain a Normal Function of Gastrointestinal Tract" (3779), and "Contributes to Body Defences against External Agents" (ID 3467) Pursuant to Article 13(1) of Regulation (EC) No 1924/2006. Available online: https://www.efsa.europa.eu/en/efsajournal/pub/2033 (accessed on 5 August 2020).
44. EFSA. Panel on Dietetic Products. *EFSA J.* **2011**, *9*, 2033–2058.
45. Scotece, M.; Gomez, R.; Conde, J.; Lopez, V.; Gomez-Reino, J.J.; Lago, F.; Smith, A.B., 3rd; Gualillo, O. Further evidence for the anti-inflammatory activity of oleocanthal: Inhibition of MIP-1alpha and IL-6 in J774 macrophages and in ATDC5 chondrocytes. *Life Sci.* **2012**, *91*, 1229–1235. [CrossRef]
46. Beauchamp, G.K.; Keast, R.S.; Morel, D.; Lin, J.; Pika, J.; Han, Q.; Lee, C.H.; Smith, A.B.; Breslin, P.A. Phytochemistry: Ibuprofen-like activity in extra-virgin olive oil. *Nature* **2005**, *437*, 45–46. [CrossRef]
47. Lanza, B.; Ninfali, P. Antioxidants in Extra Virgin Olive Oil and Table Olives: Connections between Agriculture and Processing for Health Choices. *Antioxidants* **2020**, *9*, 41. [CrossRef]

48. Carnevale, R.; Nocella, C.; Cammisotto, V.; Bartimoccia, S.; Monticolo, R.; D'Amico, A.; Stefanini, L.; Pagano, F.; Pastori, D.; Cangemi, R.; et al. Antioxidant activity from extra virgin olive oil via inhibition of hydrogen peroxide-mediated NADPH-oxidase 2 activation. *Nutrition* **2018**, *55–56*, 36–40. [CrossRef]
49. Jemai, H.; Fki, I.; Bouaziz, M.; Bouallagui, Z.; El Feki, A.; Isoda, H.; Sayadi, S. Lipid-lowering and antioxidant effects of hydroxytyrosol and its triacetylated derivative recovered from olive tree leaves in cholesterol-fed rats. *J. Agric. Food Chem.* **2008**, *56*, 2630–2636. [CrossRef]
50. Cao, K.; Xu, J.; Zou, X.; Li, Y.; Chen, C.; Zheng, A.; Li, H.; Li, H.; Szeto, I.M.; Shi, Y.; et al. Hydroxytyrosol prevents diet-induced metabolic syndrome and attenuates mitochondrial abnormalities in obese mice. *Free Radic. Biol. Med.* **2014**, *67*, 396–407. [CrossRef]
51. Verhoeven, V.; Van der Auwera, A.; Van Gaal, L.; Remmen, R.; Apers, S.; Stalpaert, M.; Wens, J.; Hermans, N. Can red yeast rice and olive extract improve lipid profile and cardiovascular risk in metabolic syndrome?: A double blind, placebo controlled randomized trial. *BMC Complement. Altern. Med.* **2015**, *15*, 52. [CrossRef]
52. Hermans, M.P.; Lempereur, P.; Salembier, J.P.; Maes, N.; Albert, A.; Jansen, O.; Pincemail, J. Supplementation Effect of a Combination of Olive (*Olea europea* L.) Leaf and Fruit Extracts in the Clinical Management of Hypertension and Metabolic Syndrome. *Antioxidants* **2020**, *9*, 872. [CrossRef]
53. Kannel, W.B.; Wilson, P.W. Efficacy of lipid profiles in prediction of coronary disease. *Am. Heart J.* **1992**, *124*, 768–774. [CrossRef]
54. Nam, B.H.; Kannel, W.B.; D'Agostino, R.B. Search for an optimal atherogenic lipid risk profile: From the Framingham Study. *Am. J. Cardiol.* **2006**, *97*, 372–375. [CrossRef]
55. Alfaddagh, A.; Martin, S.S.; Leucker, T.M.; Michos, E.D.; Blaha, M.J.; Lowenstein, C.J.; Jones, S.R.; Toth, P.P. Inflammation and cardiovascular disease: From mechanisms to therapeutics. *Am. J. Prev. Cardiol.* **2020**, *4*, 100130. [CrossRef]
56. Libby, P. Inflammation in atherosclerosis. *Arterioscler. Thromb. Vasc. Biol.* **2012**, *32*, 2045–2051. [CrossRef]
57. Ridker, P.M.; Rifai, N.; Stampfer, M.J.; Hennekens, C.H. Plasma concentration of interleukin-6 and the risk of future myocardial infarction among apparently healthy men. *Circulation* **2000**, *101*, 1767–1772. [CrossRef]
58. Bermudez, E.A.; Rifai, N.; Buring, J.; Manson, J.E.; Ridker, P.M. Interrelationships among circulating interleukin-6, C-reactive protein, and traditional cardiovascular risk factors in women. *Arterioscler. Thromb. Vasc. Biol.* **2002**, *22*, 1668–1673. [CrossRef]
59. Lucas, L.; Russell, A.; Keast, R. Molecular mechanisms of inflammation. Anti-inflammatory benefits of virgin olive oil and the phenolic compound oleocanthal. *Curr. Pharm. Des.* **2011**, *17*, 754–768. [CrossRef]
60. Tousoulis, D.; Antoniades, C.; Stefanadis, C. Assessing inflammatory status in cardiovascular disease. *Heart* **2007**, *93*, 1001–1007. [CrossRef]
61. Pearson, T.A.; Mensah, G.A.; Alexander, R.W.; Anderson, J.L.; Cannon, R.O., 3rd; Criqui, M.; Fadl, Y.Y.; Fortmann, S.P.; Hong, Y.; Myers, G.L.; et al. Markers of inflammation and cardiovascular disease: Application to clinical and public health practice: A statement for healthcare professionals from the Centers for Disease Control and Prevention and the American Heart Association. *Circulation* **2003**, *107*, 499–511. [CrossRef]
62. Nezu, T.; Hosomi, N.; Aoki, S.; Matsumoto, M. Carotid Intima-Media Thickness for Atherosclerosis. *J. Atheroscler. Thromb.* **2016**, *23*, 18–31. [CrossRef]
63. Afari, M.E.; Bhat, T. Neutrophil to lymphocyte ratio (NLR) and cardiovascular diseases: An update. *Expert Rev. Cardiovasc. Ther.* **2016**, *14*, 573–577. [CrossRef]
64. Kurtul, A.; Ornek, E. Platelet to Lymphocyte Ratio in Cardiovascular Diseases: A Systematic Review. *Angiology* **2019**, *70*, 802–818. [CrossRef]
65. Malm, C.J.; Hansson, E.C.; Akesson, J.; Andersson, M.; Hesse, C.; Shams Hakimi, C.; Jeppsson, A. Preoperative platelet function predicts perioperative bleeding complications in ticagrelor-treated cardiac surgery patients: A prospective observational study. *Br. J. Anaesth.* **2016**, *117*, 309–315. [CrossRef] [PubMed]
66. He, Z.; Li, D.; Xu, Y.; Wang, H.; Gao, J.; Zhang, Z.; Chen, K. Prognostic significance of metastatic lymph node ratio in patients with gastric cancer after curative gastrectomy: A single-center retrospective study. *Scand. J. Gastroenterol.* **2022**, *57*, 832–841. [CrossRef] [PubMed]
67. Li, H.; Zhou, Y.; Ma, Y.; Han, S.; Zhou, L. The prognostic value of the platelet-to-lymphocyte ratio in acute coronary syndrome: A systematic review and meta-analysis. *Kardiol. Pol.* **2017**, *75*, 666–673. [CrossRef]
68. Gong, S.; Gao, X.; Xu, F.; Shang, Z.; Li, S.; Chen, W.; Yang, J.; Li, J. Association of lymphocyte to monocyte ratio with severity of coronary artery disease. *Medicine* **2018**, *97*, e12813. [CrossRef]
69. Touboul, P.J.; Labreuche, J.; Bruckert, E.; Schargrodsky, H.; Prati, P.; Tosetto, A.; Hernandez-Hernandez, R.; Woo, K.S.; Silva, H.; Vicaut, E.; et al. HDL-C, triglycerides and carotid IMT: A meta-analysis of 21,000 patients with automated edge detection IMT measurement. *Atherosclerosis* **2014**, *232*, 65–71. [CrossRef]
70. Zhang, W.R.; Parikh, C.R. Biomarkers of Acute and Chronic Kidney Disease. *Annu. Rev. Physiol.* **2019**, *81*, 309–333. [CrossRef]
71. Piepoli, M.F.; Hoes, A.W.; Agewall, S.; Albus, C.; Brotons, C.; Catapano, A.L.; Cooney, M.T.; Corra, U.; Cosyns, B.; Deaton, C.; et al. 2016 European Guidelines on cardiovascular disease prevention in clinical practice: The Sixth Joint Task Force of the European Society of Cardiology and Other Societies on Cardiovascular Disease Prevention in Clinical Practice (constituted by representatives of 10 societies and by invited experts) Developed with the special contribution of the European Association for Cardiovascular Prevention & Rehabilitation (EACPR). *Eur. Heart. J.* **2016**, *37*, 2315–2381. [CrossRef]
72. Pang, K.L.; Chin, K.Y. The Biological Activities of Oleocanthal from a Molecular Perspective. *Nutrients* **2018**, *10*, 570. [CrossRef]

73. Perez Banasco, V.; Gil-Cunquero, J.M.; Borrego, F.J.; Grasso, M.; Segura, P.; Warletta, F.; Lozano, J.L.; Costa, L.A.; Torres, J.; Gaforio, J.J.; et al. Preliminary study on efficacy and tolerance of a "coupage" of olive oil in patients with chronic kidney disease. Nutritonal evaluation. *Nefrologia* **2007**, *27*, 472–481.
74. Rondanelli, M.; Talluri, J.; Peroni, G.; Donelli, C.; Guerriero, F.; Ferrini, K.; Riggi, E.; Sauta, E.; Perna, S.; Guido, D. Beyond Body Mass Index. Is the Body Cell Mass Index (BCMI) a useful prognostic factor to describe nutritional, inflammation and muscle mass status in hospitalized elderly?: Body Cell Mass Index links in elderly. *Clin. Nutr.* **2018**, *37*, 934–939. [CrossRef]

nutrients

MDPI

Article

Adherence to Mediterranean Diet and Soluble Klotho Level: The Value of Food Synergy in Aging

Shou-En Wu [1], Ying-Jen Chen [2] and Wei-Liang Chen [3,4,5,*]

1 Department of Dermatology, Tri-Service General Hospital, School of Medicine, National Defense Medical Center, Taipei 11490, Taiwan
2 Department of Ophthalmology, Tri-Service General Hospital, School of Medicine, National Defense Medical Center, Taipei 11490, Taiwan
3 Division of Family Medicine, Department of Family and Community Medicine, Tri-Service General Hospital, School of Medicine, National Defense Medical Center, Taipei 11490, Taiwan
4 Division of Geriatric Medicine, Department of Family and Community Medicine, Tri-Service General Hospital, School of Medicine, National Defense Medical Center, Taipei 11490, Taiwan
5 Department of Biochemistry, National Defense Medical Center, Taipei 11490, Taiwan
* Correspondence: weiliang0508@gmail.com; Tel.: +886-2-8792-3311 (ext. 16567); Fax: +886-2-8792-7057

Abstract: Diets for healthy aging have long been an intriguing issue. The current study makes a head-to-head comparison of four dietary patterns and their associations with soluble Klotho (s-Klotho) levels, an aging-related marker. The dietary data of 7906 subjects were obtained from the National Health and Nutrition Examination Survey 2007–2016. Each participant was given a score or was grouped according to four dietary patterns, namely the Mediterranean adherence diet score (MDS), the low-carbohydrate-diet score, a low-fat diet, and a low-carbohydrate diet. Subsequently, the associations with s-Klotho were examined using linear regression analyses. In addition, we calculated the odds ratio (OR) for aging in different dietary patterns, taking the lowest quartile of s-Klotho as a reference for aging. The MDS was the only dietary pattern that revealed a relationship with s-Klotho levels. The positive association (β coefficient: 9.41, $p < 0.001$) remained significant when dividing the MDS into tertiles (Tertile 2: β coefficient: 36.87, $p < 0.001$; Tertile 3: β coefficient: 45.92, $p < 0.001$) and grouping participants into subsets by sex, age, and BMI. A lower OR for aging was observed in higher MDS groups (Tertile 2: OR = 0.86, $p = 0.026$; Tertile 3: OR = 0.77, $p < 0.001$). However, when analyzed separately, merely three out of nine components of the MDS, namely alcohol consumption (β coefficient: 42.54, $p < 0.001$), fruit (β coefficient: 11.59, $p = 0.029$), and dairy products (β coefficient: 8.55, $p = 0.032$), showed a significant association with s-Klotho. The Mediterranean diet adopts a food-based approach, which has the merit of valuing the complex interactions between foods and their constituents, and further brings benefits to healthy aging.

Keywords: soluble Klotho; Mediterranean diet; low-carbohydrate diet; low-fat diet; aging

1. Introduction

Diet plays a crucial role in determining lifespan. Scientists have worked unceasingly on exploring a life-extending dietary pattern which grants health and wellness. Distinct dietary patterns show strengths in different aspects. For instance, the Mediterranean diet, which highlights monounsaturated fat (mainly virgin and extra-virgin olive oil) and a moderate intake of alcohol [1], has been demonstrated to reduce overall mortality [2], cardiovascular events [3], and the incidence of cancer [4]. Low-carbohydrate and low-fat diets have both been reported to bring positive effects to weight loss and a reduction in cardiovascular events [5,6]. In this research, we are committed to investigating a dietary pattern that brings the most benefits to healthy aging with the use of an anti-aging biomarker, soluble Klotho (s-Klotho) [7]. The Klotho gene and the Klotho protein it encodes have attracted scientists' attention by virtue of the involvement of many pathways in the aging process. It regulates phosphate homeostasis [8], insulin-like growth factor 1 [9], and Wnt signaling pathways [10], while also protecting cells from oxidative stress and cell senescence [11]. s-Klotho is cleaved from the extracellular domain of membrane klotho and enters circulation to exert biological functions. With regard to the association between diet and s-Klotho, the number of studies is small. The main ones were published by the same group of researchers, who enrolled 74 middle-aged sedentary Spanish adults into their studies, revealing an inverse association with alcohol consumption [12], a weak positive association with dietary inflammation index [13], and a negative association in adherence to the Mediterranean diet, which disappeared after controlling for lean mass index [14]. Nevertheless, their studies were limited to small amounts of participants and reflected only certain age groups (45–65 years old).

To the best of our knowledge, this is the first study to make head-to head comparisons of different dietary patterns and aging, represented by the level of s-Klotho. The relatively large number of participants in our study represent the general population of the United States (US), and therefore may provide a more comprehensive view of the interactions between diet and healthy aging.

2. Materials and Methods

2.1. Study Design and Participants

The data of this study were retrieved from the National Health and Nutrition Examination Survey (NHANES) 2007–2016 [15]. The NHANES is a vital program administered by the National Center for Health Statistics (NCHS), which is part of the Centers for Disease Control and Prevention (CDC) that is responsible for the protection of public health and safety in the US. The NHANES continuously collects health and nutritional data of adults and children in the US and releases its dataset in two-year cycles with the aim of providing researchers with representative statistics of the general US population. The NHANES was conducted according to the guidelines of the Declaration of Helsinki, and study protocol was approved by the NCHS Institutional Review Board. It combined in-house interviews and physical examinations at a mobile examination center (MEC), and written informed consent was provided by each participant at the time of household interview.

For the present study, the main research subject, s-Klotho, was available in the NHANES 2007–2016; hence, we focused on dietary datasets from those years. There were 40,617 individuals investigated in years 2007–2016, and 13,765 of them had data of s-Klotho levels. Afterwards, we inspected the data files of dietary recall interviews, and further excluded those with incomplete data (n = 5859). Finally, 7906 subjects were eligible for further analyses. A diagram depicting the design process of our study is provided in Figure 1.

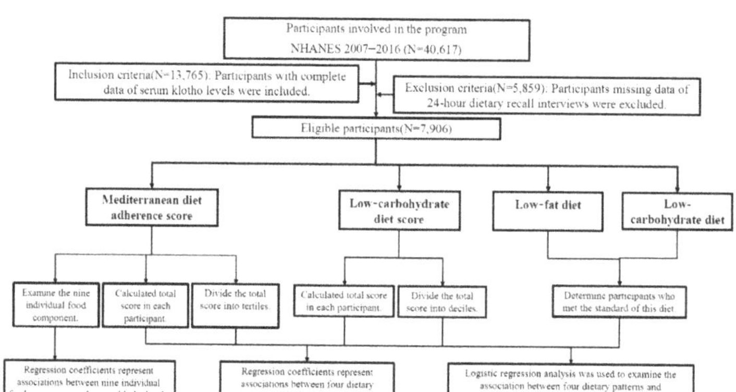

Figure 1. Flow chart of study population selection.

2.2. Dietary Data

The dietary assessment of the NHANES was collected via a 24 h dietary recall method. Since 2002, two rounds of recall were carried out for comprehensive evaluation. Trained interviewers conducted the first dietary recall in-person at the MEC, and the second recall was scheduled 3–10 days later by telephone. This study adopted data from the first round of recall due to the some loss to follow-up in the second round. The dietary recalls in the NHANES were a portion of What We Eat in America, a primary project administered by the Food Surveys Research Group (FSRG), which is a part of the US Department of Agriculture, Agricultural Research Service. Other projects held by the FSRG were used in our study to examine the dietary information of our NHANES participants. The USDA Food and Nutrient Database for Dietary Studies (FNDDS) was used to convert individual food and beverages reported by participants into gram amounts or portion sizes in order to estimate their nutrient values [16]. Another specific database, the Food Patterns Equivalents Database (FPED), integrates individual food in the FNDDS and constructs 37 food and beverage groupings according to the 2015–2020 Dietary Guidelines for Americans recommendations [17]. We utilized FPED 2007–2008, 2009–2010, 2011–2012, 2013–2014, and 2015–2016 [18–22] for the calculation of the Mediterranean diet score.

2.3. Mediterranean Diet Adherence Score

The Mediterranean diet adherence score (MDS) in our study was calculated using a literature-based adherence score proposed by Sofi et al. [23]. It was composed of nine food components, which are fruit, vegetables, legumes, cereals, fish, meat and meat products, dairy products, alcohol, and olive oil. Each component was assigned a score of "0", "1", or "2", and adding up all components gave a final MDS, ranging from 0 to 18. Higher scores reflect a better adherence to the Mediterranean dietary pattern, which are not fully equivalent to a higher intake of each component. For instance, a higher intake of meat and dairy products produces lower scores, while a moderate consumption of alcohol (1–2 alcohol unit/day) generates the highest score, followed by little (<1 alcohol unit/day) and excessive consumption (>2 alcohol unit/day). The categorization of 37 food components in the FPED into the MDS refers to a previous study that conducted a diet investigation in the NHANES 2011–2014 [24]. Some modifications were made to apply the units of measurement in the FPED to the scale constructed by Sofi et al. First, fruit, vegetables, and dairy products were calculated aggregately as cup equivalent (CE) intakes in the FPED. Modified fruit scores were <1 CE/d = "0", ≥1 CE/d = "1", and ≥2 Ces/d = "2"; modified vegetable scores were <0.5 CE/d = "0", ≥0.5 CE/d = "1", and ≥1 CE/d = "2"; and modified dairy product scores were >1.5 Ces/d CE = "0", 1–1.5 Ces/d = "1", and <1.5 Ces/d = "2". Secondly, olive oil was presented in grams in the FPED; therefore, we transformed scores into <14 g/d = "0", ≥14 g/d = "1", and ≥28 g/d Ces/d = "2". Other component scores complied with the original calculation proposed by Sofi et al. For further analysis, we also computed the 1st, 2nd, and 3rd tertile of the total MDS score. Details are shown in Table A1.

2.4. Low-Carbohydrate-Diet Score

The low-carbohydrate-diet (LCD) score was developed previously [25]. In brief, the three macronutrients (carbohydrate, protein, and fat) were calculated as a percentage (%) of total daily energy intake, and further divided into 11 strata. Scores were assigned from "0" to "10" to each stratum, but in a different ordered sequence. In the lowest stratum of intake, protein and fat scored "0", while carbohydrate scored "10". In other words, the scores for protein and fat were ranked in an ascending order according to the percentage of intake, while carbohydrate was ranked in a descending order. Summing up the scores of the three macronutrients gave an overall score ranging from "0" to "30", which was the final LCD score. For further analysis, we also computed the 1st, 5th, and 10th decile of the total LCD score. Details are shown in Table A1.

2.5. Low-Fat Diet and Low-Carbohydrate Diet

The low-fat diet was defined following the American Heart Association Dietary Guidelines [26], which recommended that <30% of total daily calorie intake come from fats. The low-carbohydrate (low-carb) diet in our study adopted the definition from the American Academy of Family Physicians [27], which specified a low-carb diet as containing <20% of total daily calorie intake from carbohydrates. Details are shown in Table A1.

2.6. Measurement of s-Klotho Levels

According to the NHANES Laboratory/Medical Technologists Procedures Manual [28], s-Klotho levels were examined using the IBL ELISA kit (Immuno-Biological Laboratories, Gunma, Japan). Duplicate tests of the sample yielded 3.8% and 3.4% for the inter-assay coefficients of variation. The reference range for s-Klotho was 285.8 to 1638.6 pg/mL.

2.7. Covariates

Self-reported demographic information was obtained in household interviews. The computation of body mass index used the formula: kg/m^2 (weight in kilograms, height in meters squared). A positive smoking history was determined by smoking at least 100 cigarettes in life. The subjects' history of medical conditions, including congestive heart failure, coronary heart disease, angina, diabetes, and hypertension were acquired by asking the participants if they were ever told by doctors or other health professional that they had the aforementioned condition.

2.8. Statistical Analyses

The software used for analysis was SPSS (IBM Corp. Released 2013. IBM SPSS Statistics for Windows, Version 22.0. Armonk, NY, USA: IBM Corp.). Linear regression analyses were used to examine the association, and β coefficients provided an estimate of the strength of the relationship. Odds ratios (ORs) were calculated by logistic regression analyses. In the present study, they evaluated the association between exposure (scoring in different dietary pattern) and outcome (aging, represented by the lowest quartile of s-Klotho levels). In all analyses, results were regarded as significant when p values were less than 0.05. Three adjustment models were provided in each analysis: Model 1 = unadjusted; Model 2 = adjusted for adjusted for age, sex, body mass index, and race/ethnicity; Model 3 = Model 2 + adjusted for history of angina, congestive heart failure, coronary heart disease, diabetes mellitus, hypertension, and smoking status. Model 2 reckoned with the effect of general health conditions, and Model 3 further considered the impact of common aging-related diseases.

3. Results

3.1. Characteristics of Participants

Demographic, laboratory, and dietary information are presented in Table 1. The mean age of the participants was 57.77 ± 10.92 years old. The mean MDS and LCD scores were 6.72 ± 2.12 and 14.98 ± 7.19, respectively. The mean percentage of daily calorie intake from carbohydrates, protein, and fats were 49%, 16%, and 34%, respectively.

Table 1. Characteristics of participants.

Characteristics	Total Participants (n = 7906)
[2] Continuous variables	
Age (years)	57.77 ± 10.92
[1] BMI (kg/m^2)	29.67 ± 6.54
Klotho (pg/mL)	861.17 ± 311.55
Mediterranean diet score	6.72 ± 2.12
Low-carbohydrate diet score	14.98 ± 7.19

Table 1. *Cont.*

Characteristics	Total Participants (n = 7906)
Daily carbohydrate intake (gm)/Percentage of calories from carbohydrate	245.50 ± 116.27 (49%)
Daily protein intake (gm)/Percentage of calories from protein	78.67 ± 39.30 (16%)
Daily fat intake (gm)/Percentage of calories from fat	76.10 ± 43.96 (34%)
Daily calorie intake (kcal)	2020.97 ± 923.62
[3] Categorical variables	
Sex	
Men	3910 (49.5%)
Women	3996 (50.5%)
Race	
Mexican American	1225 (15.5%)
Other Hispanic	855 (10.8%)
Non-Hispanic White	3704 (46.9%)
Non-Hispanic Black	1619 (20.5%)
Other race, including multi-racial	503 (6.4%)
History of congestive heart failure	312 (3.9%)
History of coronary heart disease	392 (5%)
History of angina	254 (3.2%)
History of diabetes mellitus	6705 (84.8%)
History of hypertension	5433 (68.7%)
Smoking history	3987 (50.4%)

[1] BMI: body mass index. [2] Values in the continuous variables were expressed as mean and standard deviation. [3] Values in the categorical variables were expressed in number and percentage (%).

3.2. Associations between Different Dietary Patterns and s-Klotho Levels

We observed a positive association between the MDS and s-Klotho levels, as shown in Table 2. When calculated as a total score, the β coefficient (95% CI) was 9.41 (6.08–12.74), indicating a 9.41 pg/mL rise in s-Klotho levels per 1-score increase in the MDS ($p < 0.001$) in the unadjusted model. The adjusted model also revealed a significant positive correlation (both $p < 0.001$). When calculated as scores divided into tertiles, the higher tertiles revealed a stronger association with s-Klotho levels compared to the lowest tertile (Tertile 2: β coefficient (95% CI) = 36.87(19.17–54.57), $p < 0.001$; Tertile 3: β coefficient (95% CI) = 45.92 (28.01–63.83), $p < 0.001$). By comparison, the other three dietary patterns did not reveal a significant relationship with s-Klotho levels.

3.3. Association between Different Dietary Patterns and Aging

s-Klotho levels were demonstrated to be inversely associated with age in previous studies [29,30]. Accordingly, we reason that the lowest quartile of s-Klotho levels correlates with a higher likelihood of aging. As shown in Table 3, logistic regression analyses were used to calculate the ORs for aging (represented by quartile 1 of s-Klotho) in different dietary scores. In the MDS and the LCD score, the reference groups were the lowest tertile and decile, while in the low-fat diet and the low-carb diet, ORs were compared to those who did not meet the standards mentioned in the previous section. The results of the MDS revealed that ORs gradually decreased from tertile 2 to 3, and both were less than 1, indicating protective effects from aging in higher MDS groups (Tertile 2 of MDS: OR = 0.86, $p = 0.026$; Tertile 3 of MDS: OR = 0.77, $p < 0.001$ compared to Tertile 1). The other three dietary patterns did not disclose significant results.

Table 2. Linear regression analyses for the associations between different dietary patterns and serum klotho levels.

		[1] MDS				[2] LCD Score					
		Total Score	Tertile			Total Score	Decile			Low-Fat Diet	[3] Low-Carb Diet
			1	2	3		1	5	10		
Model 1	β coefficient (95% CI)	9.41 (6.08, 12.74)	Ref.	36.87 (19.17, 54.57)	45.92 (28.01, 63.83)	−0.366 (−1.355, 0.623)	Ref.	1.45 (−19.82, 22.72)	−6.32 (−28.30, 15.67)	−2.16 (−16.97, 12.66)	−96.08 (−202.49, 10.32)
	p value	<0.001	Ref.	<0.001	<0.001	0.468	Ref.	0.894	0.573	0.775	0.077
Model 2	β coefficient (95% CI)	9.62 (6.29, 12.95)	Ref.	37.38 (19.76, 55.01)	46.79 (28.87, 64.72)	−0.116 (−1.106, 0.873)	Ref.	5.24 (−15.91, 26.40)	−1.16 (−14.58, 31.66)	−2.58 (−17.37, 12.21)	−95.37 (−201.14, 10.39)
	p value	<0.001	Ref.	<0.001	<0.001	0.818	Ref.	0.627	0.917	0.732	0.077
Model 3	β coefficient (95% CI)	9.01 (5.67, 12.34)	Ref.	35.92 (18.33, 53.51)	43.42 (25.50, 61.34)	−0.200 (−1.188, 0.788)	Ref.	3.76 (−17.34, 24.85)	−2.56 (−24.48, 19.35)	−1.80 (−16.56, 12.97)	−103.54 (−208.98, 1.89)
	p value	<0.001	Ref.	<0.001	<0.001	0.691	Ref.	0.727	0.819	0.811	0.054

[1] MDS: Mediterranean diet adherence score; [2] LCD score: low-carbohydrate-diet score; [3] Low-carb diet: low-carbohydrate diet. Model 1 = unadjusted. Model 2 = adjusted for age, sex, body mass index, and race/ethnicity. Model 3 = Model 2 + adjusted for history of angina, congestive heart failure, coronary heart disease, diabetes mellitus, hypertension, and smoking history.

Table 3. Odds ratios (95% confidence intervals) for lowest quartile of serum Klotho levels (represents aging) in various dietary patterns.

		[1] MDS			[2] LCD Score				
		Tertile			Decile			Low-Fat Diet	[3] Low-Carb Diet
		1	2	3	1	5	10		
Model 1	OR (95% CI)	Ref.	0.86 (0.76, 0.98)	0.77 (0.68, 0.88)	Ref.	0.97 (0.83, 1.13)	0.96 (0.82, 1.13)	1.01 (0.91, 1.13)	1.50 (0.73, 3.11)
	p value	Ref.	0.026	<0.001	Ref.	0.653	0.648	0.867	0.271
Model 2	OR (95% CI)	Ref.	0.85 (0.75, 0.97)	0.76 (0.66, 0.86)	Ref.	0.95 (0.81, 1.11)	0.94 (0.80, 1.11)	1.01 (0.91, 1.13)	1.52 (0.73, 3.15)
	p value	Ref.	0.017	<0.001	Ref.	0.512	0.478	0.929	0.260
Model 3	OR (95% CI)	Ref.	0.86 (0.75, 0.98)	0.77 (0.67, 0.88)	Ref.	0.96 (0.82, 1.12)	0.95 (0.81, 1.12)	1.01 (0.89, 1.12)	1.58 (0.76, 3.29)
	p value	Ref.	0.024	<0.001	Ref.	0.956	0.949	0.933	0.217

[1] MDS: Mediterranean diet adherence score; [2] LCD score: low-carbohydrate-diet score; [3] Low-carb diet: low-carbohydrate diet. Model 1 = unadjusted. Model 2 = adjusted for age, sex, body mass index, and race/ethnicity. Model 3 = Model 2 + adjusted for history of angina, congestive heart failure, coronary heart disease, diabetes mellitus, hypertension, and smoking history.

3.4. Associations across Tertiles of MDS and s-Klotho Levels in Subgroups

Owing to the significant relationship revealed in the MDS, either calculated as the total score or in tertiles, we were interested in whether the correlation was still present in specific groups. In Table 4, we sorted participants by sex, age, and BMI and examined the relationship by linear regression analyses. In men, the β coefficients were higher in tertile 3 (β coefficient: 43.48, 95% CI = 20.39–66.56, $p < 0.001$) than tertile 2 (β coefficient: 26.62, 95% CI = 4.18–49.05, $p = 0.020$). Meanwhile, in women, the β coefficients were of a similar value in tertile 2 (β coefficient: 41.01, 95% CI = 13.34–68.69, $p = 0.004$) and 3 (β coefficient: 40.28, 95% CI = 12.63–67.94, $p = 0.004$). In addition, a stronger relationship with s-Klotho (presented as a higher β coefficient value) appeared in women compared to men. When sorted by age, older adults (≥ 65 years old) revealed a stronger relationship with s-Klotho. In the unadjusted model, the younger group had a β coefficient = 33.44 and 48.38 in tertile 2 and 3, respectively, while the older group had a β coefficient = 55.30 and 55.75 in tertile 2 and 3, respectively. When sorted by BMI, participants with a greater BMI (≥30) presented a stronger relationship with s-Klotho. In the unadjusted model, participants with a lower BMI had a β coefficient = 29.98 and 40.56 in tertile 2 and 3, respectively, while the older group had a β coefficient = 46.82 and 53.69 in tertile 2 and 3, respectively. It is noteworthy that all subgroups revealed statistically significant results.

Table 4. Associations across tertiles of Mediterranean diet score and serum Klotho levels in subgroups.

		Tertile 1 of [1] MDS	Tertile 2 of MDS	Tertile 3 of MDS
		Sorted by sex		
		Men		
Model 1	β coefficient (95% CI)	Ref.	26.62 (4.18, 49.05)	43.48 (20.39, 66.56)
	p value	Ref.	0.020	<0.001
Model 2	β coefficient (95% CI)	Ref.	29.73 (7.34, 52.13)	49.59 (26.45, 72.73)
	p value	Ref.	0.009	<0.001
Model 3	β coefficient (95% CI)	Ref.	27.81 (5.47, 50.16)	45.31 (22.16, 68.47)
	p value	Ref.	0.015	<0.001
		Women		
Model 1	β coefficient (95% CI)	Ref.	41.01 (13.34, 68.69)	40.28 (12.63, 67.94)
	p value	Ref.	0.004	0.004
Model 2	β coefficient (95% CI)	Ref.	45.34 (17.79, 72.89)	45.01 (17.43, 72.59)
	p value	Ref.	0.001	0.001
Model 3	β coefficient (95% CI)	Ref.	43.22 (15.75, 70.69)	41.23 (13.67, 68.79)
	p value	Ref.	0.002	0.003
		Sorted by age		
		<65 years old		
Model 1	β coefficient (95% CI)	Ref.	33.44 (12.83, 54.05)	48.38 (27.29, 69.48)
	p value	Ref.	0.001	<0.001
Model 2	β coefficient (95% CI)	Ref.	31.58 (11.01, 52.15)	45.22 (24.09, 66.35)
	p value	Ref.	0.003	<0.001
Model 3	β coefficient (95% CI)	Ref.	30.59 (10.09, 51.09)	40.19 (19.07, 61.32)
	p value	Ref.	0.003	<0.001

Table 4. *Cont.*

		Tertile 1 of [1] MDS	Tertile 2 of MDS	Tertile 3 of MDS
		≥65 years old		
Model 1	β coefficient (95% CI)	Ref.	55.30 (20.99, 89.62)	55.75 (21.85, 89.65)
	p value	Ref.	0.002	0.001
Model 2	β coefficient (95% CI)	Ref.	53.87 (19.54, 88.21)	52.40 (18.43, 86.38)
	p value	Ref.	0.002	0.003
Model 3	β coefficient (95% CI)	Ref.	51.03 (16.68, 85.38)	49.61 (15.54, 83.68)
	p value	Ref.	0.004	0.004
		Sorted by BMI		
		BMI < 30		
Model 1	β coefficient (95% CI)	Ref.	29.98 (6.66, 53.32)	40.56 (16.93, 64.19)
	p value	Ref.	0.012	0.001
Model 2	β coefficient (95% CI)	Ref.	31.09 (7.86, 54.31)	40.98 (17.31, 64.66)
	p value	Ref.	0.009	0.001
Model 3	β coefficient (95% CI)	Ref.	27.93 (4.74, 51.11)	36.67 (12.97, 60.38)
	p value	Ref.	0.018	0.002
		BMI ≥ 30		
Model 1	β coefficient (95% CI)	Ref.	46.82 (19.67, 73.97)	53.69 (26.25, 81.13)
	p value	Ref.	0.001	<0.001
Model 2	β coefficient (95% CI)	Ref.	45.52 (18.42, 72.61)	54.14 (26.68, 81.59)
	p value	Ref.	0.001	<0.001
Model 3	β coefficient (95% CI)	Ref.	46.29 (19.27, 73.31)	51.86 (24.46, 79.26)
	p value	Ref.	0.001	<0.001

[1] MDS: Mediterranean diet adherence score. Model 1 = unadjusted. Model 2 = adjusted for age, sex, body mass index, and race/ethnicity. Model 3 = Model 2 + adjusted for history of angina, congestive heart failure, coronary heart disease, diabetes mellitus, hypertension, and smoking history.

3.5. Associations between Nine Individual Food Components of MDS and s-Klotho Levels

We further investigated in nine individual food components of the MDS to examine which ones showed a significant association with s-Klotho. Figure 2 presents a forest plot of the β coefficient, which discloses the degree of change in s-Klotho levels for each 1-score increase in individual components. Among the nine, only three components revealed significant results. The most notable one was alcohol consumption, with a β coefficient of 42.54 (95% CI = 32.09–52.99, $p < 0.001$). The other two were fruit (β coefficient: 11.59, 95% CI = 1.21–21.97, $p = 0.029$) and dairy products (β coefficient: 8.55, 95% CI = 0.73–16.37, $p = 0.032$).

Owing to the result that most components did not reveal a significant relationship with s-Klotho when viewed separately, we calculated the change of mean s-Klotho levels in the total MDS, as shown in Figure 3. We combined the extreme maximum and minimum scores due to the scant number in these groups (scores 0 and 1 combined into ≤1, and scores 12–18 combined into ≥12). A steady upward trend can be observed from the lowest to the highest MDS group ($p < 0.001$), demonstrating that the positive association between the MDS and s-Klotho levels is revealed only when viewed as a whole.

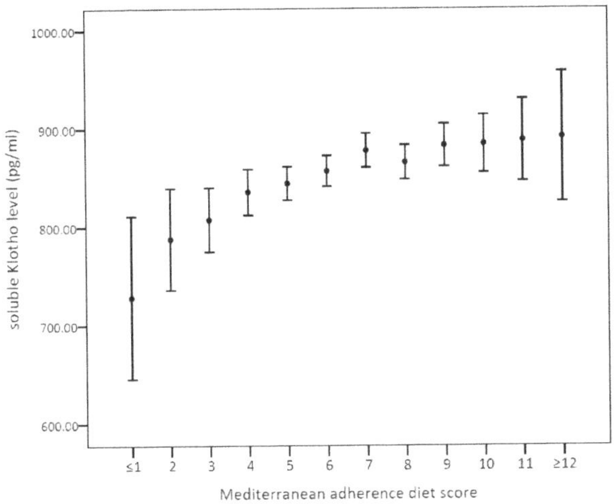

Figure 2. A line chart showing the change of mean s-Klotho levels in Mediterranean diet adherence score from the lowest (score ≤ 1) to the highest (score ≥ 12).

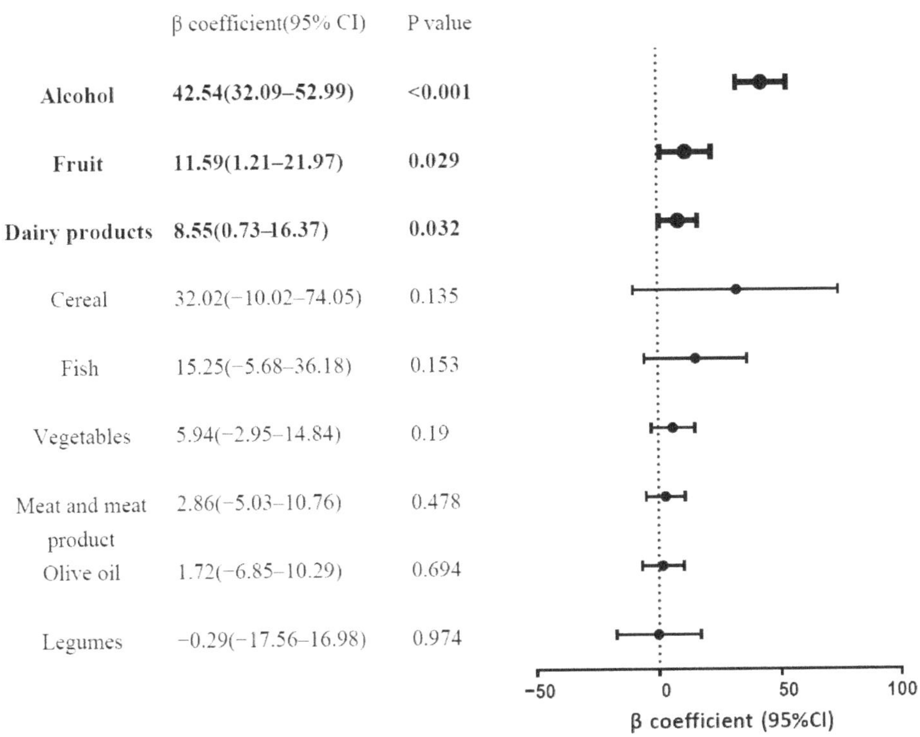

Figure 3. Forest plot of β coefficients presenting the association between nine components in the Mediterranean diet adherence score and s-Klotho levels as outcome. The β coefficient discloses the degree of change in s-Klotho levels for each 1-score increase in an individual component. Components that revealed significant associations are highlighted in bold.

4. Discussion

The current study highlights the positive association between the MDS and s-Klotho levels, and the association remains significant in all subgroups, including men and women, the young and the old, and the obese and the non-obese. In addition, on the assumption that the lowest quartile of s-Klotho correlates to aging, a higher MDS indicates protective effects against aging. On the other hand, the other three dietary pattern of interest, namely the LCD, low-fat diet, and low-carb diet failed to show any association with s-Klotho or aging.

The Mediterranean diet and healthy aging have been widely discussed in the literature. The first direct evidence regarding lifespan was demonstrated in a study collected in Greek villages, showing a one-unit increase in diet score related to a 17% reduction in overall mortality [31]. Subsequently, studies conducted outside the Mediterranean region, where people generally followed the spirit of the Mediterranean diet but did not rigorously follow the traditional version, also revealed a significantly lower mortality risk [32,33]. Mechanisms that have been validated as a contribution to its protective property include its antioxidant and anti-inflammatory capacity [34], lipid-lowering effects [35], and improvement in insulin sensitivity [36].

Evidence for the relationship between carbohydrates and lifespan is conflicting in humans. A low-carbohydrate diet is reported to bring benefits to weight loss [5], coronary heart disease [37], and diabetes mellitus [38], but several studies showed increased mortality in adults consuming low-carbohydrate–high-protein diets [39,40]. One study, however, showed no clear association with mortality [41]. Other studies in different organisms targeting carbohydrates and lifespan revealed varied results. In *C. elegans*, the restriction of glucose availability was proved to extend lifespan [42]. On the contrary, strategies of increasing the carbohydrate-to-protein ratio were demonstrated to maximize life expectancy in Drosophila [43] and mice [44]. With regard to dietary lipids, a low-fat diet contributes to weight loss [45], but recent evidence points out the importance of collaboratively controlling glycemic load [46] and total calorie intake [47]. In addition, specific lipids induce heterogeneous effects. For instance, a polyunsaturated fatty acid-supplemented diet extends the lifespan in *C. elegans* [48] but shortens the lifespan in mice [49]. Researchers have proposed the possibility that fatty acid compositions on cellular membranes are essential factors in the determination of longevity [50] rather than dietary lipids. Our study, however, found no significant association with s-Klotho levels in either the LCD or low-carb diet or low-fat diet. Discordant results may be attributed to the complex cellular mechanisms linking diet and aging, and centering on a portion of a single macronutrient could not draw solid conclusions.

The findings of the association between individual food components of the MDS and s-Klotho levels echo previous studies investigating the association with all-cause mortality. A meta-analysis that summarized the results from 16 Mediterranean diet studies, with respect to longevity, reported that the excess relative risk was the highest for moderate alcohol intake (−14%), followed by fruit (−12%) [51]. The summary relative risk (RR) in association with all-cause mortality also revealed that the most notable inverse association was with alcohol intake (RR = 0.86) and fruit (RR = 0.88). By contrast, other components revealed minimal association (RR ranged from 0.94–1.07), or even null association, for legumes (RR = 1.00) and fish intake (RR = 1.01). Another review article compared the potential benefits of the Mediterranean diet or its components toward cardiovascular disease [52]. They concluded that, despite each component yielding protective effects to a certain extent, none of them proved to be as beneficial as the whole Mediterranean diet for the primary and secondary prevention of cardiovascular disease. Our study, although with a different research outcome, revealed consistent findings with merely three components presenting significant associations. The favorable impacts brought by the Mediterranean diet can be well explained by the concept of "food synergy", which emphasizes the stronger health benefits lying in a total diet rather than individual foods or food constituents [53,54]. Several advantages have been proposed. A synergetic dietary pattern serves a buffer effect in which each constituent is balanced, rather than an excessive intake of a single one. Furthermore, the physical and chemical interactions between various foods and with the body system, which is specifically termed "the food matrix", are essential in overall health [55].

The concept of food synergy not only delineates the findings that the Mediterranean diet is more powerful as a whole, but also illustrates the results that the Mediterranean diet is the only diet in our study that correlates with s-Klotho levels. The feature that distinguishes the Mediterranean diet from the other three is that it is a food-based approach rather than a nutrient-based approach, which has been proposed to be a fundamental strategy that gives the full picture of the complex metabolic interrelations between foods. Scientists argue that, despite the fact that identifying single food or nutrient provides a better understanding in several cases, a comprehensive knowledge of food and its relationship with general health should be underpinned by an integrated model, the "whole food-oriented research" [56] or "nutritional geometry" [57]. The Mediterranean diet, being a pyramid-shaped eating pattern that comprises a large base of plant foods, a middle layer of fish, poultry, and dairy products, and an apex of red meat products and sweets, has the merit of stressing the assembly of foods and an adequate amount of each. In comparison to other macronutrient-based diets, it provides a blended diet that values the constituents and nutrients of each food, whether abundant or scarce, playing a vital role in the multidimensional framework of nutrition. This accounts for the main reason why the Mediterranean diet shows significant results in all analyses.

Another issue that deserves attention is how the 'type' and 'amount' of alcohol have an influence on Klotho and ageing. In the Mediterranean diet, the overall intake is more emphasized, with studies supporting the notion that controlling the amount, irrespective of the beverage source, brings protective effects [58,59]. However, there is evidence illustrating that red wine may somehow show a more potent capability of cardiovascular protection [60,61]. Others have argued that this phenomenon can observed in countries that habitually consume wine rather than other alcoholic beverages, terming it the 'French paradox' [62,63]. To date, these observational results remain an issue for debate. From the present study, we can only tell that consuming alcohol in moderation correlates with higher s-Klotho levels, but a conclusion regarding the differences between types of alcohol cannot be drawn due to a lack of corresponding data.

Some limitations in the present study should be acknowledged. First, some modifications were made to the calculation of the MDS due to different units of measurements in the original version of the MDS by Sofi et al. [23] and the accessible dietary data in the NHANES. One previous NHANES study on the Mediterranean diet [24] encountered the same predicament, and we referred to their conversion methods in the hopes of minimizing the statistical error. Secondly, causal inference in cross-sectional studies, e.g., the NHANES, is hard to approach. Associations could be observed between exposures and outcomes, but the direction of cause and effect within is difficult to determine in practice. Further research is needed to verify the underlying cause of the association.

5. Conclusions

In the present study, the MDS revealed a positive association with s-Klotho levels, an anti-aging biomarker, while the other three dietary patterns, namely the LCD, low-fat diet, and low-carb diet showed null association. The association remained significant when participants were grouped into subsets by sex, age, and BMI. In addition, the association disappeared in six out of nine components in the MDS when viewed separately. The Mediterranean diet differs from the other three by offering a combination of foods instead of stressing the individual macronutrients, which embodies the spirit of "food synergy" that values the complex interactions between food and its constituents. Future studies are warranted to investigate how diets influence s-Klotho levels and other aging-related biomarkers.

Author Contributions: Conceptualization, S.-E.W. and W.-L.C.; methodology, W.-L.C.; software, Y.-J.C. and W.-L.C.; validation, S.-E.W. and W.-L.C.; formal analysis, S.-E.W. and W.-L.C.; investigation, S.-E.W. and W.-L.C.; resources, Y.-J.C. and W.-L.C.; data curation, S.-E.W. and W.-L.C.; writing—original draft preparation, S.-E.W.; writing—review and editing, S.-E.W. and W.-L.C.; visualization, S.-E.W. and W.-L.C.; supervision, W.-L.C. All authors have read and agreed to the published version of the manuscript.

Funding: This research received no external funding.

Institutional Review Board Statement: Data of this study was retrieved from the National Health and Nutrition Examination Survey (NHANES) 2007–2016. NHANES was conducted according to the guidelines of Declaration of Helsinki, and study protocol was approved by the NCHS Institutional Review Board (Continuation of Protocol #2005-06, Continuation of Protocol #2005-06, and Protocol #2011-17). It combines in-house interviews and physical examinations at mobile examination center (MEC), and written informed consents are provided by each participant at the time of household interview.

Informed Consent Statement: The National Health and Nutrition Examination Survey (NHANES) is a publicly available data set and all participants in the NHANES provide written informed consent, consistent with approval from the National Center for Health Statistics Research Ethics Review Board (NCHS ERB).

Data Availability Statement: The datasets generated and analyzed during the current study are publicly available from the NHANES website. (https://wwwn.cdc.gov/nchs/nhanes/nhanes3/default.aspx, accessed on 12 July 2022).

Conflicts of Interest: The authors declare no conflict of interest.

Appendix A

Table A1. The definition and calculation method of four dietary patterns in the present study.

	Mediterranean Adherence Diet Score (MDS)				Low-Carbohydrate-Diet Score (LCD)			Low-Fat Diet	Low-Carbohydrate Diet
Definition	A score ranging from 0–18 by adding up nine components. Each component is assigned a score of "0", "1", or "2" according to the amount of intake.				A score ranging from 0–30 by adding up individual scores of three macronutrients, carbohydrate, protein, and fat. Each macronutrient was calculated as a percentage (%) of total daily energy intake, and further divided into 11 strata.			<30% of total daily calorie intake from fat	<20% of total daily calorie intake from carbohydrate
Calculation method	Scores	0	1	2	Scores	Carbohydrate	Protein/Fat		
	Fruit	<1 CE/d	≥1 CE/d	≥2 CE/d	0	11th stratum	1st stratum		
	Vegetables 1 portion = 70 g = 2.5 oz	<0.5 CE/d	≥0.5 CE/d	≥1 CE/d	1	10th stratum	2nd stratum		
	Cereals 1 portion = 130 g = 4.6 oz	<4.6 oz/d	4.6–6.9 oz/d	>6.9 oz/d	2	9th stratum	3rd stratum		
	Fish 1 portion = 100 g = 3.5 oz	<3.5 oz/wk	3.5–8.75 oz/wk	>8.75 oz/wk	3	8th stratum	4th stratum		
	Meat product 1 portion = 80 g = 2.8 oz	>4.2 oz/d	2.8–4.2 oz/d	<2.8 oz/d	4	7th stratum	5th stratum		
	Dairy products	>1.5 CE/d	1–1.5 CE/d	<1 CE/d	5	6th stratum	6th stratum		
	Alcohol (mL/day) 1 AU = 12 g	>2 AU/d	<1 AU/d	1–2 AU/d	6	5th stratum	7th stratum		
	Olive oil (gm)	<14 g/d	≥14 g/d	≥28 g/d	7	4th stratum	8th stratum		
	CE = cup equivalent intakes; d = day; wk = week; gm = gram; mL = milliliter; oz = ounce				8	3rd stratum	9th stratum		
					9	2nd stratum	10th stratum		
					10	1st stratum	11th stratum		
References	Previous literature by Sofi et al. [23]				Previous literature by Halton et al. [25]			American Heart Association Dietary Guidelines [5]	American Academy of Family Physicians [26]

References

1. Capurso, C.; Bellanti, F.; Lo Buglio, A.; Vendemiale, G. The Mediterranean Diet Slows Down the Progression of Aging and Helps to Prevent the Onset of Frailty: A Narrative Review. *Nutrients* **2019**, *12*, 35. [CrossRef] [PubMed]
2. Soltani, S.; Jayedi, A.; Shab-Bidar, S.; Becerra-Tomás, N.; Salas-Salvadó, J. Adherence to the Mediterranean Diet in Relation to All-Cause Mortality: A Systematic Review and Dose-Response Meta-Analysis of Prospective Cohort Studies. *Adv. Nutr.* **2019**, *10*, 1029–1039. [CrossRef]
3. Tang, C.; Wang, X.; Qin, L.Q.; Dong, J.Y. Mediterranean Diet and Mortality in People with Cardiovascular Disease: A Meta Analysis of Prospective Cohort Studies. *Nutrients* **2021**, *13*, 2623. [CrossRef]
4. Morze, J.; Danielewicz, A.; Przybyłowicz, K.; Zeng, H.; Hoffmann, G.; Schwingshackl, L. An updated systematic review and meta-analysis on adherence to mediterranean diet and risk of cancer. *Eur. J. Nutr.* **2021**, *60*, 1561–1586. [CrossRef] [PubMed]
5. Chawla, S.; Tessarolo Silva, F.; Amaral Medeiros, S.; Mekary, R.A.; Radenkovic, D. The Effect of Low-Fat and Low-Carbohydrate Diets on Weight Loss and Lipid Levels: A Systematic Review and Meta-Analysis. *Nutrients* **2020**, *12*, 3774. [CrossRef] [PubMed]
6. Shan, Z.; Guo, Y.; Hu, F.B.; Liu, L.; Qi, Q. Association of Low-Carbohydrate and Low-Fat Diets With Mortality Among US Adults *JAMA Intern. Med.* **2020**, *180*, 513–523. [CrossRef] [PubMed]
7. Xiao, N.M.; Zhang, Y.M.; Zheng, Q.; Gu, J. Klotho is a serum factor related to human aging. *Chin. Med. J.* **2004**, *117*, 742–747.
8. Fernández-Fernández, B.; Valiño-Rivas, L.; Sánchez-Niño, M.D.; Ortiz, A. Albuminuria Downregulation of the Anti-Aging Factor Klotho: The Missing Link Potentially Explaining the Association of Pathological Albuminuria with Premature Death. *Adv. Ther.* **2020**, *37*, 62–72. [CrossRef]
9. Olejnik, A.; Franczak, A.; Krzywonos-Zawadzka, A.; Kałużna-Oleksy, M.; Bil-Lula, I. The Biological Role of Klotho Protein in the Development of Cardiovascular Diseases. *BioMed Res. Int.* **2018**, *2018*, 5171945. [CrossRef]
10. Saar-Kovrov, V.; Donners, M.; van der Vorst, E.P.C. Shedding of Klotho: Functional Implications in Chronic Kidney Disease and Associated Vascular Disease. *Front. Cardiovasc. Med.* **2020**, *7*, 617842. [CrossRef]
11. Daneshgar, N.; Dai, D.F. ROS, Klotho and mTOR in cardiorenal aging. *Aging* **2020**, *12*, 19830–19831. [CrossRef] [PubMed]
12. Jurado-Fasoli, L.; Amaro-Gahete, F.J.; De-la, O.A.; Gutiérrez, Á.; Castillo, M.J. Alcohol consumption and S-Klotho plasma levels in sedentary healthy middle-aged adults: A cross sectional study. *Drug Alcohol Depend.* **2019**, *194*, 107–111. [CrossRef] [PubMed]
13. Jurado-Fasoli, L.; Castillo, M.J.; Amaro-Gahete, F.J. Dietary Inflammatory Index and S-Klotho Plasma Levels in Middle-Aged Adults. *Nutrients* **2020**, *12*, 281. [CrossRef]
14. Jurado-Fasoli, L.; Amaro-Gahete, F.J.; De-la, O.A.; Martinez-Tellez, B.; Ruiz, J.R.; Gutiérrez, Á.; Castillo, M.J. Adherence to the Mediterranean diet, dietary factors, and S-Klotho plasma levels in sedentary middle-aged adults. *Exp. Gerontol.* **2019**, *119*, 25–32. [CrossRef]
15. Centers for Disease Control and Prevention, National Center for Health Statistics. National Health and Nutrition Examination Survey. Available online: http://www.cdc.gov/nchs/nhanes/about_nhanes (accessed on 12 July 2022).
16. Beltsville, M.A.R.S.; Food Surveys Research Group. USDA Food and Nutrient Database for Dietary Studies. Available online: https://www.ars.usda.gov/northeast-area/beltsville-md-bhnrc/beltsville-human-nutrition-research-center/food-surveys-research-group/docs/fndds/ (accessed on 12 July 2022).
17. DeSalvo, K.B.; Olson, R.; Casavale, K.O. Dietary guidelines for Americans. *JAMA* **2016**, *315*, 457–458. [CrossRef]
18. Bowman, S.; Clemens, J.; Friday, J.; Thoerig, R.; Shimizu, M.; Barrows, B.; Moshfegh, A. *Food Patterns Equivalents Database 2007–2008: Methodology and User Guide*; US Department of Agriculture, Agricultural Research Service: Beltsville, MD, USA, 2013.
19. Bowman, S.; Clemens, J.; Thoerig, R.; Friday, J.; Shimizu, M.; Moshfegh, A. Food Patterns Equivalents Database 2009–2010: Methodology and User Guide. US Department of Agriculture, Agricultural Research Service, Beltsville Human Nutrition Research Center. Available online: http://www.ars.usda.gov/ba/bhnrc/fsrg (accessed on 12 July 2022).
20. Bowman, S.; Clemens, J.; Friday, J.; Thoerig, R.; Moshfegh, J. *Food Patterns Equivalents Database 2011–2012: Methodology and User Guide. Food Surveys Research Group, Beltsville Human Nutrition Research Center*; Agricultural Research Service, US Department of Agriculture: Beltsville, MD, USA, 2014.
21. Bowman, S.; Clemens, J.; Friday, J.; Lynch, K.; Moshfegh, A. *Food Patterns Equivalents Database 2013–2014: Methodology and User Guide*; Food Surveys Research Group: Beltsville, MD, USA, 2017.
22. Bowman, S.; Clemens, J.; Shimizu, M.; Friday, J.; Moshfegh, A. *Food Patterns Equivalents Database 2015–2016: Methodology and User Guide*; US Department of Agriculture: Beltsville, MD, USA, 2018.
23. Sofi, F.; Macchi, C.; Abbate, R.; Gensini, G.F.; Casini, A. Mediterranean diet and health status: An updated meta-analysis and a proposal for a literature-based adherence score. *Public Health Nutr.* **2014**, *17*, 2769–2782. [CrossRef]
24. Taylor, M.K.; Mahnken, J.D.; Sullivan, D.K. NHANES 2011-2014 Reveals Cognition of US Older Adults may Benefit from Better Adaptation to the Mediterranean Diet. *Nutrients* **2020**, *12*, 1929. [CrossRef]
25. Halton, T.L.; Willett, W.C.; Liu, S.; Manson, J.E.; Albert, C.M.; Rexrode, K.; Hu, F.B. Low-carbohydrate-diet score and the risk of coronary heart disease in women. *N. Engl. J. Med.* **2006**, *355*, 1991–2002. [CrossRef]
26. Krauss, R.M.; Eckel, R.H.; Howard, B.; Appel, L.J.; Daniels, S.R.; Deckelbaum, R.J.; Erdman, J.W., Jr.; Kris-Etherton, P.; Goldberg, I.J.; Kotchen, T.A.; et al. AHA Dietary Guidelines: Revision 2000: A statement for healthcare professionals from the Nutrition Committee of the American Heart Association. *Circulation* **2000**, *102*, 2284–2299. [CrossRef]
27. Last, A.R.; Wilson, S.A. Low-carbohydrate diets. *Am. Fam. Physician* **2006**, *73*, 1942–1948.

28. Centers for Disease Control and Prevention, National Center for Health Statistics. National Health and Nutrition Examination Survey. Laboratory Procedures Manual. 2011. Available online: https://www.cdc.gov/nchs/data/nhanes/nhanes_11_12/2011-12_laboratory_procedures_manual.pdf (accessed on 12 July 2022).
29. Yamazaki, Y.; Imura, A.; Urakawa, I.; Shimada, T.; Murakami, J.; Aono, Y.; Hasegawa, H.; Yamashita, T.; Nakatani, K.; Saito, Y.; et al. Establishment of sandwich ELISA for soluble alpha-Klotho measurement: Age-dependent change of soluble alpha-Klotho levels in healthy subjects. *Biochem. Biophys. Res. Commun.* **2010**, *398*, 513–518. [CrossRef] [PubMed]
30. Pedersen, L.; Pedersen, S.M.; Brasen, C.L.; Rasmussen, L.M. Soluble serum Klotho levels in healthy subjects. Comparison of two different immunoassays. *Clin. Biochem.* **2013**, *46*, 1079–1083. [CrossRef] [PubMed]
31. Trichopoulou, A.; Kouris-Blazos, A.; Wahlqvist, M.L.; Gnardellis, C.; Lagiou, P.; Polychronopoulos, E.; Vassilakou, T.; Lipworth, L.; Trichopoulos, D. Diet and overall survival in elderly people. *BMJ* **1995**, *311*, 1457–1460. [CrossRef] [PubMed]
32. Fung, T.T.; Rexrode, K.M.; Mantzoros, C.S.; Manson, J.E.; Willett, W.C.; Hu, F.B. Mediterranean diet and incidence of and mortality from coronary heart disease and stroke in women. *Circulation* **2009**, *119*, 1093–1100. [CrossRef] [PubMed]
33. Knoops, K.T.; de Groot, L.C.; Kromhout, D.; Perrin, A.E.; Moreiras-Varela, O.; Menotti, A.; van Staveren, W.A. Mediterranean diet, lifestyle factors, and 10-year mortality in elderly European men and women: The HALE project. *JAMA* **2004**, *292*, 1433–1439. [CrossRef] [PubMed]
34. Billingsley, H.E.; Carbone, S. The antioxidant potential of the Mediterranean diet in patients at high cardiovascular risk: An in-depth review of the PREDIMED. *Nutr. Diabetes* **2018**, *8*, 13. [CrossRef]
35. Formisano, E.; Pasta, A.; Cremonini, A.L.; Di Lorenzo, I.; Sukkar, S.G.; Pisciotta, L. Effects of a Mediterranean Diet, Dairy, and Meat Products on Different Phenotypes of Dyslipidemia: A Preliminary Retrospective Analysis. *Nutrients* **2021**, *13*, 1161. [CrossRef]
36. Mirabelli, M.; Chiefari, E.; Arcidiacono, B.; Corigliano, D.M.; Brunetti, F.S.; Maggisano, V.; Russo, D.; Foti, D.P.; Brunetti, A. Mediterranean Diet Nutrients to Turn the Tide against Insulin Resistance and Related Diseases. *Nutrients* **2020**, *12*, 1066. [CrossRef]
37. Jimenez-Torres, J.; Alcalá-Diaz, J.F.; Torres-Peña, J.D.; Gutierrez-Mariscal, F.M.; Leon-Acuña, A.; Gómez-Luna, P.; Fernández-Gandara, C.; Quintana-Navarro, G.M.; Fernandez-Garcia, J.C.; Perez-Martinez, P.; et al. Mediterranean Diet Reduces Atherosclerosis Progression in Coronary Heart Disease: An Analysis of the CORDIOPREV Randomized Controlled Trial. *Stroke* **2021**, *52*, 3440–3449. [CrossRef]
38. Milenkovic, T.; Bozhinovska, N.; Macut, D.; Bjekic-Macut, J.; Rahelic, D.; Velija Asimi, Z.; Burekovic, A. Mediterranean Diet and Type 2 Diabetes Mellitus: A Perpetual Inspiration for the Scientific World. A Review. *Nutrients* **2021**, *13*, 1307. [CrossRef]
39. Lagiou, P.; Sandin, S.; Weiderpass, E.; Lagiou, A.; Mucci, L.; Trichopoulos, D.; Adami, H.O. Low carbohydrate-high protein diet and mortality in a cohort of Swedish women. *J. Intern. Med.* **2007**, *261*, 366–374. [CrossRef]
40. Trichopoulou, A.; Psaltopoulou, T.; Orfanos, P.; Hsieh, C.C.; Trichopoulos, D. Low-carbohydrate-high-protein diet and long-term survival in a general population cohort. *Eur. J. Clin. Nutr.* **2007**, *61*, 575–581. [CrossRef] [PubMed]
41. Nilsson, L.M.; Winkvist, A.; Eliasson, M.; Jansson, J.H.; Hallmans, G.; Johansson, I.; Lindahl, B.; Lenner, P.; Van Guelpen, B. Low-carbohydrate, high-protein score and mortality in a northern Swedish population-based cohort. *Eur. J. Clin. Nutr.* **2012**, *66*, 694–700. [CrossRef] [PubMed]
42. Lee, S.J.; Murphy, C.T.; Kenyon, C. Glucose shortens the life span of *C. elegans* by downregulating DAF-16/FOXO activity and aquaporin gene expression. *Cell Metab.* **2009**, *10*, 379–391. [CrossRef] [PubMed]
43. Bruce, K.D.; Hoxha, S.; Carvalho, G.B.; Yamada, R.; Wang, H.D.; Karayan, P.; He, S.; Brummel, T.; Kapahi, P.; Ja, W.W. High carbohydrate-low protein consumption maximizes Drosophila lifespan. *Exp. Gerontol.* **2013**, *48*, 1129–1135. [CrossRef]
44. Solon-Biet, S.M.; Walters, K.A.; Simanainen, U.K.; McMahon, A.C.; Ruohonen, K.; Ballard, J.W.; Raubenheimer, D.; Handelsman, D.J.; Le Couteur, D.G.; Simpson, S.J. Macronutrient balance, reproductive function, and lifespan in aging mice. *Proc. Natl. Acad. Sci. USA* **2015**, *112*, 3481–3486. [CrossRef]
45. Kendall, A.; Levitsky, D.A.; Strupp, B.J.; Lissner, L. Weight loss on a low-fat diet: Consequence of the imprecision of the control of food intake in humans. *Am. J. Clin. Nutr.* **1991**, *53*, 1124–1129. [CrossRef]
46. Ebbeling, C.B.; Leidig, M.M.; Feldman, H.A.; Lovesky, M.M.; Ludwig, D.S. Effects of a low-glycemic load vs low-fat diet in obese young adults: A randomized trial. *JAMA* **2007**, *297*, 2092–2102. [CrossRef] [PubMed]
47. Noakes, M.; Keogh, J.B.; Foster, P.R.; Clifton, P.M. Effect of an energy-restricted, high-protein, low-fat diet relative to a conventional high-carbohydrate, low-fat diet on weight loss, body composition, nutritional status, and markers of cardiovascular health in obese women. *Am. J. Clin. Nutr.* **2005**, *81*, 1298–1306. [CrossRef]
48. O'Rourke, E.J.; Kuballa, P.; Xavier, R.; Ruvkun, G. ω-6 Polyunsaturated fatty acids extend life span through the activation of autophagy. *Genes Dev.* **2013**, *27*, 429–440. [CrossRef]
49. Tsuduki, T.; Honma, T.; Nakagawa, K.; Ikeda, I.; Miyazawa, T. Long-term intake of fish oil increases oxidative stress and decreases lifespan in senescence-accelerated mice. *Nutrition* **2011**, *27*, 334–337. [CrossRef] [PubMed]
50. Hulbert, A.J. Metabolism and longevity: Is there a role for membrane fatty acids? *Integr. Comp. Biol.* **2010**, *50*, 808–817. [CrossRef] [PubMed]
51. Eleftheriou, D.; Benetou, V.; Trichopoulou, A.; La Vecchia, C.; Bamia, C. Mediterranean diet and its components in relation to all-cause mortality: Meta-analysis. *Br. J. Nutr.* **2018**, *120*, 1081–1097. [CrossRef] [PubMed]

52. Widmer, R.J.; Flammer, A.J.; Lerman, L.O.; Lerman, A. The Mediterranean diet, its components, and cardiovascular disease. *Am. J. Med.* **2015**, *128*, 229–238. [CrossRef]
53. Jacobs, D.R., Jr.; Gross, M.D.; Tapsell, L.C. Food synergy: An operational concept for understanding nutrition. *Am. J. Clin. Nutr.* **2009**, *89*, 1543s–1548s. [CrossRef]
54. Jacobs, D.R., Jr.; Steffen, L.M. Nutrients, foods, and dietary patterns as exposures in research: A framework for food synergy. *Am. J. Clin. Nutr.* **2003**, *78*, 508s–513s. [CrossRef]
55. Aguilera, J.M. The food matrix: Implications in processing, nutrition and health. *Crit. Rev. Food Sci. Nutr.* **2019**, *59*, 3612–3629. [CrossRef]
56. Jacobs, D.R., Jr.; Tapsell, L.C. Food, not nutrients, is the fundamental unit in nutrition. *Nutr. Rev.* **2007**, *65*, 439–450. [CrossRef]
57. Simpson, S.J.; Le Couteur, D.G.; Raubenheimer, D. Putting the balance back in diet. *Cell* **2015**, *161*, 18–23. [CrossRef]
58. Martínez-González, M.A.; Sánchez-Villegas, A. The emerging role of Mediterranean diets in cardiovascular epidemiology: Monounsaturated fats, olive oil, red wine or the whole pattern? *Eur. J. Epidemiol.* **2004**, *19*, 9–13. [CrossRef]
59. Imhof, A.; Woodward, M.; Doering, A.; Helbecque, N.; Loewel, H.; Amouyel, P.; Lowe, G.D.; Koenig, W. Overall alcohol intake, beer, wine, and systemic markers of inflammation in western Europe: Results from three MONICA samples (Augsburg, Glasgow, Lille). *Eur. Heart J.* **2004**, *25*, 2092–2100. [CrossRef] [PubMed]
60. van der Gaag, M.S.; Ubbink, J.B.; Sillanaukee, P.; Nikkari, S.; Hendriks, H.F. Effect of consumption of red wine, spirits, and beer on serum homocysteine. *Lancet* **2000**, *355*, 1522. [CrossRef]
61. Mukamal, K.J.; Conigrave, K.M.; Mittleman, M.A.; Camargo, C.A., Jr.; Stampfer, M.J.; Willett, W.C.; Rimm, E.B. Roles of drinking pattern and type of alcohol consumed in coronary heart disease in men. *N. Engl. J. Med.* **2003**, *348*, 109–118. [CrossRef] [PubMed]
62. Martínez-González, M.A.; Gea, A.; Ruiz-Canela, M. The Mediterranean Diet and Cardiovascular Health. *Circ. Res.* **2019**, *124*, 779–798. [CrossRef]
63. Fragopoulou, E.; Antonopoulou, S. The French paradox three decades later: Role of inflammation and thrombosis. *Clin. Chim. Acta Int. J. Clin. Chem.* **2020**, *510*, 160–169. [CrossRef]

nutrients

MDPI

Review

Linking Migraine to Gut Dysbiosis and Chronic Non-Communicable Diseases

Manuela Di Lauro [1], Cristina Guerriero [1], Kevin Cornali [1], Maria Albanese [1,2], Micaela Costacurta [3], Nicola Biagio Mercuri [1,2], Nicola Di Daniele [1,4] and Annalisa Noce [1,5,*]

1 Department of Systems Medicine, University of Rome Tor Vergata, 00133 Rome, RM, Italy; manuela.dilauro@ptvonline.it (M.D.L.); cristinaguerriero@hotmail.it (C.G.); cornali.kevin@hotmail.it (K.C.); maria.albanese@hotmail.it (M.A.); mercurin@med.uniroma2.it (N.B.M.); didaniele@med.uniroma2.it (N.D.D.)

2 Neurology Unit, Headache Center, Tor Vergata University Hospital, 00133 Rome, RM, Italy

3 Department of Surgical Sciences, University of Rome Tor Vergata, 00133 Rome, RM, Italy; micaela.costacurta@uniroma2.it

4 Fondazione Leonardo per le Scienze Mediche Onlus, Policlinico Abano, 35031 Abano Terme, PD, Italy

5 UOSD Nephrology and Dialysis, Policlinico Tor Vergata, 00133 Rome, RM, Italy

* Correspondence: annalisa.noce@uniroma2.it; Tel.: +39-0620902191

Abstract: In the world, migraine is one of the most common causes of disability in adults. To date, there is no a single cause for this disorder, but rather a set of physio-pathogenic triggers in combination with a genetic predisposition. Among the factors related to migraine onset, a crucial role seems to be played by gut dysbiosis. In fact, it has been demonstrated how the intestine is able to modulate the central nervous system activities, through the gut–brain axis, and how gut dysbiosis can influence neurological pathologies, including migraine attacks. In this context, in addition to conventional pharmacological treatments for migraine, attention has been paid to an adjuvant therapeutic strategy based on different nutritional approaches and lifestyle changes able to positively modulate the gut microbiota composition. In fact, the restoration of the balance between the different gut bacterial species, the reconstruction of the gut barrier integrity, and the control of the release of gut-derived inflammatory neuropeptides, obtained through specific nutritional patterns and lifestyle changes, represent a possible beneficial additive therapy for many migraine subtypes. Herein, this review explores the bi-directional correlation between migraine and the main chronic non-communicable diseases, such as diabetes mellitus, arterial hypertension, obesity, cancer, and chronic kidney diseases, whose link is represented by gut dysbiosis.

Keywords: migraine; chronic non-communicable diseases; gut microbiota; nutritional approaches; lifestyle changes

1. Introduction

Migraine is a complex neurological disorder that triggers a particular type of headache, characterized by unilateral, pulsating, and moderate–severe pain, which generally worsens with physical activity and is associated with other symptoms, such as nausea, vomiting, and photophonophobia [1]. With an estimated global prevalence of 14.7% [2], the World Health Organization (WHO) listed migraine among the top ten causes of disabilities worldwide [3]; it is in first place if we consider people younger than 50 years old [4]. Women are 3–4 times more affected than men and show more disabling and drug-resistant, attacks and this consequently provokes a great socio-economic burden [5–7]. About 3% of the patients, suffering from episodic migraine, evolves every year towards a more complex clinical picture of chronic migraine. In this latter condition, patients should suffer a monthly migraine of about 15 or more days, in the last three months [8].

The main trigger factors of this migraine progression are hormonal pathways, psychological syndromes, drugs assumption, environmental factors, and nutritional habits (Figure 1).

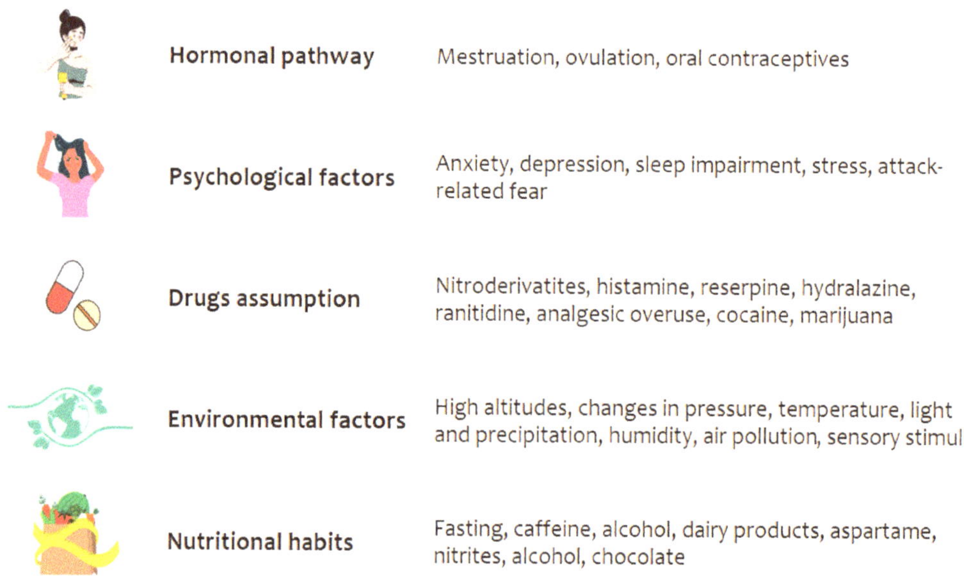
Hormonal pathway
Mestruation, ovulation, oral contraceptives
Psychological factors
Anxiety, depression, sleep impairment, stress, attack-related fear
Drugs assumption
Nitroderivatites, histamine, reserpine, hydralazine, ranitidine, analgesic overuse, cocaine, marijuana
Environmental factors
High altitudes, changes in pressure, temperature, light and precipitation, humidity, air pollution, sensory stimuli
Nutritional habits
Fasting, caffeine, alcohol, dairy products, aspartame, nitrites, alcohol, chocolate

Figure 1. Common trigger factors for migraine development and chronicization.

In women, migraine can be linked to the fluctuations in sexual reproductive hormones. In fact, decreased estrogens in the late luteal phase of the menstrual cycle lead to an increased permeability of blood vessels to prostaglandins, becoming a migraine trigger [9]. On the contrary, elevated estrogen levels are associated with more frequent pain attacks, especially with aura [10]. For this reason and for a higher stroke risk, associated with aura, the use of oral contraceptives is still restricted by the current guidelines in those women affected by this headache subtype [11]. The most frequently experienced psychological factors associated with this pathological condition are (i) anxiety, which seems to have a shared genetic basis with a migraine [12,13]; (ii) depression [12,14], characterized by a low availability of 5-hydroxytryptamine (5-HT), an increased sensitivity of trigeminovascular pathways [15], the hypofunction of the dopaminergic system [14], a down-regulation of the GABAergic system, and decreased estrogen levels; (iii) stress [16], namely, previous and recurrent stressful events that have been shown to be correlated with migraine onset and its chronicization [17]; and (iv) an excessive fear of migraine attacks, which refers to the fear of a headache occurring and that can worsen the disease course [18]. Even the use of some psychoactive drugs can be an important provoking agent for migraine generation, including nitroderivates, histamine, reserpine, hydralazine, and ranitidine, as well as cocaine and marijuana [19–23].

Notably, the overuse of analgesic or other abortive pain medications (i.e., triptans) is the major clinical factor of a migraine worsening, inducing a particular condition, known as "medication overuse headache" [24]. Among the environmental factors that can lead to the migraine development are high altitudes, changes in the atmospheric pressure, temperature, light and precipitation, humidity, air pollution, and sensory stimuli, such as olfactory and visual ones [25]. Impaired sleep patterns can also promote migraine attacks, particularly in young adults [26]. Other important migraine triggers are nutritional habits and certain foods, including fasting, caffeine, natural sweeteners (such as aspartame), nitrites of preserved meats, biogenic monoamines of alcohol, chocolate and dairy products (such as cheese and yogurt), and monosodium glutamate [25].

Migraine is frequently associated with chronic non-communicable diseases (CNCDs), such as diabetes mellitus (DM), arterial hypertension (AH), obesity, and cancer and chronic kidney disease (CKD). Moreover, CNCDs are themselves both the cause and consequence of a negative change in the gut microbiota composition, called "dysbiosis" [27–29].

In this regard, in addition to pharmacological treatments, a new adjuvant therapeutic strategy able to counteract migraine can be represented by different nutritional approaches able to modulate the gut microbiota composition and gut–brain axis [30].

The term "microbiota" means a very wide community consisting of bacteria, viruses, fungi, Archea, and unicellular eukaryotes. The term "microbiome", instead, indicates a set of genetic patrimonies of microorganisms, which constitute it [31].

The microbial component and its genetic patrimonies are affected by lifestyle, dietetic habits, and other external factors, such as the environment. Therefore, the gut microbiota is a dynamic system that is in constant evolution [32] and is also composed by the vascular gut barrier [33]. The latter is a fundamental coating system able to control epithelium permeability and the passage of potentially pathogenic molecules and bacteria into the bloodstream [34,35]. Therefore, the microbiota can be defined as a "meta-organ", namely, it is a structure that anatomically is not a part of the organism; however, it accompanies human phylogenetic evolution [36,37].

The aim of this narrative review is to analyze the possible correlation between migraine and gut microbiota dysbiosis and the possible relationship between migraine and CNCDs. Moreover, we examine the possible nutritional approaches and lifestyle changes able to positively modulate gut microbiota composition, reducing migraine frequency and intensity.

2. Materials and Methods

In order to achieve the review's aim, a literature search was conducted using three databases (PubMed, Scopus, and Cochrane Library), until August 2023. The search was limited to peer-reviewed journals, written in the English language, and the search terms were "migraine" in combination with "gut microbiota", AND "chronic degenerative non communicable diseases", AND "diabetes mellitus", AND "Arterial Hypertension", AND "obesity", AND "cancer", AND "chronic kidney disease", AND "Mediterranean Diet", AND "Ketogenic Diet", AND "probiotics", AND "physical exercises", AND "vitamins", AND "iron", AND "polyphenols", AND "electrolytes", AND "histamine".

3. The Gut Microbiota Physiological Composition

The first studies related to the discovery of the microbiota date back to the beginning of the twentieth century, when a student of Pasteur, Elie Metchnikov [38] explored the theme of symbiotic bacteria in organisms, unlike Pasteur who focused his attention mainly on pathogenic ones. Metchinikov described the beneficial effects of lactic ferments on the bacterial flora and health host [38]. Subsequent studies have pointed out the presence of these bacteria that are involved in the absorption of nutrients as well as in immune system modulation [39,40]. In the 1990s, for the first time, the "gut–brain axis" was highlighted, namely, how the microbiota exerted a physiological role in the maintenance of host health [41].

The human microbiota is characterized by a high bacterial density, with a metagenome that in the adult is 150-times larger than the overall human genetic pattern [42]. It is an ecosystem composed by a set of ecological niches in close contact with the intestinal mucosa, forming an area of 250–400 m^2 [37]. A more precise view of the complexity of the gut microbiota has been made in recent years, thanks to the metagenomic data.

Although there is a wide variety of symbiotic microorganisms, among the 160 species present in the human intestine, of which at least 57 are common to all individuals, the most widespread microbial phyla are only 4: Bacteroides, Firmicutes, Actinobacteri, and Proteobacteria. The first two are present in a higher quantity; in fact, they constitute about 90% of the human gut microbiota [43,44].

The microbiota is an extremely heterogeneous and complex system, strongly modulated by external factors (Figure 2).

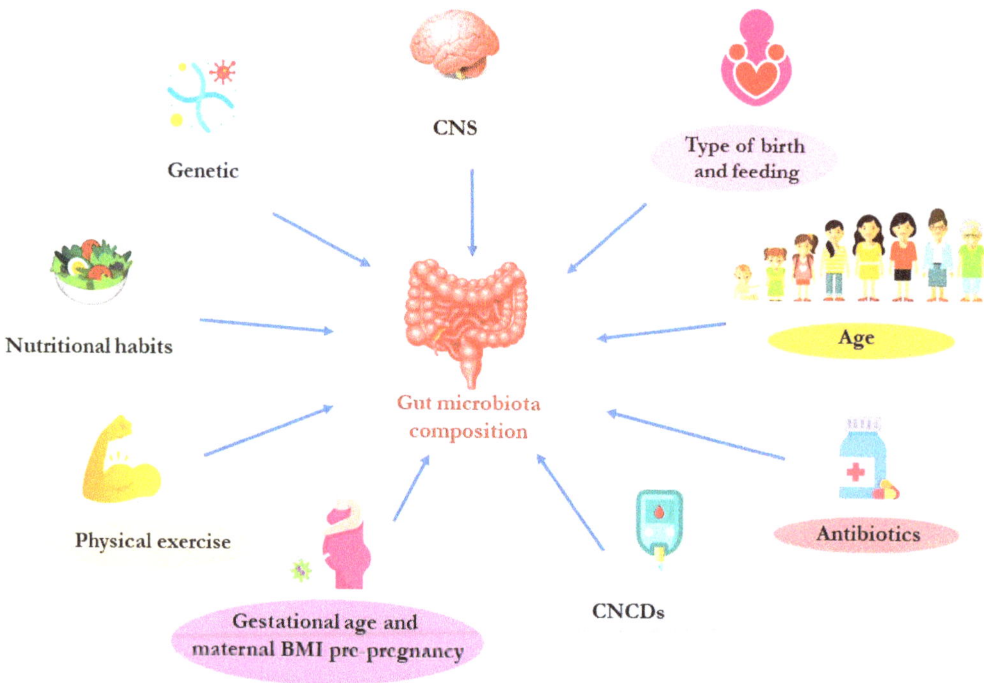

Figure 2. Main factors that can influence the gut microbiota composition. Abbreviation: BMI, body mass index; CNCDs, chronic non-communicable diseases; CNS, central nervous system.

The composition of the gut microbiota changes in relation to age. In fact, recent studies reported that the microbiota begins to colonize the intestinal tract during intrauterine life [45,46]. In this regard, it has been demonstrated that placental microbiota can influence, during pregnancy, correct fetal growth and development [47]. The maintenance of a correct placental eubiosis is influenced by the nutritional habits of the mother during pregnancy. In particular, a diet rich in fats may induce the placental dysbiosis that has been associated with a high risk of developing metabolic syndrome in adults [48]. Moreover, placenta dysbiosis can damage the maternal hypothalamic–pituitary–adrenal (HPA) axis and can influence the circulating levels of 5-HT, inducing possible damage to fetal neuronal development [49]. In a child's gastrointestinal (GI) tract, Bifidobacteria are the most abundant bacteria [50]. In adulthood, the bacterial composition appears to be greater both in terms of the number of microorganisms and the diversification of the taxa (called α-diversity). The gut microbiota α-diversity reflects the variability of species within the human intestine. Recent studies have highlighted how it is directly related to host health and how a poor α-diversity is associated with various CNCDs [51,52]. The gut microbiota changes that are observed in relation to age are mainly due to the switch from a liquid to a solid diet [53]. This switch causes the enrichment of bacterial flora, especially the families of *Lachnospiraceae* and *Ruminococcaceae* [43]. Throughout life, dietary habits influence the composition of the gut microbiota. Scientific studies have reported that bacteria belonging to the genus Clostridium (the main producers of butyrate, a short-chain fatty acid—SCFA) are more present in subjects following a Mediterranean diet (MD), while the subjects that follow a Western diet show fewer bacteria responsible for the degradation of fibers, such as Prevotella and Succinivibrio [54,55]. In the elderly, gut microbiota composition is less variable due to the reduction in food variety in the diet and the reduction in fiber intake, which results in a decrease in Firmicutes, (among these, the *Clostridium* cluster XIVa and *Feacalibacterium prausnitzii* are involved in saccharolytic fermentation), and in an increase in Proteobacteria [56]. This induces the reduced availability of SCFAs that, in turn, contributes to the aging and increased activity of proteolytic fermentation [57]. This phenomenon induces an enhanced production of gut-derived toxins, such as trimethylamine N-oxide (TMAO), p-cresyl sulfate (p-CS), indoxyl sulfate (IS), and indole-3 acetic acid (IAA). Moreover, an increase in proteolytic fermentation triggers low-grade chronic systemic inflammation, a factor related to the onset and progression of CNCDs and sarcopenia [27,58,59].

Other factors that influence the gut microbiota's qualitative and quantitative compositions are (i) gestational age; (ii) antibiotic therapy, mostly in the perinatal period; (iii) mode of childbirth (vaginal or cesarean); (iv) type of feeding (breast feeding, artificial or mixed, composition and timing of complementary feeding); (v) pre-pregnancy body mass index (BMI); and maternal body weight increase during pregnancy [60,61].

(i) *Gestational age.* An interesting study analyzed the gut microbiota's possible differences in full-term and in pre-term deliveries. Full-term infants are characterized by a greater abundance of *Bacteroides,* while pre-term infants show a greater abundance of *Lactobacillus* [62].
(ii) *Antibiotic therapy, especially in the perinatal period.* Antibiotics, especially broad-spectrum ones, qualitatively and quantitatively alter the gut microbiota's composition [63]. Studies conducted on mice suggested complex mechanisms (endocrine and neurocrine) involved in the signaling between gut microbiota and the brain, which were induced by an excessive use of antibiotics, especially in children [64]. In fact, an excessive use of antibiotics promotes the gut colonization of *Clostridium difficile* [65], an opportunistic pathogen that can cause diarrhea, specifically in the case of the simultaneous intake of drugs that reduce the gut microbiota α-diversity [66,67].
(iii) *Mode of childbirth.* It has been shown that the microbiota of natural births is dominated by bacterial genera, such as *Bacteroides* (Bacteroidetes), bifidobacteria (Actinobatteria), lactobacilli (Firmicutes), and enterobacteria (Proteobacteria). On the contrary, the microbial pattern of Caesarean births is instead characterized by a qualitative–quantitative alteration in the gut microbiota's composition [68]. Additionally, Caesarean births lack the Bacteroides species until 18 months of age, due to non-exposure to the maternal vaginal microbiota [69].
(iv) *Type of feeding.* The α-diversity appears to be lower in breastfed infants compared to formula-fed infants, and the gut microbiota composition shows differences. *Bifidobacterium* and Bacteroides are more abundant in breastfed infants, while Streptococcus and Enterococcus are more abundant in formula-fed infants [70].
(v) *Pre-pregnancy BMI and maternal body weight gain during pregnancy.* A recent study pointed out the differences in maternal gut microbiota composition based on pre-pregnancy weight and gestational weight gain. In fact, overweight/obese mothers, before pregnancy, are characterized by the presence of some taxa, such as the *Christensenellaceae* family and the genera *Lachnospira, Parabacteroides, Bifidobacterium,* and *Blautia.* Moreover, overweight or obese women before pregnancy show less α-diversity compared to non-overweight/non-obese women. This gut microbiota maternal pattern seems to not be related to the global differences in the infant gut microbiota within the first two years of life [71].

Recent studies demonstrated that physical activity is also able to modulate the gut microbiota, in terms of the composition and function [72]. On the contrary, physical inactivity has been repeatedly associated with alterations in the bacterial composition of the gut microbiota [73,74]. In particular, as described in the following paragraph, physical exercise is able to improve the body's composition, positively modulating the gut microbiota pattern and stimulating SCFAs production [75]. Nevertheless, the benefits obtained during a period of continuous physical activity are lost if you return to a sedentary condition [76].

Furthermore, as previously described, CNCDs are, at the same time, both the cause and consequence of gut microbiota dysbiosis [32,77]. For example, in CKD patients, there is an alteration in gut permeability, which allows the passage of bacteria and bacterial material from the gut to the bloodstream. This phenomenon induces a chronic inflammatory state that exacerbates CKD itself. In CKD patients, an accumulation and increased production of gut-derived toxins can be observed (such as IS, TMAO, and p-CS, IAA). These toxins are associated with an increase in cardiovascular (CV) risk [27].

4. Migraine and Gut Dysbiosis

In recent decades, the literature demonstrates that the gut microbiota is involved in central nervous system (CNS) activities [78]. Over time, several studies have investigated and defined some of the mechanisms through which the brain is able to connect itself to the gut, defining the "gut–brain axis" [79].

The importance of this axis has been mainly highlighted in the studies that evaluated the causes underlying neurodegenerative and psychiatric diseases and neurodevelopment [80,81]. In particular, the CNS can influence the gut environment impacting on some intestinal functions, such as the regulation of gut movements, excretions, and the immune system [82]. The interaction between the intestine and brain is confirmed by a gut microbiota modification, which can impact on the CNS's different functions [64,83].

The brain communicates with the intestine through numerous "roads" [64], such as (i) the immune system; (ii) SCFAs; (iii) the autonomic nervous system (vagal nerve); (iv) tryptophan metabolism, the precursor of the neurotransmitter serotonin; (v) neurotransmitters; (vi) gastric peptides produced by specialized endocrine cells, whose release is influenced by the microbiota itself; and (vii) the HPA axis [30,84].

Therefore, the intestine can be considered as the "second brain", as it produces a series of neurotransmitters, such as serotonin and histamine [85]. Several studies demonstrated that low levels of cerebral serotonin were strongly associated with migraine. In particular, migraineurs have higher levels of cerebral serotonin during an acute pain attack compared with the periods between attacks [86,87]. In this regard, a symptomatic migraine-specific class of drugs commonly used in the clinical practice are triptans, serotonin-receptor agonists that can "recreate" an optimal brain neurotransmitter concentration by reducing the inflammation and, consequentially, the pain. Unfortunately, these medications are characterized by several side effects, such as cardiovascular dysfunction, GI disorders, muscle aches, drowsiness, tingling, and dermatological disorders [88].

Moreover, it was demonstrated that chronic headache patients presented higher histamine concentrations than healthy subjects, either during or between migraine attacks [89]. Previous studies have focused on the effects of antihistamines in the pain treatment behind the proven histamine's role as a potent migraine trigger. However, this evidence is of a poor quality and often limited by frequent undesirable adverse events (i.e., excessive somnolence). Although there are positive reports about histamine H3-receptor agonists (H3Rs) that seem to effectively inhibit the histamine release in the CNS, they are not very credible because they are based on subtherapeutic analgesic dosages [90,91].

As previously described, nausea and vomiting are symptoms commonly associated with migraine. Moreover, patients with frequent migraine attacks often present GI symptoms, such as reflux, diarrhea, and constipation [92]. Starting from this observation, Camara-Lemarroy et al. highlighted the relationship between migraine and GI disorders [93]. This statement is strengthened by the fact that inflammatory bowel disease patients often suffer from migraine [94]. Gut dysbiosis seems to play a key role in the pathogenesis of migraine, since this intestinal alteration seems to induce an increased production of gut-derived inflammatory cytokines that can modulate the HPA axis [95]. Furthermore, these gut-derived inflammatory cytokines, in turn, appear to be involved in the modulation of vagus nerve activity, which, among other functions, innervates the intestinal free fatty acid-receptor 3. This receptor seems to be involved in the metabolic pathway of SCFAs [96]. Therefore, the mechanisms underlying the interaction between the gut microbiota and migraine are supported by several studies that highlight the direct and indirect evidence [97]. The former includes the fact that gut dysbiosis, associated with an impaired production of SCFAs, induces the release of pro-inflammatory cytokines, such as tumor necrosis factor (TNF)-α. The latter, in animal models, seems to regulate migraine-like pain [98]. The second ones are deduced from the scientific studies that suggest that nutritional approaches, use of probiotics, and stimulation of the vagus nerve can represent new therapeutic strategies for migraine, based on gut microbiota modulation [99–101]. Therefore, it is evident that there is a correlation between the gut microbiota and migraine. In fact, numerous studies both conducted on animal models and clinical trials highlighted a gut microbiota alteration in migraine patients compared to the healthy subjects. In this regard, it is important to understand whether the possible comorbidities (such as CNCDs) inducing dysbiosis can be a trigger for migraine and, at the same time, whether specific nutritional approaches or lifestyle changes can represent a valid and innovative adjuvant therapy for the treatment of migraine.

5. Migraine and Its Correlation with Chronic Non-Communicable Diseases

The bi-directional correlation between migraine and the main CNCDs is already described in the literature, even if the mechanisms underlying this correlation are not fully clarified. A possible link between these pathological conditions could be represented by gut microbiota alteration, that is, by a condition known as dysbiosis. In fact, as widely described in the previous paragraphs, gut microbiota dysbiosis appears to represent both an important trigger for the onset of migraine and for its chronic development and, in turn, seems to be induced by the migraine itself. This relationship is possible thanks to the gut–brain axis, which allows the communication between the two organs. At the same time, an alteration in the gut microbiota has been broadly described in the literature in CNCDs patients. In fact, gut dysbiosis can be involved both in CNCDs progression and in chronic migraine onset in CNCDs patients (Figure 3). In this context, lifestyle changes and healthy nutritional approaches, capable of restoring gut eubiosis, can represent a valid adjuvant therapy to simultaneously improve the symptoms and the clinical evolution of the migraine and, consequently, the CNCDs' clinical course.

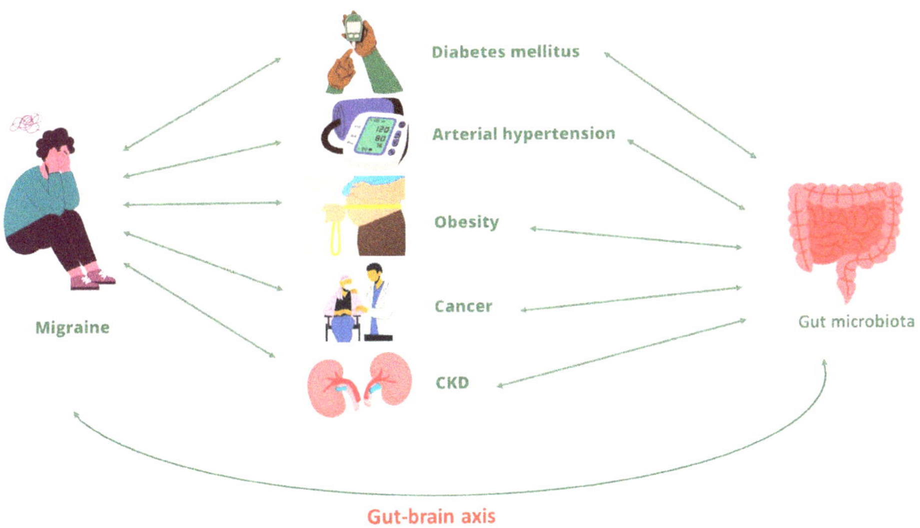

Figure 3. Correlation between migraine and chronic non-communicable diseases. Abbreviation: CKD, chronic kidney diseases.

5.1. Diabetes Mellitus and Migraine

The correlation between DM and migraine is currently controversial [102]. Some epidemiological studies suggest that migraine can be considered a non-traditional risk factor for DM onset and progression [103,104]. In fact, a study demonstrated that migraine attacks in DM patients may be related to the episodes of hypoglycemia that these patients often manifest. Moreover, it was supposed that a possible treatment able to counteract migraine episodes was optimal glycemic control with a contextual reduction in hypoglycemic episodes [102].

Moreover, at the same time, the insulin resistance that characterizes type-2 diabetes mellitus patients has been associated with migraine development. In particular, insulin resistance seems capable of significantly prolonging migraine attacks, but not their severity [105]. A possible explanation for this last correlation could be that insulin resistance, at the brain level, can lead to an impaired release of neurotransmitters. Moreover, insulin resistance and high blood glucose levels can cause a systemic inflammatory response that spreads to the peripheral and central nervous systems, inducing the neuroinflammation phenomenon [106,107]. In turn, neuroinflammation can damage the blood–brain barrier [108].

On the contrary, other studies showed an inverse correlation between these two pathological conditions, considering type-1 DM a protective factor against migraine. Although the exact mechanisms that underline this indirect relationship have not yet been sufficiently elucidated, it has been proposed that similarities in the genetic and biochemical pathways and in lifestyle could account for this [109–111]. To corroborate this observation, a recent epidemiological study conducted on over 70,000 French women highlighted a lower risk of developing type-2 DM in women with migraine compared to those without a migraine history [112].

5.2. Arterial Hypertension and Migraine

AH and headaches have been linked to each other in the medical literature [113]. In fact, it is well known how a hypertensive crisis, namely, a sudden increase in blood pressure, can occur with abrupt headaches [114]. Migraine and AH may share common mechanisms, such as endothelial dysfunction (ED), a deficiency of autonomic CV regulation, and renin–angiotensin–aldosterone system (RAAS) involvement [114]. Preventive anti-migraine effects were described for several antihypertensive drugs, such as beta-blockers, angiotensin-converting enzyme inhibitors, and angiotensin II-receptor blockers [115]. ED may be both one of the factors that increase the cerebrovascular and CV risks in migraine subjects and a determinant cause of AH development [116]. Nitric oxide (NO) plays a pivotal role in the pathogenesis of migraine; in fact, it is involved in the regulation of cerebral and extra-cerebral cranial blood flows and artery size. In migraineurs, the arteries are hypersensitive to NO, and it has been hypothesized that this phenomenon is one of the main triggers of migraine attacks [117].

Moreover, the RAAS can be another factor responsible for the clinical correlation between migraine and AH [118]. This might explain why some angiotensin-converting enzyme inhibitors and angiotensin II-receptor blockers are effective in preventing migraine, regardless of the presence of AH [119]. Notably, the presence of AH in a migraine patient increases the CV risk [120].

5.3. Obesity and Migraine

The WHO defines obesity as a condition characterized by an excessive presence of adipose tissue in the human body that induces a significant increase in CV mortality and morbidity in both sexes [121]. Obesity is commonly considered a consequence of excessive calorie intake, compared to energy expenditure, and the decrease in physical activity, very common habits in Western societies [122].

The clinical evidence shows that obesity can intensify the risk of episodic and chronic migraine and that the body weight reduction in obese subjects can decrease the intensity, frequency, and duration of migraine attacks [123].

The link between obesity and headaches is attributed to shared pathophysiological features [124]. For example, obese adult subjects showed increased calcitonin gene-related peptide (CGRP) plasma levels, which were also elevated in migraine patients [125]. Furthermore, an increase in proinflammatory cytokines, such as interleukin (IL)-6 and TNF-α, was reported in obese individuals and in the acute headache phase [126].

5.4. Cancer and Migraine

For most cancer types, there is no evidence to support a link between increased oncological risks in migraineurs [127], except for tumors of a neurological origin of which migraine can often represent the onset symptom. In contrast, a lower prevalence of GI cancers in migraine subjects has been described, compared to those without migraine [128].

Moreover, cancer patients may present an amplified risk of developing migraine. It is very important to recognize migraine causes in order to treat them promptly and exclude the presence of secondary headache causes (i.e., brain metastasis) [129]. Migraine induces a negative impact on the quality of life of cancer patients and, showing a very broad etiology, makes its diagnosis difficult [130]. For cancer patients, any change in pharmacological treatments, including chemotherapy, can trigger headaches [131].

5.5. CKD and Migraine

Several epidemiological studies have highlighted a direct correlation between CKD and migraine onset, even if the mechanisms underlying this correlation remain partially known. A study conducted by Wang et al. evaluated CKD incidence in a group of subjects with normal renal functions suffering from chronic migraine, compared to a group of subjects without migraine. The authors showed that CKD incidence was higher in subjects suffering from chronic migraine than in the control group. In particular, male gender, age, and nonsteroidal anti-inflammatory drugs (NSAIDs) abuse appeared to be independent risk factors for CKD onset [132]. This correlation seemed to be associated with ED secondary to a migraine, which would increase the risk of developing CKD [133]. Other factors that can lead to CKD onset in chronic migraine patients are blood pressure fluctuations and coexisting comorbidities [134]. A study evaluated the possible genetic link between the two pathological conditions; although, no overall genetic correlation was found, four specific genomic regions were identified that appeared to be related to the common pathogenic mechanisms underlying both migraine and CKDs. These mechanisms appeared to involve the cardiovascular system and endothelial function [133].

Hemodialysis-related migraine has been described in the literature. In fact, hemodialysis patients often suffer from headaches during or after hemodialysis (HD) treatment. The headache usually occurs in the first hour of an HD session and it resolves after a maximum of 72 h after HD treatment [135]. This phenomenon can be related to the electrolyte imbalance and blood pressure fluctuations that occur during dialysis treatment [136].

6. Possible Nutritional Approaches and Lifestyle Changes to Counteract Migraine

Proper nutrition patterns and a healthy lifestyle are useful to prevent and alleviate headache symptoms. This issue has a very ancient origin [137]. In fact, Ippocrate was aware of the relationship between the consumption of some foods and the onset of migraine [138]. Indeed, there are many foods that can cause painful attacks because they contain substances that are able to alter intracranial blood circulation [139], inducing vasodilation–vasoconstriction imbalance and a consequent headache. In this context, a healthy diet may represent a valid preventive therapeutic strategy for migraine [140].

6.1. Mediterranean Diet

The MD can be defined as a model of dietary habits adopted by the populations living in the Mediterranean area [141]. It is characterized by a high consumption of fresh fruit and vegetables, legumes, and complex carbohydrates, accompanied by a moderate consumption of seafoods and extra virgin olive oil (EVOO), as the main source of fats, and by a moderate consumption of wine [141]. There are numerous clinical studies that highlight how MD is able to reduce the risk of CNCDs onset and slow down their progression [142]. MD may also be considered an adjuvant approach to fight migraine in this patient population [143].

A meta-analysis highlighted the potential role of the MD in the fight against major neurodegenerative diseases [144]. This diet is rich in polyunsaturated fatty acids (PUFAs) and monounsaturated fatty acids (MUFAs) that seem to prevent the onset of Alzheimer's and Parkinson's diseases [145]. Moreover, the intake of PUFAs and specifically of eicosapentaenoic acid (EPA) seem to have antidepressant effects [146]. A recent meta-analysis analyzed 26 randomized double-blind placebo-controlled trials, highlighting the beneficial effects on the depression symptoms of EPA intake, at a dosage of $\leq$1 g/day, compared to a placebo [147]. Furthermore, as PUFAs are the main lipid-forming cerebral cortex, they are able to play an important role in higher cognitive processes and in learning [148].

Moreover, the MD is rich in polyphenols, vitamins C, E, B12, and B9, and carotenoids, and it is therefore able to counteract oxidative stress (OS) and lipid peroxidation, exerting cardioprotective and neuroprotective effects [149].

The MD seems to reduce chronic migraine symptoms [143]. In fact, a recent clinical study conducted on subjects aged between 18–64 years, who suffered from chronic migraines, highlighted how those who had a poor adherence to the MD developed more severe and frequent migraine attacks, compared to those who had a high adherence to the MD [150]. This symptom reduction appeared to be associated with the systemic inflammation decrease, mediated by MD typical foods. A Western diet, on the other hand, rich in pro-inflammatory foods, seems to be associated with an increase in migraine symptoms [151,152]. These associations seem to be related to the gut microbiota modification induced by the different nutritional patterns. In fact, it is known that the Western diet, characterized by a high dietary intake of salt, increases the *Firmicutes/Bacteroidetes* ratio, providing the conditions for gut dysbiosis. The latter induces a reduction in SCFA-producing bacteria, losing their important beneficial functions for the host [55]. On the other hand, the MD seems capable of positively modulating the gut microbiota by increasing its α-diversity [153].

The Western diet, rich in saturated fatty acids, is characterized by an increase in proteolytic fermentation, which leads to the production of gut-derived toxins, as previously described. Instead, the MD is characterized by an enhancement of saccharolytic fermentation that stimulates SCFAs production [27].

6.2. The Ketogenic Diet

The ketogenic diet (KD) was initially used as an adjuvant treatment for drug-resistant epilepsy and, to date, it is also widely used for rapid weight loss [154]. Its effects on neurodegenerative diseases, cognitive functions, and autistic spectrum disorders have also been studied. This nutritional approach is characterized by a high lipid intake, the right amounts of proteins, and a low energy intake from carbohydrates. The objective of KD is to reduce glycolysis and to stimulate the formation of endogenous ketones through the oxidation of fatty acids [155].

The increased concentration of ketones leads to a state of ketosis, so that these molecules take the place of glucose and can be used as the primary energy source by the brain. The KD can protect the brain from OS and can normalize the neuronal bioenergetics through the stimulation of mitochondrial biogenesis and the stabilization of synaptic functions [156].

The first piece of evidence that the KD was able to alleviate the symptoms of migraine dates back to the beginning of the last century. Since then, numerous clinical studies have been conducted on patients suffering from chronic headaches. These studies have shown that, through different mechanisms, the KD is able to reduce systemic inflammation [157] and OS [158] at the level of the CNS, and to positively modulate the gut microbiota [159], reducing the symptoms of migraine [160–162].

6.3. Probiotic and Prebiotic Supplementations

The WHO has defined probiotics as "living micro-organisms" capable of creating benefits to human health when administered in adequate quantities [163]. The main prebiotics belong to genera Lactobacilli and Bifidobacteria and their effects depend on the species and the strain, for example, *Lactobacillus rhamnosus* seems to be very effective in the treatment of GI disorders, such as infectious diarrhea in children, or in the prevention of antibiotic-induced diarrhea [164,165].

Probiotic integration can modulate chronic migraine symptoms [32,166]. The possible mechanisms of action are unclear and may include the stimulation of SCFAs production, the improvement of gut epithelial integrity, and the decrease in inflammation by the suppression of the kappa-B nuclear factor (NF-κB) pathway, lowering the levels of proinflammatory cytokines [167]. Probiotics can also increase the rate of gastric emptying and attenuate gastric stasis, a GI disorder commonly present in patients with migraine [168]. Several studies have shown that probiotics assumption can rebalance the gut microbiota's composition, improve gut permeability, and prevent the onset of neurological disorders, such as migraine [169].

In some subjects, even some food allergies and intolerances can trigger migraine attacks. Conversely, a decrease in gut permeability can provide relief from migraine. Therefore, probiotics, thanks to an improvement of gut barrier functions, can also have beneficial effects on headache patients. New clinical studies are necessary to confirm this hypothesis [124,170].

Prebiotics are described as undigested substances capable of selectively stimulating the growth and/or the activity of one or a limited number of symbiotic intestinal bacteria. Prebiotics supplementation is able to restore gut eubiosis and can promote a reduction in migraine attacks [171]. Many studies focus on the effects induced by the two main prebiotics, galactogosharides (GOSs) and fructooligosaccharides (FOSs), demonstrating how these organic substances are able to reduce neuroinflammation and brain OS [172,173]. GOSs and FOSs seem to stimulate brain functions and synaptic plasticity towards the brain neurotrophic factor and receptors for N-methyl-D-aspartic acid (NMDA) [174].

6.4. *Physical Activity*

Physical activity, at the doses recommended by the WHO, seems to improve the quality of life. In particular, the WHO recommends a daily moderate-intensity aerobic physical activity of at least 150–300 min, or 75–150 min of vigorous-intensity aerobic physical activity for adults [175]. This physical activity seems to improve muscle mass, cardiorespiratory fitness, and bone health, and it appears to reduce the risks of AH, CV diseases, DM, various types of cancer (including breast and colon cancers), and depression [176]. Regarding this latter aspect, the mechanisms whereby physical exercise exerts its beneficial neurological effects are numerous, which include the regulation of the HPA axis, the promotion of an anti-inflammatory state, and the increase in neuroplasticity [177]. It is interesting to note that physical exercise can determine changes in the gut microbiota's composition, restoring homeostasis and regulating energy expenditure [178]. Low-intensity physical exercise can affect GI tract functions, reducing the intestinal transit time and, thus, the contact time between pathogens and the GI mucus layer [179].

Adapted physical activity can represent a valid non-pharmacological strategy for the clinical management of patients affected by CNCDs [180]. In fact, these patients, as previously illustrated, present an alteration in the gut microbiota, which induces and amplifies the chronic inflammatory state, which is, in turn, responsible for CNCDs progression [181]. Numerous studies suggest that adapted physical activity in CNCDs patients is able to both qualitatively and quantitatively modulate the gut microbiota's composition, exerting important benefits on the patient's quality of life and reducing CV risk [74]. Physical activity increases the abundance of gut microbiota bacteria and improves its quality (Figure 4) [182]. Studies on animal models suggest that physical activity is able to increase the abundance of the genus *Bacteroidetes* and decrease the genus *Firmicutes*, with a consequent reduction in the *Firmicutes*/*Bacteroidetes* ratio, improving the quality of the gut microbiota composition [74].

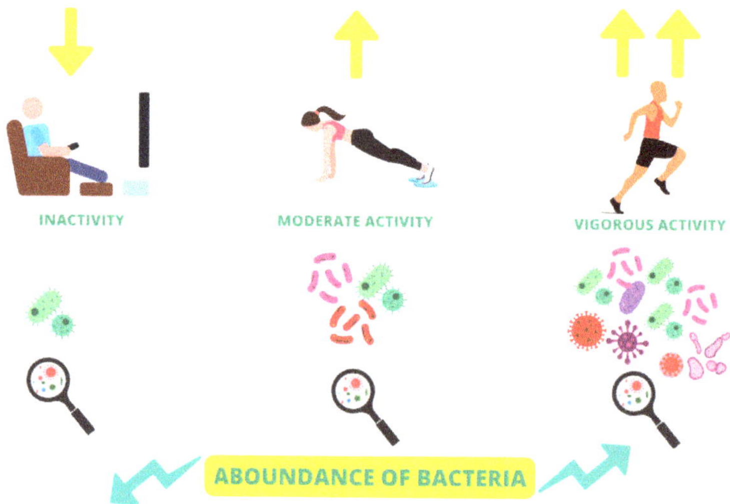

Figure 4. Modulation of gut microbiota composition and α-diversity by the physical activity degree.

Thanks to the positive modulation of the gut microbiota by physical exercise, the latter, especially the aerobic type, seems able to prevent the onset of chronic migraine, rather than being able to reduce the symptoms of chronic headaches already existing. Several clinical studies, in fact, have highlighted how sedentary subjects are more likely to develop chronic migraine compared to active subjects [183]. On the other hand, other clinical studies showed that, in subjects who already suffered from migraine, intense physical exercise led to the exacerbation of this disorder [184].

6.5. Vitamin D Supplementation

It is well known that a vitamin D deficiency is associated with chronic pain, depression, and some neurological disorders [185]. The brain is characterized by an abundance of receptors for vitamin D and there is evidence of the non-skeletal role of vitamin D in the mechanisms that regulate inflammation, immunity, and neurotransmitter metabolism [186]. Vitamin D blood levels are related to sun exposure (depending on the latitude and outdoor activities), dietary intake, and genetic components [187]. Migraine patients tend to avoid sunlight because of photophobia during migraine attacks. Moreover, it is known that reduced physical activity and a sedentary lifestyle, conducted indoors, greatly increase the risk of vitamin D deficiency [188].

Several studies have reported that vitamin D low-serum levels may be associated with an increased risk of migraines/headaches [189]. In addition, it has been suggested that the prevalence of a deficiency/insufficiency of vitamin D may be greater in patients suffering from migraines/headaches when compared with subjects without headaches [190].

6.6. Other Vitamin Supplementations

In patients with very intense migraine, a lack of vitamin B12 is often observed [191]. Vitamin B12 deficiency in association with hyperhomocysteinemia causes damage to endothelial cells, increasing free radical levels, which may be related to migraine episode generation [192]. Recent studies suggested that a vitamin B12 deficiency in chronic migraine can be induced by the frequent use of analgesics, which may alter vitamin B12 absorption [193].

Furthermore, studies on riboflavin have shown that the intake of this vitamin is effective in the prophylaxis of migraine, thus reducing the frequency of attacks [194].

Emerging evidence shows the statistically significant role of thiamine (vitamin B1) in migraine mitigation [195,196]. Thiamine has been shown to be particularly important in the regulation of brain levels of serotonin; abnormalities in the function of serotonin seem to be directly involved in the pathophysiology of migraine [86].

Vitamin K2 supplementation can also play a potential role in patients with migraine [197].

6.7. Iron Supplementation

Dietary iron is the primary source of iron in the body [198]. Dietary iron intake has different effects on migraine in women of different ages, and these different effects may be due to age-related menstrual changes [199]. Higher serum levels of ferritin in women over 50 years of age may have a protective effect against migraine [200]. The recommended dietary allowance (RDA) for iron is 18 mg/day for females; however, as evidenced by numerous scientific studies, the average dietary intake of iron for women aged 20 to 50 years old is lower than the RDA [201].

To verify the frequency of migraine attacks in patients with iron deficiency anemia, a study was conducted on 127 subjects who underwent validated tests on migraine, anxiety, depression, and quality of life. The results obtained showed that almost 80% of patients suffered from recurring headaches and that they were often smokers and showed low hemoglobin levels and low mean corpuscular volume values. Moreover, most patients with an iron deficiency presented depression, anxiety, and a poor quality of life [202].

6.8. Polyphenol-Rich Foods Consumption

Polyphenols are important constituents of plant-based foods, closely related to the main sensory and beneficial properties of fruit, vegetables, and their derivatives. Polyphenols can be classified into four main categories (flavonoids, phenolic acids, stilbenes, and lignans) based on the number of phenolic rings and other structural elements that bind these rings together [203]. A diet rich in polyphenols, especially flavanones and lignans, has been associated in the literature with reduced migraine severity. A lower intake of phenols and flavonoids, on the other hand, seems to correlate with more severe migraine attacks. Encouraging the consumption of polyphenol-rich foods, such as fruit, vegetables, and EVOO, can represent a valid adjuvant strategy to counteract migraine [204]. The beneficial analgesic action of polyphenols seems to be mainly exerted by their antioxidant properties. Indeed, the literature studies suggest that OS may play a significant role in the pathogenesis of migraine. The antioxidant compounds contained in foods seem to be able to prevent OS by inhibiting the initiation and propagation of the oxidative chain reaction, which is at the basis of the migraine attack [205].

One of the most controversial polyphenol-rich foods related to migraine onset is chocolate (rich in catechins, flavonols, anthocyanins, and procyanidins). Numerous studies have evaluated the possibility that the consumption of chocolate can stimulate migraine attack onset in subjects who are predisposed to it; however, the pathophysiological mechanisms underlying this correlation have not been elucidated and there is currently insufficient evidence to establish if chocolate is a real migraine trigger [206].

6.9. Magnesium Supplementation

Magnesium is an essential mineral that plays an important role in nerve function [207]. Recent studies have shown, for the general population, a lower average magnesium consumption level than the dietary recommendations, suggesting that a low intake of magnesium may be associated with migraine and that a good percentage of migraine subjects may suffer from a magnesium deficiency [208]. Magnesium inhibits neuronal overexcitation and vasospasm, reduces the formation of inflammatory substances, and improves mitochondrial oxidative phosphorylation and serotonin receptor transmission [209]. At present, most studies on magnesium as a possible preventive treatment for migraine are limited to oral food supplements, not considering magnesium-rich foods [208]. However, most of these oral food supplements have several limitations and side effects, such as GI disorders, nephrolithiasis, and an increased risk of CV disease [210].

6.10. Abstention from Histamine-Rich Food Consumption

Histamine (2-[3H-imidazol-4-yl]ethanamine) activation causes a number of vascular phenomena, which can result in a migraine attack [90,211]. Histamine is a substance that is regularly produced by our body within immune cells [212]. It is a chemical mediator within our body that performs two important functions: a mediator of inflammatory and allergic reactions and a neurotransmitter [212]. Several host factors, in addition to genetic factors, may influence histamine/receptor effects, including the gut microbiota composition, gender, aging, autoimmune diseases, cancer, and pulmonary diseases [213].

Histamine is also a biogenic amine that can be found in many foods; in particular, it may be present in high levels in those foods, often referred to as triggers of migraine in susceptible individuals [214]. The relationship between the diet and migraine has long been controversial and it based on the association between the consumption of certain foods and the manifestation of migraine pain [215]. Many of the foods in question are potentially rich in biologically active amines: histamine, tyramine, and others [216]. Because of the genetic origin, some subjects produce low levels of diaminossidase (DAO) and this means that an excess of histamine is not neutralized and it causes, among other issues, migraine [217]. Mutations involving genes responsible for producing DAO (AOC1 on chromosome 7) can increase the susceptibility to histamine-intolerance development [218]. Some drugs, including NSAIDS, antidepressants, immunomodulators, antiarrhythmics, and other substances (e.g., acetylcysteine, clavulan acid, metoclopramide, and verapamil), may decrease the threshold of tolerance to histamines [219]. Alcohol consumption, in particular, red wine, is a powerful inhibitor of DAO because it also contains, in addition to high levels of histamine, other classes of biogenic amines, such as tyramine and sulfites, which compete with the histamine for binding to the active site of the enzyme [220].

7. Conclusions

Migraine development seems to be partially related to the condition of gut dysbiosis. In fact, it can lead to a reduction in SCFAs production and to a concomitant increase in gut-derived inflammatory cytokines, which can influence CNS activities and, in turn, cause migraine. Moreover, there seems to be a bi-directional correlation between migraine and the risk of CNCDs onset and progression, where the gut microbiota plays a pivotal role.

Besides, numerous studies highlight an association between specific nutritional patterns and lifestyles related to gut eubiosis restoration and the prevention of migraine attacks. Therefore, healthy nutritional habits (such as a MD), an appropriate choice of foods both in quantitative and qualitative terms, oral food supplements administration (such as prebiotics and probiotics), and a constant physical exercise seem to be effective adjuvant strategies for migraine prevention.

The main limitations of this narrative review are certainly to be found in the lacking of this scientific field. In fact, the literature and clinical trials, regarding the link between CNCDs and migraine and the possible role played by gut dysbiosis, are limited and, above all, controversial. To better clarify these possible correlations, it would be useful to perform randomized clinical trials on CNCDs patients with migraine, evaluating the potential presence of gut dysbiosis and monitoring how it can influence the progression of these pathological conditions. Moreover, it would be interesting to examine the positive impacts of possible therapeutic approaches, based on a personalized diet and oral food supplements, formulated *ad hoc*.

Author Contributions: Conceptualization, A.N.; writing—original draft preparation, M.D.L., C.G. and K.C.; writing—review and editing, M.A., M.C. and A.N.; visualization, M.D.L. and C.G.; supervision, N.B.M., N.D.D. and A.N. All authors have read and agreed to the published version of the manuscript.

Funding: This research received no external funding.

Institutional Review Board Statement: Not applicable.

Informed Consent Statement: Not applicable.

Data Availability Statement: Not applicable.

Acknowledgments: We would like to thank Gabriella Venafro for the English language revision.

Conflicts of Interest: The authors declare no conflict of interest.

Abbreviations

5-HT	5-hydroxytryptamine
AH	Arterial Hypertension
BDNF	Brain Neurotrophic Factor
BMI	Body Mass Index
CGRP	Calcitonin Gene-Related Peptide
CKD	Chronic Kidney Disease
CNCDs	Chronic Non-Communicable Diseases
CNS	Central Nervous System
CV	Cardiovascular
DAO	Diaminossidase
DM	Dibetes Mellitus
ED	Endothelial Dysfunction
EPA	Aicosapentaenoic Acid
EVOO	Extra Virgin Olive Oil
FOSs	Fructooligosaccharides
GI	Gastrointestinal
GOSs	Galactogosharides
HPA	Hypothalamic–Pituitary–Adrenal
H3R	Histamine H3 Receptor Agonist
IAA	Indole 3 Acetic Acid
IL	Interleukin
IS	Indoxyl Sulphate
KD	Ketogenic Diet
MD	Mediteranean Diet
MUFAs	Monounsaturated Fatty Acids
NF-κB	Kappa-B Nuclear Factor
NMDA	N-Methyl-D-Aspartic Acid
NO	Nitric Oxide
NSAIDs	Nonsteroidal Anti-Inflammatory Drugs
OS	Oxidative Stress
p-CS	P-Cresyl Sulfate
PUFAs	Polyunsaturated Fatty Acids
RAAS	Renin–Angiotensin–Aldosterone System
RDA	Recommended Dietary Allowance
SCFAs	Short Chain Fatty Acids
TMAO	Trimethylamine N-Oxide
TNF	Tumor Necrosis Factor
WHO	World Health Organization

References

1. Burstein, R.; Noseda, R.; Borsook, D. Migraine: Multiple processes, complex pathophysiology. *J. Neurosci.* **2015**, *35*, 6619–6629. [CrossRef] [PubMed]
2. Stovner, L.J.; Hagen, K.; Linde, M.; Steiner, T.J. The global prevalence of headache: An update, with analysis of the influences of methodological factors on prevalence estimates. *J. Headache Pain* **2022**, *23*, 34. [CrossRef] [PubMed]
3. Steiner, T.J.; Stovner, L.J.; Vos, T.; Jensen, R.; Katsarava, Z. Migraine is first cause of disability in under 50s: Will health politicians now take notice? *J. Headache Pain* **2018**, *19*, 17. [CrossRef] [PubMed]

4. Cieza, A.; Causey, K.; Kamenov, K.; Hanson, S.W.; Chatterji, S.; Vos, T. Global estimates of the need for rehabilitation based on the Global Burden of Disease study 2019: A systematic analysis for the Global Burden of Disease Study 2019. *Lancet* **2021**, *396*, 2006–2017. [CrossRef] [PubMed]
5. Rossi, M.F.; Tumminello, A.; Marconi, M.; Gualano, M.R.; Santoro, P.E.; Malorni, W.; Moscato, U. Sex and gender differences in migraines: A narrative review. *Neurol. Sci.* **2022**, *43*, 5729–5734. [CrossRef]
6. Sacco, S.; Lampl, C.; van den Brink, A.M.; Caponnetto, V.; Braschinsky, M.; Ducros, A.; Little, P.; Pozo-Rosich, P.; Reuter, U.; de la Torre, E.R.; et al. Burden and attitude to resistant and refractory migraine: A survey from the European Headache Federation with the endorsement of the European Migraine & Headache Alliance. *J. Headache Pain* **2021**, *22*, 39. [CrossRef]
7. Tonini, M.C.; Fiorencis, A.; Iannacchero, R.; Zampolini, M.; Cappuccio, A.; Raddino, R.; Grillo, E.; Albanese, M.; Allais, G.; Bassano, M.A.; et al. Narrative Medicine to integrate patients', caregivers' and clinicians' migraine experiences: The DRONE multicentre project. *Neurol. Sci.* **2021**, *42*, 5277–5288. [CrossRef]
8. Burch, R.C.; Buse, D.C.; Lipton, R.B. Migraine: Epidemiology, Burden, and Comorbidity. *Neurol. Clin.* **2019**, *37*, 631–649. [CrossRef]
9. Paredes, S.; Cantillo, S.; Candido, K.D.; Knezevic, N.N. An Association of Serotonin with Pain Disorders and Its Modulation by Estrogens. *Int. J. Mol. Sci.* **2019**, *20*, 5729. [CrossRef]
10. Calhoun, A.H.; Batur, P. Combined hormonal contraceptives and migraine: An update on the evidence. *Cleve. Clin. J. Med.* **2017**, *84*, 631–638. [CrossRef]
11. Calhoun, A.H. Hormonal Contraceptives and Migraine With Aura-Is There Still a Risk? *Headache* **2017**, *57*, 184–193. [CrossRef] [PubMed]
12. Lee, A.; Syed, Y.Y. Estetrol/Drospirenone: A Review in Oral Contraception. *Drugs* **2022**, *82*, 1117–1125. [CrossRef] [PubMed]
13. Gasparini, C.F.; Smith, R.A.; Griffiths, L.R. Genetic and biochemical changes of the serotonergic system in migraine pathobiology. *J. Headache Pain* **2017**, *18*, 20. [CrossRef] [PubMed]
14. Zhang, Q.; Shao, A.; Jiang, Z.; Tsai, H.; Liu, W. The exploration of mechanisms of comorbidity between migraine and depression. *J. Cell Mol. Med.* **2019**, *23*, 4505–4513. [CrossRef] [PubMed]
15. Peres, M.F.P.; Mercante, J.P.P.; Tobo, P.R.; Kamei, H.; Bigal, M.E. Anxiety and depression symptoms and migraine: A symptom-based approach research. *J. Headache Pain* **2017**, *18*, 37. [CrossRef]
16. Stubberud, A.; Buse, D.C.; Kristoffersen, E.S.; Linde, M.; Tronvik, E. Is there a causal relationship between stress and migraine? Current evidence and implications for management. *J. Headache Pain* **2021**, *22*, 155. [CrossRef]
17. Radat, F. Stress and migraine. *Rev. Neurol.* **2013**, *169*, 406–412. [CrossRef]
18. Klan, T.; Diezemann-Prossdorf, A.; Guth, A.L.; Gaul, C.; Witthoft, M. Fear of migraine attacks: Diagnosis and treatment. *Schmerz* **2023**, 1–8. [CrossRef]
19. Tepper, S.J. Medication-overuse headache. *Continuum* **2012**, *18*, 807–822. [CrossRef]
20. Tfelt-Hansen, P.C.; Tfelt-Hansen, J. Nitroglycerin headache and nitroglycerin-induced primary headaches from 1846 and onwards: A historical overview and an update. *Headache* **2009**, *49*, 445–456. [CrossRef]
21. Lance, J.W. 5-Hydroxytryptamine and its role in migraine. *Eur. Neurol.* **1991**, *31*, 279–281. [CrossRef]
22. Connor, J.P.; Stjepanovic, D.; Budney, A.J.; Le Foll, B.; Hall, W.D. Clinical management of cannabis withdrawal. *Addiction* **2022**, *117*, 2075–2095. [CrossRef] [PubMed]
23. Farooque, U.; Okorie, N.; Kataria, S.; Shah, S.F.; Bollampally, V.C. Cocaine-Induced Headache: A Review of Pathogenesis, Presentation, Diagnosis, and Management. *Cureus* **2020**, *12*, e10128. [CrossRef] [PubMed]
24. Takahashi, T.T.; Ornello, R.; Quatrosi, G.; Torrente, A.; Albanese, M.; Vigneri, S.; Guglielmetti, M.; Maria De Marco, C.; Dutordoir, C.; Colangeli, E.; et al. Medication overuse and drug addiction: A narrative review from addiction perspective. *J. Headache Pain* **2021**, *22*, 32. [CrossRef] [PubMed]
25. Marmura, M.J. Triggers, Protectors, and Predictors in Episodic Migraine. *Curr. Pain Headache Rep.* **2018**, *22*, 81. [CrossRef]
26. Minen, M.T.; Begasse De Dhaem, O.; Kroon Van Diest, A.; Powers, S.; Schwedt, T.J.; Lipton, R.; Silbersweig, D. Migraine and its psychiatric comorbidities. *J. Neurol. Neurosurg. Psychiatry* **2016**, *87*, 741–749. [CrossRef]
27. Noce, A.; Marchetti, M.; Marrone, G.; Di Renzo, L.; Di Lauro, M.; Di Daniele, F.; Albanese, M.; Di Daniele, N.; De Lorenzo, A. Link between gut microbiota dysbiosis and chronic kidney disease. *Eur. Rev. Med. Pharmacol. Sci.* **2022**, *26*, 2057–2074. [CrossRef]
28. Noce, A.; Marrone, G.; Di Daniele, F.; Ottaviani, E.; Wilson Jones, G.; Bernini, R.; Romani, A.; Rovella, V. Impact of Gut Microbiota Composition on Onset and Progression of Chronic Non-Communicable Diseases. *Nutrients* **2019**, *11*, 1073. [CrossRef]
29. Ceppa, F.A.; Izzo, L.; Sardelli, L.; Raimondi, I.; Tunesi, M.; Albani, D.; Giordano, C. Human Gut-Microbiota Interaction in Neurodegenerative Disorders and Current Engineered Tools for Its Modeling. *Front. Cell Infect. Microbiol.* **2020**, *10*, 297. [CrossRef]
30. Cryan, J.F.; O'Riordan, K.J.; Cowan, C.S.M.; Sandhu, K.V.; Bastiaanssen, T.F.S.; Boehme, M.; Codagnone, M.G.; Cussotto, S.; Fulling, C.; Golubeva, A.V.; et al. The Microbiota-Gut-Brain Axis. *Physiol. Rev.* **2019**, *99*, 1877–2013. [CrossRef]
31. Matijasic, M.; Mestrovic, T.; Paljetak, H.C.; Peric, M.; Baresic, A.; Verbanac, D. Gut Microbiota beyond Bacteria-Mycobiome, Virome, Archaeome, and Eukaryotic Parasites in IBD. *Int. J. Mol. Sci.* **2020**, *21*, 2668. [CrossRef] [PubMed]
32. Hills, R.D., Jr.; Pontefract, B.A.; Mishcon, H.R.; Black, C.A.; Sutton, S.C.; Theberge, C.R. Gut Microbiome: Profound Implications for Diet and Disease. *Nutrients* **2019**, *11*, 1613. [CrossRef] [PubMed]

33. Gonzalez-Sarrias, A.; Romo-Vaquero, M.; Garcia-Villalba, R.; Cortes-Martin, A.; Selma, M.V.; Espin, J.C. The Endotoxemia Marker Lipopolysaccharide-Binding Protein is Reduced in Overweight-Obese Subjects Consuming Pomegranate Extract by Modulating the Gut Microbiota: A Randomized Clinical Trial. *Mol. Nutr. Food Res.* **2018**, *62*, e1800160. [CrossRef] [PubMed]
34. Bjorksten, B. The gut microbiota: A complex ecosystem. *Clin. Exp. Allergy* **2006**, *36*, 1215–1217. [CrossRef] [PubMed]
35. Chakaroun, R.M.; Massier, L.; Kovacs, P. Gut Microbiome, Intestinal Permeability, and Tissue Bacteria in Metabolic Disease: Perpetrators or Bystanders? *Nutrients* **2020**, *12*, 1082. [CrossRef] [PubMed]
36. Rodriguez, J.M.; Murphy, K.; Stanton, C.; Ross, R.P.; Kober, O.I.; Juge, N.; Avershina, E.; Rudi, K.; Narbad, A.; Jenmalm, M.C.; et al. The composition of the gut microbiota throughout life, with an emphasis on early life. *Microb. Ecol. Health Dis.* **2015**, *26*, 26050. [CrossRef] [PubMed]
37. Thursby, E.; Juge, N. Introduction to the human gut microbiota. *Biochem. J.* **2017**, *474*, 1823–1836. [CrossRef]
38. Mackowiak, P.A. Recycling metchnikoff: Probiotics, the intestinal microbiome and the quest for long life. *Front. Public Health* **2013**, *1*, 52. [CrossRef]
39. Belkaid, Y.; Hand, T.W. Role of the microbiota in immunity and inflammation. *Cell* **2014**, *157*, 121–141. [CrossRef]
40. Rowland, I.; Gibson, G.; Heinken, A.; Scott, K.; Swann, J.; Thiele, I.; Tuohy, K. Gut microbiota functions: Metabolism of nutrients and other food components. *Eur. J. Nutr.* **2018**, *57*, 1–24. [CrossRef]
41. Miller, I. The gut-brain axis: Historical reflections. *Microb. Ecol. Health Dis.* **2018**, *29*, 1542921. [CrossRef] [PubMed]
42. Wang, W.L.; Xu, S.Y.; Ren, Z.G.; Tao, L.; Jiang, J.W.; Zheng, S.S. Application of metagenomics in the human gut microbiome. *World J. Gastroenterol.* **2015**, *21*, 803–814. [CrossRef] [PubMed]
43. Rinninella, E.; Raoul, P.; Cintoni, M.; Franceschi, F.; Miggiano, G.A.D.; Gasbarrini, A.; Mele, M.C. What is the Healthy Gut Microbiota Composition? A Changing Ecosystem across Age, Environment, Diet, and Diseases. *Microorganisms* **2019**, *7*, 14. [CrossRef]
44. Bull, M.J.; Plummer, N.T. Part 1: The Human Gut Microbiome in Health and Disease. *Integr. Med.* **2014**, *13*, 17–22.
45. Walker, R.W.; Clemente, J.C.; Peter, I.; Loos, R.J.F. The prenatal gut microbiome: Are we colonized with bacteria in utero? *Pediatr. Obes.* **2017**, *12* (Suppl. 1), 3–17. [CrossRef]
46. Tanaka, M.; Nakayama, J. Development of the gut microbiota in infancy and its impact on health in later life. *Allergol. Int.* **2017**, *66*, 515–522. [CrossRef] [PubMed]
47. Nyangahu, D.D.; Jaspan, H.B. Influence of maternal microbiota during pregnancy on infant immunity. *Clin. Exp. Immunol.* **2019**, *198*, 47–56. [CrossRef] [PubMed]
48. Easton, Z.J.W.; Regnault, T.R.H. The Impact of Maternal Body Composition and Dietary Fat Consumption upon Placental Lipid Processing and Offspring Metabolic Health. *Nutrients* **2020**, *12*, 3031. [CrossRef]
49. Kapoor, A.; Dunn, E.; Kostaki, A.; Andrews, M.H.; Matthews, S.G. Fetal programming of hypothalamo-pituitary-adrenal function: Prenatal stress and glucocorticoids. *J. Physiol.* **2006**, *572*, 31–44. [CrossRef]
50. Arboleya, S.; Watkins, C.; Stanton, C.; Ross, R.P. Gut Bifidobacteria Populations in Human Health and Aging. *Front. Microbiol.* **2016**, *7*, 1204. [CrossRef]
51. Manor, O.; Dai, C.L.; Kornilov, S.A.; Smith, B.; Price, N.D.; Lovejoy, J.C.; Gibbons, S.M.; Magis, A.T. Health and disease markers correlate with gut microbiome composition across thousands of people. *Nat. Commun.* **2020**, *11*, 5206. [CrossRef] [PubMed]
52. Pickard, J.M.; Zeng, M.Y.; Caruso, R.; Nunez, G. Gut microbiota: Role in pathogen colonization, immune responses, and inflammatory disease. *Immunol. Rev.* **2017**, *279*, 70–89. [CrossRef] [PubMed]
53. Hagerty, S.L.; Hutchison, K.E.; Lowry, C.A.; Bryan, A.D. An empirically derived method for measuring human gut microbiome alpha diversity: Demonstrated utility in predicting health-related outcomes among a human clinical sample. *PLoS ONE* **2020**, *15*, e0229204. [CrossRef] [PubMed]
54. Conlon, M.A.; Bird, A.R. The impact of diet and lifestyle on gut microbiota and human health. *Nutrients* **2014**, *7*, 17–44. [CrossRef]
55. Canale, M.P.; Noce, A.; Di Lauro, M.; Marrone, G.; Cantelmo, M.; Cardillo, C.; Federici, M.; Di Daniele, N.; Tesauro, M. Gut Dysbiosis and Western Diet in the Pathogenesis of Essential Arterial Hypertension: A Narrative Review. *Nutrients* **2021**, *13*, 1162. [CrossRef]
56. Kim, S.; Jazwinski, S.M. The Gut Microbiota and Healthy Aging: A Mini-Review. *Gerontology* **2018**, *64*, 513–520. [CrossRef]
57. Salazar, N.; Arboleya, S.; Fernandez-Navarro, T.; de Los Reyes-Gavilan, C.G.; Gonzalez, S.; Gueimonde, M. Age-Associated Changes in Gut Microbiota and Dietary Components Related with the Immune System in Adulthood and Old Age: A Cross-Sectional Study. *Nutrients* **2019**, *11*, 1765. [CrossRef]
58. Lin, X.; Liang, W.; Li, L.; Xiong, Q.; He, S.; Zhao, J.; Guo, X.; Xiang, S.; Zhang, P.; Wang, H.; et al. The Accumulation of Gut Microbiome-derived Indoxyl Sulfate and P-Cresyl Sulfate in Patients With End-stage Renal Disease. *J. Ren. Nutr.* **2022**, *32*, 578–586. [CrossRef]
59. Noce, A.; Marrone, G.; Ottaviani, E.; Guerriero, C.; Di Daniele, F.; Pietroboni Zaitseva, A.; Di Daniele, N. Uremic Sarcopenia and Its Possible Nutritional Approach. *Nutrients* **2021**, *13*, 147. [CrossRef]
60. Raspini, B.; Vacca, M.; Porri, D.; De Giuseppe, R.; Calabrese, F.M.; Chieppa, M.; Liso, M.; Cerbo, R.M.; Civardi, E.; Garofoli, F.; et al. Early Life Microbiota Colonization at Six Months of Age: A Transitional Time Point. *Front. Cell. Infect. Microbiol.* **2021**, *11*, 590202. [CrossRef]
61. Zhou, L.; Xiao, X. The role of gut microbiota in the effects of maternal obesity during pregnancy on offspring metabolism. *Biosci. Rep.* **2018**, *38*, BSR20171234. [CrossRef] [PubMed]

62. Fouhy, F.; Watkins, C.; Hill, C.J.; O'Shea, C.A.; Nagle, B.; Dempsey, E.M.; O'Toole, P.W.; Ross, R.P.; Ryan, C.A.; Stanton, C. Perinata factors affect the gut microbiota up to four years after birth. *Nat. Commun.* **2019**, *10*, 1517. [CrossRef] [PubMed]
63. Ramirez, J.; Guarner, F.; Bustos Fernandez, L.; Maruy, A.; Sdepanian, V.L.; Cohen, H. Antibiotics as Major Disruptors of Gu Microbiota. *Front. Cell. Infect. Microbiol.* **2020**, *10*, 572912. [CrossRef]
64. Carabotti, M.; Scirocco, A.; Maselli, M.A.; Severi, C. The gut-brain axis: Interactions between enteric microbiota, central and enteric nervous systems. *Ann. Gastroenterol.* **2015**, *28*, 203–209. [PubMed]
65. Perez-Cobas, A.E.; Moya, A.; Gosalbes, M.J.; Latorre, A. Colonization Resistance of the Gut Microbiota against Clostridium difficile. *Antibiotics* **2015**, *4*, 337–357. [CrossRef]
66. Langdon, A.; Crook, N.; Dantas, G. The effects of antibiotics on the microbiome throughout development and alternative approaches for therapeutic modulation. *Genome Med.* **2016**, *8*, 39. [CrossRef]
67. Elvers, K.T.; Wilson, V.J.; Hammond, A.; Duncan, L.; Huntley, A.L.; Hay, A.D.; van der Werf, E.T. Antibiotic-induced changes in the human gut microbiota for the most commonly prescribed antibiotics in primary care in the UK: A systematic review. *BMJ Open* **2020**, *10*, e035677. [CrossRef]
68. Coelho, G.D.P.; Ayres, L.F.A.; Barreto, D.S.; Henriques, B.D.; Prado, M.; Passos, C.M.D. Acquisition of microbiota according to the type of birth: An integrative review. *Rev. Lat. Am. Enfermagem.* **2021**, *29*, e3446. [CrossRef]
69. Mitchell, C.M.; Mazzoni, C.; Hogstrom, L.; Bryant, A.; Bergerat, A.; Cher, A.; Pochan, S.; Herman, P.; Carrigan, M.; Sharp, K.; et al Delivery Mode Affects Stability of Early Infant Gut Microbiota. *Cell Rep. Med.* **2020**, *1*, 100156. [CrossRef]
70. Ma, J.; Li, Z.; Zhang, W.; Zhang, C.; Zhang, Y.; Mei, H.; Zhuo, N.; Wang, H.; Wang, L.; Wu, D. Comparison of gut microbiota in exclusively breast-fed and formula-fed babies: A study of 91 term infants. *Sci. Rep.* **2020**, *10*, 15792. [CrossRef]
71. Stanislawski, M.A.; Dabelea, D.; Wagner, B.D.; Sontag, M.K.; Lozupone, C.A.; Eggesbo, M. Pre-pregnancy weight, gestational weight gain, and the gut microbiota of mothers and their infants. *Microbiome* **2017**, *5*, 113. [CrossRef] [PubMed]
72. Dorelli, B.; Galle, F.; De Vito, C.; Duranti, G.; Iachini, M.; Zaccarin, M.; Preziosi Standoli, J.; Ceci, R.; Romano, F.; Liguori, G.; et al Can Physical Activity Influence Human Gut Microbiota Composition Independently of Diet? A Systematic Review. *Nutrients* **2021**, *13*, 1890. [CrossRef] [PubMed]
73. Dziewiecka, H.; Buttar, H.S.; Kasperska, A.; Ostapiuk-Karolczuk, J.; Domagalska, M.; Cichon, J.; Skarpanska-Stejnborn, A Physical activity induced alterations of gut microbiota in humans: A systematic review. *BMC Sports Sci. Med. Rehabil.* **2022**, *14*, 122. [CrossRef] [PubMed]
74. Noce, A.; Tranchita, E.; Marrone, G.; Grazioli, E.; Di Lauro, M.; Murri, A.; Vanni, G.; Della Morte Canosci, D.; Di Daniele, N.; Parisi, A.; et al. The possible role of physical activity in the modulation of gut microbiota in chronic kidney disease and its impact on cardiovascular risk: A narrative review. *Eur. Rev. Med. Pharmacol. Sci.* **2023**, *27*, 3733–3746. [CrossRef] [PubMed]
75. Aragon-Vela, J.; Solis-Urra, P.; Ruiz-Ojeda, F.J.; Alvarez-Mercado, A.I.; Olivares-Arancibia, J.; Plaza-Diaz, J. Impact of Exercise on Gut Microbiota in Obesity. *Nutrients* **2021**, *13*, 3999. [CrossRef]
76. Katzmarzyk, P.T. Physical activity, sedentary behavior, and health: Paradigm paralysis or paradigm shift? *Diabetes* **2010**, *59*, 2717–2725. [CrossRef]
77. Vijay, A.; Valdes, A.M. Role of the gut microbiome in chronic diseases: A narrative review. *Eur. J. Clin. Nutr.* **2022**, *76*, 489–501. [CrossRef]
78. Ojeda, J.; Avila, A.; Vidal, P.M. Gut Microbiota Interaction with the Central Nervous System throughout Life. *J. Clin. Med.* **2021**, *10*, 1299. [CrossRef]
79. Martin, C.R.; Osadchiy, V.; Kalani, A.; Mayer, E.A. The Brain-Gut-Microbiome Axis. *Cell. Mol. Gastroenterol. Hepatol.* **2018**, *6*, 133–148. [CrossRef]
80. Novellino, F.; Sacca, V.; Donato, A.; Zaffino, P.; Spadea, M.F.; Vismara, M.; Arcidiacono, B.; Malara, N.; Presta, I.; Donato, G. Innate Immunity: A Common Denominator between Neurodegenerative and Neuropsychiatric Diseases. *Int. J. Mol. Sci.* **2020**, *21*, 1115. [CrossRef]
81. Maiuolo, J.; Gliozzi, M.; Musolino, V.; Carresi, C.; Scarano, F.; Nucera, S.; Scicchitano, M.; Oppedisano, F.; Bosco, F.; Ruga, S.; et al. The Contribution of Gut Microbiota-Brain Axis in the Development of Brain Disorders. *Front. Neurosci.* **2021**, *15*, 616883. [CrossRef]
82. Kappeter, A.; Sipos, D.; Varga, A.; Vigvari, S.; Halda-Kiss, B.; Peterfi, Z. Migraine as a Disease Associated with Dysbiosis and Possible Therapy with Fecal Microbiota Transplantation. *Microorganisms* **2023**, *11*, 2083. [CrossRef] [PubMed]
83. Zhu, X.; Han, Y.; Du, J.; Liu, R.; Jin, K.; Yi, W. Microbiota-gut-brain axis and the central nervous system. *Oncotarget* **2017**, *8*, 53829–53838. [CrossRef] [PubMed]
84. Socala, K.; Doboszewska, U.; Szopa, A.; Serefko, A.; Wlodarczyk, M.; Zielinska, A.; Poleszak, E.; Fichna, J.; Wlaz, P. The role of microbiota-gut-brain axis in neuropsychiatric and neurological disorders. *Pharmacol. Res.* **2021**, *172*, 105840. [CrossRef] [PubMed]
85. Ochoa-Reparaz, J.; Kasper, L.H. The Second Brain: Is the Gut Microbiota a Link between Obesity and Central Nervous System Disorders? *Curr. Obes. Rep.* **2016**, *5*, 51–64. [CrossRef] [PubMed]
86. Hamel, E. Serotonin and migraine: Biology and clinical implications. *Cephalalgia* **2007**, *27*, 1293–1300. [CrossRef]
87. Deen, M.; Christensen, C.E.; Hougaard, A.; Hansen, H.D.; Knudsen, G.M.; Ashina, M. Serotonergic mechanisms in the migraine brain—A systematic review. *Cephalalgia* **2017**, *37*, 251–264. [CrossRef]
88. Ferrari, M.D.; Goadsby, P.J.; Roon, K.I.; Lipton, R.B. Triptans (serotonin, 5-HT1B/1D agonists) in migraine: Detailed results and methods of a meta-analysis of 53 trials. *Cephalalgia* **2002**, *22*, 633–658. [CrossRef]

89. Heatley, R.V.; Denburg, J.A.; Bayer, N.; Bienenstock, J. Increased plasma histamine levels in migraine patients. *Clin. Allergy* **1982**, *12*, 145–149. [CrossRef]
90. Worm, J.; Falkenberg, K.; Olesen, J. Histamine and migraine revisited: Mechanisms and possible drug targets. *J. Headache Pain* **2019**, *20*, 30. [CrossRef]
91. Yuan, H.; Silberstein, S.D. Histamine and Migraine. *Headache* **2018**, *58*, 184–193. [CrossRef] [PubMed]
92. Aamodt, A.H.; Stovner, L.J.; Hagen, K.; Zwart, J.A. Comorbidity of headache and gastrointestinal complaints. The Head-HUNT Study. *Cephalalgia* **2008**, *28*, 144–151. [CrossRef] [PubMed]
93. Camara-Lemarroy, C.R.; Rodriguez-Gutierrez, R.; Monreal-Robles, R.; Marfil-Rivera, A. Gastrointestinal disorders associated with migraine: A comprehensive review. *World J. Gastroenterol.* **2016**, *22*, 8149–8160. [CrossRef] [PubMed]
94. Chang, F.Y.; Lu, C.L. Irritable bowel syndrome and migraine: Bystanders or partners? *J. Neurogastroenterol. Motil.* **2013**, *19*, 301–311. [CrossRef]
95. Zanos, T.P.; Silverman, H.A.; Levy, T.; Tsaava, T.; Battinelli, E.; Lorraine, P.W.; Ashe, J.M.; Chavan, S.S.; Tracey, K.J.; Bouton, C.E. Identification of cytokine-specific sensory neural signals by decoding murine vagus nerve activity. *Proc. Natl. Acad. Sci. USA* **2018**, *115*, E4843–E4852. [CrossRef]
96. Cook, T.M.; Gavini, C.K.; Jesse, J.; Aubert, G.; Gornick, E.; Bonomo, R.; Gautron, L.; Layden, B.T.; Mansuy-Aubert, V. Vagal neuron expression of the microbiota-derived metabolite receptor, free fatty acid receptor (FFAR3), is necessary for normal feeding behavior. *Mol. Metab.* **2021**, *54*, 101350. [CrossRef]
97. Crawford, J.; Liu, S.; Tao, F. Gut microbiota and migraine. *Neurobiol. Pain* **2022**, *11*, 100090. [CrossRef]
98. Tang, Y.; Liu, S.; Shu, H.; Yanagisawa, L.; Tao, F. Gut Microbiota Dysbiosis Enhances Migraine-Like Pain Via TNFalpha Upregulation. *Mol. Neurobiol.* **2020**, *57*, 461–468. [CrossRef]
99. David, L.A.; Materna, A.C.; Friedman, J.; Campos-Baptista, M.I.; Blackburn, M.C.; Perrotta, A.; Erdman, S.E.; Alm, E.J. Host lifestyle affects human microbiota on daily timescales. *Genome Biol.* **2014**, *15*, R89. [CrossRef]
100. Singh, R.K.; Chang, H.W.; Yan, D.; Lee, K.M.; Ucmak, D.; Wong, K.; Abrouk, M.; Farahnik, B.; Nakamura, M.; Zhu, T.H.; et al. Influence of diet on the gut microbiome and implications for human health. *J. Transl. Med.* **2017**, *15*, 73. [CrossRef]
101. Ramsden, C.E.; Zamora, D.; Faurot, K.R.; MacIntosh, B.; Horowitz, M.; Keyes, G.S.; Yuan, Z.X.; Miller, V.; Lynch, C.; Honvoh, G.; et al. Dietary alteration of n-3 and n-6 fatty acids for headache reduction in adults with migraine: Randomized controlled trial. *BMJ* **2021**, *374*, n1448. [CrossRef] [PubMed]
102. Haghighi, F.S.; Rahmanian, M.; Namiranian, N.; Arzaghi, S.M.; Dehghan, F.; Chavoshzade, F.; Sepehri, F. Migraine and type 2 diabetes; is there any association? *J. Diabetes Metab. Disord.* **2015**, *15*, 37. [CrossRef]
103. Lopez-de-Andres, A.; Luis Del Barrio, J.; Hernandez-Barrera, V.; de Miguel-Diez, J.; Jimenez-Trujillo, I.; Martinez-Huedo, M.A.; Jimenez-Garcia, R. Migraine in adults with diabetes; is there an association? Results of a population-based study. *Diabetes Metab. Syndr. Obes.* **2018**, *11*, 367–374. [CrossRef] [PubMed]
104. Cheon, D.Y.; Han, K.; Yang, Y.S.; Kim, Y.; Lee, S.H.; Kim, C.; Sohn, J.H.; Oh, M.S.; Lee, B.C.; Lee, M.; et al. Associations between migraine and major cardiovascular events in type 2 diabetes mellitus. *Cardiovasc. Diabetol.* **2022**, *21*, 275. [CrossRef]
105. Bhoi, S.K.; Kalita, J.; Misra, U.K. Metabolic syndrome and insulin resistance in migraine. *J. Headache Pain* **2012**, *13*, 321–326. [CrossRef] [PubMed]
106. Ali, M.; Hussein, M.; Magdy, R.; Khamis, A.; Al-Azayem, S.A.; Othman, A.M.; Ahmed, A.; Osama, W. The potential impact of insulin resistance and metabolic syndrome on migraine headache characteristics. *BMC Neurol.* **2022**, *22*, 422. [CrossRef] [PubMed]
107. Zhang, Q.; Jin, K.; Chen, B.; Liu, R.; Cheng, S.; Zhang, Y.; Lu, J. Overnutrition Induced Cognitive Impairment: Insulin Resistance, Gut-Brain Axis, and Neuroinflammation. *Front. Neurosci.* **2022**, *16*, 884579. [CrossRef] [PubMed]
108. Van Dyken, P.; Lacoste, B. Impact of Metabolic Syndrome on Neuroinflammation and the Blood-Brain Barrier. *Front. Neurosci.* **2018**, *12*, 930. [CrossRef]
109. Hagen, K.; Asvold, B.O.; Midthjell, K.; Stovner, L.J.; Zwart, J.A.; Linde, M. Inverse relationship between type 1 diabetes mellitus and migraine. Data from the Nord-Trondelag Health Surveys 1995–1997 and 2006–2008. *Cephalalgia* **2018**, *38*, 417–426. [CrossRef]
110. Berge, L.I.; Riise, T.; Fasmer, O.B.; Hundal, O.; Oedegaard, K.J.; Midthjell, K.; Lund, A. Does diabetes have a protective effect on migraine? *Epidemiology* **2013**, *24*, 129–134. [CrossRef]
111. Aamodt, A.H.; Stovner, L.J.; Midthjell, K.; Hagen, K.; Zwart, J.A. Headache prevalence related to diabetes mellitus. The Head-HUNT study. *Eur. J. Neurol.* **2007**, *14*, 738–744. [CrossRef] [PubMed]
112. Fagherazzi, G.; El Fatouhi, D.; Fournier, A.; Gusto, G.; Mancini, F.R.; Balkau, B.; Boutron-Ruault, M.C.; Kurth, T.; Bonnet, F. Associations between Migraine and Type 2 Diabetes in Women: Findings From the E3N Cohort Study. *JAMA Neurol.* **2019**, *76*, 257–263. [CrossRef] [PubMed]
113. Friedman, B.W.; Mistry, B.; West, J.R.; Wollowitz, A. The association between headache and elevated blood pressure among patients presenting to an ED. *Am. J. Emerg. Med.* **2014**, *32*, 976–981. [CrossRef] [PubMed]
114. Paolucci, M.; Altamura, C.; Vernieri, F. The Role of Endothelial Dysfunction in the Pathophysiology and Cerebrovascular Effects of Migraine: A Narrative Review. *J. Clin. Neurol.* **2021**, *17*, 164–175. [CrossRef] [PubMed]
115. Tronvik, E.; Stovner, L.J.; Helde, G.; Sand, T.; Bovim, G. Prophylactic treatment of migraine with an angiotensin II receptor blocker: A randomized controlled trial. *JAMA* **2003**, *289*, 65–69. [CrossRef]

116. Mahmoud, A.N.; Mentias, A.; Elgendy, A.Y.; Qazi, A.; Barakat, A.F.; Saad, M.; Mohsen, A.; Abuzaid, A.; Mansoor, H.; Mojadidi, M.K.; et al. Migraine and the risk of cardiovascular and cerebrovascular events: A meta-analysis of 16 cohort studies including 1 152 407 subjects. *BMJ Open* **2018**, *8*, e020498. [CrossRef]
117. Olesen, J. The role of nitric oxide (NO) in migraine, tension-type headache and cluster headache. *Pharmacol. Ther.* **2008**, *120*, 157–171. [CrossRef]
118. Entonen, A.H.; Suominen, S.B.; Sillanmaki, L.H.; Rautava, P.T.; Kauniskangas, K.; Mantyselka, P.T.; Sumanen, M.; Koskenvuo, M.J. Prevalent migraine as a predictor of incident hypertension. *Eur. J. Public Health* **2022**, *32*, 297–301. [CrossRef] [PubMed]
119. Gales, B.J.; Bailey, E.K.; Reed, A.N.; Gales, M.A. Angiotensin-converting enzyme inhibitors and angiotensin receptor blockers for the prevention of migraines. *Ann. Pharmacother.* **2010**, *44*, 360–366. [CrossRef]
120. Barbanti, P.; Aurilia, C.; Egeo, G.; Fofi, L. Hypertension as a risk factor for migraine chronification. *Neurol. Sci.* **2010**, *31* (Suppl. 1), S41–S43. [CrossRef]
121. Manna, P.; Jain, S.K. Obesity, Oxidative Stress, Adipose Tissue Dysfunction, and the Associated Health Risks: Causes and Therapeutic Strategies. *Metab. Syndr. Relat. Disord.* **2015**, *13*, 423–444. [CrossRef]
122. Bleich, S.; Cutler, D.; Murray, C.; Adams, A. Why is the developed world obese? *Annu. Rev. Public Health* **2008**, *29*, 273–295. [CrossRef] [PubMed]
123. Gelaye, B.; Sacco, S.; Brown, W.J.; Nitchie, H.L.; Ornello, R.; Peterlin, B.L. Body composition status and the risk of migraine: A meta-analysis. *Neurology* **2017**, *88*, 1795–1804. [CrossRef] [PubMed]
124. Arzani, M.; Jahromi, S.R.; Ghorbani, Z.; Vahabizad, F.; Martelletti, P.; Ghaemi, A.; Sacco, S.; Togha, M.; School of Advanced Studies of the European Headache Federation (EHF-SAS). Gut-brain Axis and migraine headache: A comprehensive review. *J. Headache Pain* **2020**, *21*, 15. [CrossRef] [PubMed]
125. Westgate, C.S.J.; Israelsen, I.M.E.; Jensen, R.H.; Eftekhari, S. Understanding the link between obesity and headache- with focus on migraine and idiopathic intracranial hypertension. *J. Headache Pain* **2021**, *22*, 123. [CrossRef] [PubMed]
126. Kany, S.; Vollrath, J.T.; Relja, B. Cytokines in Inflammatory Disease. *Int. J. Mol. Sci.* **2019**, *20*, 6008. [CrossRef]
127. Wu, X.; Wang, M.; Li, S.; Zhang, Y. Migraine and breast cancer risk: A meta-analysis of observational studies based on MOOSE compliant. *Medicine* **2016**, *95*, e4031. [CrossRef]
128. Elser, H.; Skajaa, N.; Ehrenstein, V.; Fuglsang, C.H.; Farkas, D.K.; Sorensen, H.T. Cancer risk in patients with migraine: A population-based cohort study in Denmark. *Headache* **2022**, *62*, 57–64. [CrossRef]
129. Chen, C.H.; Sheu, J.J.; Lin, Y.C.; Lin, H.C. Association of migraines with brain tumors: A nationwide population-based study. *J. Headache Pain* **2018**, *19*, 111. [CrossRef]
130. Goldlust, S.A.; Graber, J.J.; Bossert, D.F.; Avila, E.K. Headache in patients with cancer. *Curr. Pain Headache Rep.* **2010**, *14*, 455–464. [CrossRef]
131. Bernstein, C.A. Evaluation of headache in patients with cancer. *Cancer* **2021**, *127*, 4368–4375. [CrossRef] [PubMed]
132. Weng, S.C.; Wu, C.L.; Kor, C.T.; Chiu, P.F.; Wu, M.J.; Chang, C.C.; Tarng, D.C. Migraine and subsequent chronic kidney disease risk: A nationwide population-based cohort study. *BMJ Open* **2017**, *7*, e018483. [CrossRef] [PubMed]
133. Zhang, W.; Zhang, L.; Yang, L.; Xiao, C.; Wu, X.; Yan, P.; Cui, H.; Yang, C.; Zhu, J.; Wu, X.; et al. Migraine, chronic kidney disease and kidney function: Observational and genetic analyses. *Hum. Genet.* **2023**, *142*, 1185–1200. [CrossRef] [PubMed]
134. Rahman, A.; Segasothy, M.; Samad, S.A.; Zulfiqar, A.; Rani, M. Analgesic use and chronic renal disease in patients with headache. *Headache* **1993**, *33*, 442–445. [CrossRef] [PubMed]
135. Arnold, M. Headache Classification Committee of the International Headache Society (IHS) The International Classification of Headache Disorders, 3rd edition. *Cephalalgia* **2018**, *38*, 1–211. [CrossRef]
136. Chhaya, K.T.; Mankad, S.; Shah, M.K.; Patel, M.; Desai, D.; Desai, S.D. Headache Associated with Hemodialysis in Patients with End-Stage Renal Disease in India: A Common Yet Overlooked Comorbidity. *Ann. Indian Acad. Neurol.* **2022**, *25*, 82–87. [CrossRef]
137. Silberstein, S.D. Preventive Migraine Treatment. *Continuum* **2015**, *21*, 973–989. [CrossRef]
138. Kesserwani, H. Migraine Triggers: An Overview of the Pharmacology, Biochemistry, Atmospherics, and Their Effects on Neural Networks. *Cureus* **2021**, *13*, e14243. [CrossRef]
139. Gazerani, P. Migraine and Diet. *Nutrients* **2020**, *12*, 1658. [CrossRef]
140. Bagdy, G.; Riba, P.; Kecskemeti, V.; Chase, D.; Juhasz, G. Headache-type adverse effects of NO donors: Vasodilation and beyond. *Br. J. Pharmacol.* **2010**, *160*, 20–35. [CrossRef]
141. Lacatusu, C.M.; Grigorescu, E.D.; Floria, M.; Onofriescu, A.; Mihai, B.M. The Mediterranean Diet: From an Environment-Driven Food Culture to an Emerging Medical Prescription. *Int. J. Environ. Res. Public Health* **2019**, *16*, 942. [CrossRef] [PubMed]
142. Aridi, Y.S.; Walker, J.L.; Roura, E.; Wright, O.R.L. Adherence to the Mediterranean Diet and Chronic Disease in Australia: National Nutrition and Physical Activity Survey Analysis. *Nutrients* **2020**, *12*, 1251. [CrossRef] [PubMed]
143. Arab, A.; Khorvash, F.; Karimi, E.; Hadi, A.; Askari, G. Associations between adherence to Mediterranean dietary pattern and frequency, duration, and severity of migraine headache: A cross-sectional study. *Nutr. Neurosci.* **2023**, *26*, 1–10. [CrossRef]
144. Sofi, F.; Abbate, R.; Gensini, G.F.; Casini, A. Accruing evidence on benefits of adherence to the Mediterranean diet on health: An updated systematic review and meta-analysis. *Am. J. Clin. Nutr.* **2010**, *92*, 1189–1196. [CrossRef]
145. Alcalay, R.N.; Gu, Y.; Mejia-Santana, H.; Cote, L.; Marder, K.S.; Scarmeas, N. The association between Mediterranean diet adherence and Parkinson's disease. *Mov. Disord.* **2012**, *27*, 771–774. [CrossRef] [PubMed]

146. Liperoti, R.; Landi, F.; Fusco, O.; Bernabei, R.; Onder, G. Omega-3 polyunsaturated fatty acids and depression: A review of the evidence. *Curr. Pharm. Des.* **2009**, *15*, 4165–4172. [CrossRef] [PubMed]
147. Liao, Y.; Xie, B.; Zhang, H.; He, Q.; Guo, L.; Subramanieapillai, M.; Fan, B.; Lu, C.; McIntyre, R.S. Efficacy of omega-3 PUFAs in depression: A meta-analysis. *Transl. Psychiatry* **2019**, *9*, 190. [CrossRef]
148. Tamir, H.; Mahadik, S.P.; Rapport, M.M. Fractionation of synaptic membranes with sodium diatrizoate. *Anal. Biochem.* **1976**, *76*, 634–647. [CrossRef]
149. Azzini, E.; Polito, A.; Fumagalli, A.; Intorre, F.; Venneria, E.; Durazzo, A.; Zaccaria, M.; Ciarapica, D.; Foddai, M.S.; Mauro, B.; et al. Mediterranean Diet Effect: An Italian picture. *Nutr. J.* **2011**, *10*, 125. [CrossRef]
150. Bakirhan, H.; Yildiran, H.; Uyar Cankay, T. Associations between diet quality, DASH and Mediterranean dietary patterns and migraine characteristics. *Nutr. Neurosci.* **2022**, *25*, 2324–2334. [CrossRef]
151. Ghoreishy, S.M.; Askari, G.; Mohammadi, H.; Campbell, M.S.; Khorvash, F.; Arab, A. Associations between potential inflammatory properties of the diet and frequency, duration, and severity of migraine headaches: A cross-sectional study. *Sci. Rep.* **2022**, *12*, 2878. [CrossRef]
152. Martins, L.B.; Braga Tibaes, J.R.; Dos Santos Rodrigues, A.M.; Hassanzadeh Keshteli, A.; Karam Vono, C.; Borges, E.B.J.; Horta, P.M.; Teixeira, A.L.; Matos Ferreira, A.V. The quality and inflammatory index of the diet of patients with migraine. *Nutr. Neurosci.* **2022**, *25*, 2092–2099. [CrossRef]
153. Merra, G.; Noce, A.; Marrone, G.; Cintoni, M.; Tarsitano, M.G.; Capacci, A.; De Lorenzo, A. Influence of Mediterranean Diet on Human Gut Microbiota. *Nutrients* **2020**, *13*, 7. [CrossRef]
154. D'Andrea Meira, I.; Romao, T.T.; Pires do Prado, H.J.; Kruger, L.T.; Pires, M.E.P.; da Conceicao, P.O. Ketogenic Diet and Epilepsy: What We Know So Far. *Front. Neurosci.* **2019**, *13*, 5. [CrossRef]
155. Longo, R.; Peri, C.; Cricri, D.; Coppi, L.; Caruso, D.; Mitro, N.; De Fabiani, E.; Crestani, M. Ketogenic Diet: A New Light Shining on Old but Gold Biochemistry. *Nutrients* **2019**, *11*, 2497. [CrossRef]
156. Hall, K.D.; Chen, K.Y.; Guo, J.; Lam, Y.Y.; Leibel, R.L.; Mayer, L.E.; Reitman, M.L.; Rosenbaum, M.; Smith, S.R.; Walsh, B.T.; et al. Energy expenditure and body composition changes after an isocaloric ketogenic diet in overweight and obese men. *Am. J. Clin. Nutr.* **2016**, *104*, 324–333. [CrossRef] [PubMed]
157. Koh, S.; Dupuis, N.; Auvin, S. Ketogenic diet and Neuroinflammation. *Epilepsy Res.* **2020**, *167*, 106454. [CrossRef] [PubMed]
158. Greco, T.; Glenn, T.C.; Hovda, D.A.; Prins, M.L. Ketogenic diet decreases oxidative stress and improves mitochondrial respiratory complex activity. *J. Cereb. Blood Flow. Metab.* **2016**, *36*, 1603–1613. [CrossRef] [PubMed]
159. Paoli, A.; Mancin, L.; Bianco, A.; Thomas, E.; Mota, J.F.; Piccini, F. Ketogenic Diet and Microbiota: Friends or Enemies? *Genes* **2019**, *10*, 534. [CrossRef]
160. Borkum, J.M. Migraine Triggers and Oxidative Stress: A Narrative Review and Synthesis. *Headache* **2016**, *56*, 12–35. [CrossRef]
161. Anderson, G. Integrating Pathophysiology in Migraine: Role of the Gut Microbiome and Melatonin. *Curr. Pharm. Des.* **2019**, *25*, 3550–3562. [CrossRef]
162. Di Lorenzo, C.; Ballerini, G.; Barbanti, P.; Bernardini, A.; D'Arrigo, G.; Egeo, G.; Frediani, F.; Garbo, R.; Pierangeli, G.; Prudenzano, M.P.; et al. Applications of Ketogenic Diets in Patients with Headache: Clinical Recommendations. *Nutrients* **2021**, *13*, 2307. [CrossRef]
163. Kechagia, M.; Basoulis, D.; Konstantopoulou, S.; Dimitriadi, D.; Gyftopoulou, K.; Skarmoutsou, N.; Fakiri, E.M. Health benefits of probiotics: A review. *ISRN Nutr.* **2013**, *2013*, 481651. [CrossRef]
164. Fijan, S. Microorganisms with claimed probiotic properties: An overview of recent literature. *Int. J. Environ. Res. Public Health* **2014**, *11*, 4745–4767. [CrossRef] [PubMed]
165. Vlasova, A.N.; Kandasamy, S.; Chattha, K.S.; Rajashekara, G.; Saif, L.J. Comparison of probiotic lactobacilli and bifidobacteria effects, immune responses and rotavirus vaccines and infection in different host species. *Vet. Immunol. Immunopathol.* **2016**, *172*, 72–84. [CrossRef] [PubMed]
166. Naghibi, M.M.; Day, R.; Stone, S.; Harper, A. Probiotics for the Prophylaxis of Migraine: A Systematic Review of Randomized Placebo Controlled Trials. *J. Clin. Med.* **2019**, *8*, 1441. [CrossRef] [PubMed]
167. Caetano, M.A.F.; Castelucci, P. Role of short chain fatty acids in gut health and possible therapeutic approaches in inflammatory bowel diseases. *World J. Clin. Cases* **2022**, *10*, 9985–10003. [CrossRef]
168. van Hemert, S.; Breedveld, A.C.; Rovers, J.M.; Vermeiden, J.P.; Witteman, B.J.; Smits, M.G.; de Roos, N.M. Migraine associated with gastrointestinal disorders: Review of the literature and clinical implications. *Front. Neurol.* **2014**, *5*, 241. [CrossRef]
169. Hemarajata, P.; Versalovic, J. Effects of probiotics on gut microbiota: Mechanisms of intestinal immunomodulation and neuromodulation. *Therap. Adv. Gastroenterol.* **2013**, *6*, 39–51. [CrossRef]
170. Dai, Y.J.; Wang, H.Y.; Wang, X.J.; Kaye, A.D.; Sun, Y.H. Potential Beneficial Effects of Probiotics on Human Migraine Headache: A Literature Review. *Pain Physician* **2017**, *20*, E251–E255.
171. Bedu-Ferrari, C.; Biscarrat, P.; Langella, P.; Cherbuy, C. Prebiotics and the Human Gut Microbiota: From Breakdown Mechanisms to the Impact on Metabolic Health. *Nutrients* **2022**, *14*, 2096. [CrossRef]
172. Macfarlane, G.T.; Steed, H.; Macfarlane, S. Bacterial metabolism and health-related effects of galacto-oligosaccharides and other prebiotics. *J. Appl. Microbiol.* **2008**, *104*, 305–344. [CrossRef]
173. Divyashri, G.; Sadanandan, B.; Chidambara Murthy, K.N.; Shetty, K.; Mamta, K. Neuroprotective Potential of Non-Digestible Oligosaccharides: An Overview of Experimental Evidence. *Front. Pharmacol.* **2021**, *12*, 712531. [CrossRef]

174. Levine, E.S.; Crozier, R.A.; Black, I.B.; Plummer, M.R. Brain-derived neurotrophic factor modulates hippocampal synaptic transmission by increasing N-methyl-D-aspartic acid receptor activity. *Proc. Natl. Acad. Sci. USA* **1998**, *95*, 10235–10239. [CrossRef] [PubMed]
175. Bull, F.C.; Al-Ansari, S.S.; Biddle, S.; Borodulin, K.; Buman, M.P.; Cardon, G.; Carty, C.; Chaput, J.P.; Chastin, S.; Chou, R.; et al. World Health Organization 2020 guidelines on physical activity and sedentary behaviour. *Br. J. Sports Med.* **2020**, *54*, 1451–1462. [CrossRef]
176. Warburton, D.E.; Nicol, C.W.; Bredin, S.S. Health benefits of physical activity: The evidence. *Can. Med. Assoc. J.* **2006**, *174*, 801–809. [CrossRef] [PubMed]
177. Cerda, B.; Perez, M.; Perez-Santiago, J.D.; Tornero-Aguilera, J.F.; Gonzalez-Soltero, R.; Larrosa, M. Gut Microbiota Modification: Another Piece in the Puzzle of the Benefits of Physical Exercise in Health? *Front. Physiol.* **2016**, *7*, 51. [CrossRef] [PubMed]
178. Zhang, L.; Liu, Y.; Wang, X.; Zhang, X. Physical Exercise and Diet: Regulation of Gut Microbiota to Prevent and Treat Metabolic Disorders to Maintain Health. *Nutrients* **2023**, *15*, 1539. [CrossRef]
179. Campaniello, D.; Corbo, M.R.; Sinigaglia, M.; Speranza, B.; Racioppo, A.; Altieri, C.; Bevilacqua, A. How Diet and Physical Activity Modulate Gut Microbiota: Evidence, and Perspectives. *Nutrients* **2022**, *14*, 2456. [CrossRef]
180. Rodrigues, S.; Silva, J.M.D.; Oliveira, M.C.C.; Santana, C.M.F.; Carvalho, K.M.; Barbosa, B. Physical exercise as a non pharmacological strategy for reducing behavioral and psychological symptoms in elderly with mild cognitive impairment and dementia: A systematic review of randomized clinical trials. *Arq. Neuropsiquiatr.* **2021**, *79*, 1129–1137. [CrossRef]
181. Mizutani, T.; Ishizaka, A.; Koga, M.; Tsutsumi, T.; Yotsuyanagi, H. Role of Microbiota in Viral Infections and Pathological Progression. *Viruses* **2022**, *14*, 950. [CrossRef] [PubMed]
182. Cataldi, S.; Bonavolonta, V.; Poli, L.; Clemente, F.M.; De Candia, M.; Carvutto, R.; Silva, A.F.; Badicu, G.; Greco, G.; Fischetti, F. The Relationship between Physical Activity, Physical Exercise, and Human Gut Microbiota in Healthy and Unhealthy Subjects: A Systematic Review. *Biology* **2022**, *11*, 479. [CrossRef] [PubMed]
183. Song, T.J.; Chu, M.K. Exercise in Treatment of Migraine Including Chronic Migraine. *Curr. Pain Headache Rep.* **2021**, *25*, 14. [CrossRef] [PubMed]
184. Lippi, G.; Mattiuzzi, C.; Sanchis-Gomar, F. Physical exercise and migraine: For or against? *Ann. Transl. Med.* **2018**, *6*, 181. [CrossRef] [PubMed]
185. Song, T.J.; Chu, M.K.; Sohn, J.H.; Ahn, H.Y.; Lee, S.H.; Cho, S.J. Effect of Vitamin D Deficiency on the Frequency of Headaches in Migraine. *J. Clin. Neurol.* **2018**, *14*, 366–373. [CrossRef]
186. Eyles, D.W. Vitamin D: Brain and Behavior. *JBMR Plus* **2021**, *5*, e10419. [CrossRef]
187. Das, S.; Hasan, M.M.; Mohsin, M.; Jeorge, D.H.; Rasul, M.G.; Khan, A.R.; Gazi, M.A.; Ahmed, T. Sunlight, dietary habits, genetic polymorphisms and vitamin D deficiency in urban and rural infants of Bangladesh. *Sci. Rep.* **2022**, *12*, 3623. [CrossRef]
188. Amiri, P.; Kazeminasab, S.; Nejadghaderi, S.A.; Mohammadinasab, R.; Pourfathi, H.; Araj-Khodaei, M.; Sullman, M.J.M.; Kolahi, A.A.; Safiri, S. Migraine: A Review on Its History, Global Epidemiology, Risk Factors, and Comorbidities. *Front. Neurol.* **2021**, *12*, 800605. [CrossRef]
189. Niu, P.P.; Wang, X.; Xu, Y.M. Higher Circulating Vitamin D Levels Are Associated With Decreased Migraine Risk: A Mendelian Randomization Study. *Front. Nutr.* **2022**, *9*, 907789. [CrossRef]
190. Zandifar, A.; Masjedi, S.S.; Banihashemi, M.; Asgari, F.; Manouchehri, N.; Ebrahimi, H.; Haghdoost, F.; Saadatnia, M. Vitamin D status in migraine patients: A case-control study. *Biomed. Res. Int.* **2014**, *2014*, 514782. [CrossRef]
191. Togha, M.; Razeghi Jahromi, S.; Ghorbani, Z.; Martami, F.; Seifishahpar, M. Serum Vitamin D Status in a Group of Migraine Patients Compared With Healthy Controls: A Case-Control Study. *Headache* **2018**, *58*, 1530–1540. [CrossRef] [PubMed]
192. Acharya, U.; Gau, J.T.; Horvath, W.; Ventura, P.; Hsueh, C.T.; Carlsen, W. Hemolysis and hyperhomocysteinemia caused by cobalamin deficiency: Three case reports and review of the literature. *J. Hematol. Oncol.* **2008**, *1*, 26. [CrossRef] [PubMed]
193. Ustun Ozek, S. A study on the correlation between pain frequency and severity and vitamin B12 levels in episodic and chronic migraine. *Arq. Neuropsiquiatr.* **2022**, *80*, 586–592. [CrossRef] [PubMed]
194. D'Onofrio, F.; Raimo, S.; Spitaleri, D.; Casucci, G.; Bussone, G. Usefulness of nutraceuticals in migraine prophylaxis. *Neurol. Sci.* **2017**, *38*, 117–120. [CrossRef]
195. Faraji, H.; Paknahad, Z.; Chitsaz, A. Dietary Intake of Thiamine in Migraine Patients and Healthy Subjects: A Case-Control Study. *Clin. Nutr. Res.* **2018**, *7*, 40–47. [CrossRef]
196. Fila, M.; Chojnacki, C.; Chojnacki, J.; Blasiak, J. Nutrients to Improve Mitochondrial Function to Reduce Brain Energy Deficit and Oxidative Stress in Migraine. *Nutrients* **2021**, *13*, 4433. [CrossRef]
197. Maresz, K. Growing Evidence of a Proven Mechanism Shows Vitamin K2 Can Impact Health Conditions Beyond Bone and Cardiovascular. *Integr. Med.* **2021**, *20*, 34–38.
198. Abbaspour, N.; Hurrell, R.; Kelishadi, R. Review on iron and its importance for human health. *J. Res. Med. Sci.* **2014**, *19*, 164–174.
199. Meng, S.H.; Zhou, H.B.; Li, X.; Wang, M.X.; Kang, L.X.; Fu, J.M.; Li, X.; Li, X.T.; Zhao, Y.S. Association between Dietary Iron Intake and Serum Ferritin and Severe Headache or Migraine. *Front. Nutr.* **2021**, *8*, 685564. [CrossRef]
200. Torres-Ferrus, M.; Ursitti, F.; Alpuente, A.; Brunello, F.; Chiappino, D.; de Vries, T.; Di Marco, S.; Ferlisi, S.; Guerritore, L.; Gonzalez-Garcia, N.; et al. From transformation to chronification of migraine: Pathophysiological and clinical aspects. *J. Headache Pain* **2020**, *21*, 42. [CrossRef]

201. Liu, H.; Wang, D.; Wu, F.; Dong, Z.; Yu, S. Association between inflammatory potential of diet and self-reported severe headache or migraine: A cross-sectional study of the National Health and Nutrition Examination Survey. *Nutrition* **2023**, *113*, 112098. [CrossRef]
202. Pamuk, G.E.; Top, M.S.; Uyanik, M.S.; Koker, H.; Akker, M.; Ak, R.; Yurekli, O.A.; Celik, Y. Is iron-deficiency anemia associated with migraine? Is there a role for anxiety and depression? *Wien. Klin. Wochenschr.* **2016**, *128*, 576–580. [CrossRef]
203. Singla, R.K.; Dubey, A.K.; Garg, A.; Sharma, R.K.; Fiorino, M.; Ameen, S.M.; Haddad, M.A.; Al-Hiary, M. Natural Polyphenols: Chemical Classification, Definition of Classes, Subcategories, and Structures. *J. AOAC Int.* **2019**, *102*, 1397–1400. [CrossRef]
204. Bakirhan, H.; Pehlivan, M.; Uyar Cankay, T.; Kocak, M. Migraine severity, disability, and duration: Is a good diet quality, high intake of phytochemicals and polyphenols important? *Front. Nutr.* **2022**, *9*, 1041907. [CrossRef] [PubMed]
205. Goschorska, M.; Gutowska, I.; Baranowska-Bosiacka, I.; Barczak, K.; Chlubek, D. The Use of Antioxidants in the Treatment of Migraine. *Antioxidants* **2020**, *9*, 116. [CrossRef] [PubMed]
206. Nowaczewska, M.; Wicinski, M.; Kazmierczak, W.; Kazmierczak, H. To Eat or Not to Eat: A Review of the Relationship between Chocolate and Migraines. *Nutrients* **2020**, *12*, 608. [CrossRef] [PubMed]
207. Meng, S.H.; Wang, M.X.; Kang, L.X.; Fu, J.M.; Zhou, H.B.; Li, X.; Li, X.; Li, X.T.; Zhao, Y.S. Dietary Intake of Calcium and Magnesium in Relation to Severe Headache or Migraine. *Front. Nutr.* **2021**, *8*, 653765. [CrossRef]
208. Domitrz, I.; Cegielska, J. Magnesium as an Important Factor in the Pathogenesis and Treatment of Migraine-From Theory to Practice. *Nutrients* **2022**, *14*, 1089. [CrossRef]
209. Yamanaka, R.; Shindo, Y.; Oka, K. Magnesium Is a Key Player in Neuronal Maturation and Neuropathology. *Int. J. Mol. Sci.* **2019**, *20*, 3439. [CrossRef]
210. Li, K.; Wang, X.F.; Li, D.Y.; Chen, Y.C.; Zhao, L.J.; Liu, X.G.; Guo, Y.F.; Shen, J.; Lin, X.; Deng, J.; et al. The good, the bad, and the ugly of calcium supplementation: A review of calcium intake on human health. *Clin. Interv. Aging* **2018**, *13*, 2443–2452. [CrossRef]
211. Schnedl, W.J.; Enko, D. Histamine Intolerance Originates in the Gut. *Nutrients* **2021**, *13*, 1262. [CrossRef]
212. Branco, A.; Yoshikawa, F.S.Y.; Pietrobon, A.J.; Sato, M.N. Role of Histamine in Modulating the Immune Response and Inflammation. *Mediators Inflamm.* **2018**, *2018*, 9524075. [CrossRef]
213. Costa, F.; Beltrami, E.; Mellone, S.; Sacchetti, S.; Boggio, E.; Gigliotti, C.L.; Stoppa, I.; Dianzani, U.; Rolla, R.; Giordano, M. Genes and Microbiota Interaction in Monogenic Autoimmune Disorders. *Biomedicines* **2023**, *11*, 1127. [CrossRef] [PubMed]
214. Durak-Dados, A.; Michalski, M.; Osek, J. Histamine and Other Biogenic Amines in Food. *J. Vet. Res.* **2020**, *64*, 281–288. [CrossRef]
215. Liu, X.; Yu, Y.; Hou, L.; Yu, Y.; Wu, Y.; Wu, S.; He, Y.; Ge, Y.; Wei, Y.; Luo, Q.; et al. Association between dietary habits and the risk of migraine: A Mendelian randomization study. *Front. Nutr.* **2023**, *10*, 1123657. [CrossRef] [PubMed]
216. Ruiz-Capillas, C.; Herrero, A.M. Impact of Biogenic Amines on Food Quality and Safety. *Foods* **2019**, *8*, 62. [CrossRef]
217. Izquierdo-Casas, J.; Comas-Baste, O.; Latorre-Moratalla, M.L.; Lorente-Gascon, M.; Duelo, A.; Soler-Singla, L.; Vidal-Carou, M.C. Diamine oxidase (DAO) supplement reduces headache in episodic migraine patients with DAO deficiency: A randomized double-blind trial. *Clin. Nutr.* **2019**, *38*, 152–158. [CrossRef]
218. Okutan, G.; Ruiz Casares, E.; Perucho Alcalde, T.; Sanchez Nino, G.M.; Penades, B.F.; Terren Lora, A.; Torrente Estringana, L.; Lopez Oliva, S.; San Mauro Martin, I. Prevalence of Genetic Diamine Oxidase (DAO) Deficiency in Female Patients with Fibromyalgia in Spain. *Biomedicines* **2023**, *11*, 660. [CrossRef]
219. Brown, R.W.; Chadwick, D.R.; Bott, T.; West, H.M.; Wilson, P.; Hodgins, G.R.; Snape, C.E.; Jones, D.L. Biochar application to temperate grasslands: Challenges and opportunities for delivering multiple ecosystem services. *Biochar* **2023**, *5*, 33. [CrossRef] [PubMed]
220. Esposito, F.; Montuori, P.; Schettino, M.; Velotto, S.; Stasi, T.; Romano, R.; Cirillo, T. Level of Biogenic Amines in Red and White Wines, Dietary Exposure, and Histamine-Mediated Symptoms upon Wine Ingestion. *Molecules* **2019**, *24*, 3629. [CrossRef]

nutrients MDPI

Review

Cyclitols: From Basic Understanding to Their Association with Neurodegeneration

Maria Derkaczew [1,2,*], Piotr Martyniuk [1,2], Adam Osowski [1] and Joanna Wojtkiewicz [1,*]

[1] Department of Human Physiology and Pathophysiology, School of Medicine, Collegium Medicum, University of Warmia and Mazury, 10-082 Olsztyn, Poland; p.martyniuk@o2.pl (P.M.)
[2] Students' Scientific Club of Pathophysiologists, Department of Human Physiology and Pathophysiology, School of Medicine, University of Warmia and Mazury, 10-082 Olsztyn, Poland
* Correspondence: m.derkaczew@gmail.com (M.D.); joanna.wojtkiewicz@uwm.edu.pl (J.W.); Tel.: +48-607-654-914 (M.D.)

Abstract: One of the most common cyclitols found in eukaryotic cells—Myo-inositol (MI) and its derivatives play a key role in many cellular processes such as ion channel physiology, signal transduction, phosphate storage, cell wall formation, membrane biogenesis and osmoregulation. The aim of this paper is to characterize the possibility of neurodegenerative disorders treatment using MI and the research of other therapeutic methods linked to MI's derivatives. Based on the reviewed literature the researchers focus on the most common neurodegenerative diseases such as Alzheimer's disease, Parkinson's disease, Huntington's disease and Spinocerebellar ataxias, but there are also works describing other seldom encountered diseases. The use of MI, D-pinitol and other methods altering MI's metabolism, although research on this topic has been conducted for years, still needs much closer examination. The dietary supplementation of MI shows a promising effect on the treatment of neurodegenerative disorders and can be of great help in alleviating the accompanying depressive symptoms.

Keywords: myo-inositol; D-pinitol; inositol phosphates; neurodegenerative disorders; Alzheimer's disease; Parkinson's disease; Huntington's disease; spinocerebellar ataxias

1. Introduction

Over the centuries, plants as natural products were used to treat a multitude of diseases. These organic "drugs" contain numerous chemical particles. One of them—myo-inositol (MI) and its derivatives—play an influential role in a great number of cellular processes such as ion channel physiology, phosphate storage, signal transduction, cell wall formation, membrane biogenesis and osmoregulation as it is a forerunner of many secondary messengers in eukaryotic cells [1,2].

MI is a pivotal and fundamental element of Inositol Phosphates (IPs) and Phosphatidylinositols (PIs or PtdIns) and their various phosphates, called phosphatidylinositol phosphate lipids (PIPs). Their interconversions are conducted by crucial enzymes, which dysfunction can lead to severe abnormalities, disorders and illnesses.

The aim of this paper is to present and analyze the documented data about cyclitols' association with pathological processes such as neurodegenerative diseases. Furthermore, cyclitols themselves may be worth considering as therapeutic agents in the treatment of numerous medical conditions. Low toxicity, possible use in pregnancy, good drug tolerance, widespread presence, and easy availability speak for use of these compounds in medicine [3]. The first part of this paper presents general information concerning the sugar alcohols, inositol and its derivatives such as PIs with the detailed characterization of metabolic pathways in this particular group and selected genetic mutations concerning PIs found in the literature; then the next part of the review focuses on the exact characteristic of IPs, to finally move on to discuss the neurodegenerative diseases connected with disorders in MI metabolic pathways and its possible usage in the treatment of these diseases as well as other innovative treatment methods.

2. Sugar Alcohols

Cyclitols are monocyclic saturated hydrocarbons containing at least three hydroxyl groups, each attached to a different ring carbon atom. The other names of this group of organic compounds are sugar alcohols or polyols. Cyclitols and their derivatives are tiny organic molecules with low toxicity and neutral charge, which makes them osmoprotectants. They are formed in plants to help them survive extreme osmotic stress. That is one of the various and numerous functions that cyclitols can perform. MI, being one of the sugar alcohols and most common cyclitols in eukaryotic cells, serves as a key component of structural lipids such as IPs, PIs and PIPs [4] (Table 1).

Table 1. Structural formulas of primary cyclitols.

Cyclitol 1,2,3,4-cyclohexenetetrol	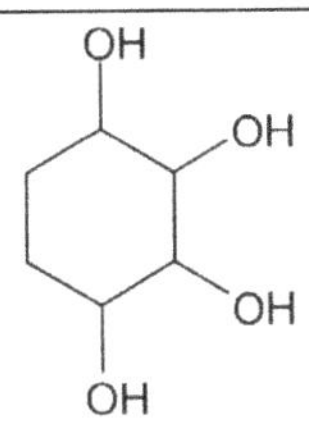
Myo-inositol	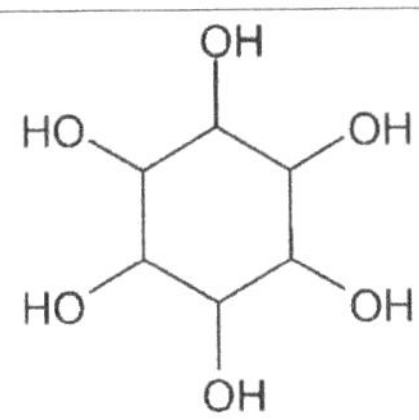
Pinitol	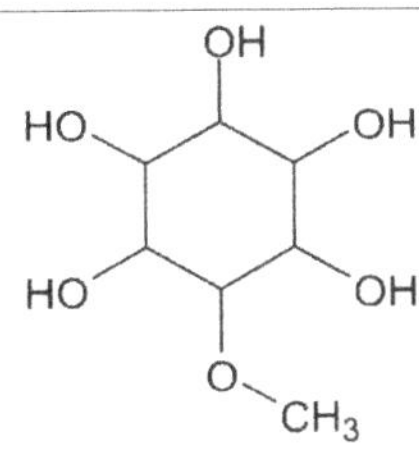

3. Inositol Characteristics

Inositol is a cyclic carbohydrate with six hydroxyl groups attached to each ring carbon. MI is one of nine inositol isomers as each hydroxyl group of the cyclohexane ring can be placed in one of two possible orientations—axial or equatorial [5]. The other eight are D-chiro-, scyllo, muco-, *cis*-, neo-, epi-, allo- and L-chiro-inositol. D-chiro- and L-chiro-inositol are two enantiomers, which means they are mirror images of each other. MI undergoes many biochemical and metabolic changes to form different stereoisomers and transforms into other more complex molecules such as IPs, PIs, PIPs, glycosyl-phosphatidylinositols (GPIs) and inositol-phosphoglycans (IPGs) (2). MI or *cis*-1,2,3,5-*trans*-4,6-cyclohexanehexol is the oldest known inositol and at the same time the most abundant one in nature [6]. It was first isolated in 1850 by Scherer from muscle extracts and named after that tissue with prefix "myo" from Greek. Other isomers that occur naturally in nature are: D-chiro-, L-chiro, scyllo-, muco- and neo-inositol [5]. Inositol is commonly called vitamin B8, which is not entirely precise due to the fact that this compound is also synthesized endogenously [7]. The functions of MI in the human body include the regulation of ion channel permeability, metabolic homeostasis, export and the translation of mRNA, stress reaction, cytoskeleton remodeling, apoptosis, fetus development, the development and function of nerves, reproductive functions, osteogenesis and metabolism of glucose and cholesterol [2,8].

4. Sources and Metabolism of MI

MI is primarily supplied with food. The highest amounts of MI can be found in plant-based products, such as grains, nuts and fruits. It is the main source of phosphorus in plant cells and is responsible for its storage [9]. MI occurs in food in its free form, but mainly in the form of phytic acid (IP_6) which is known for its both upsides and downsides. It has long been known that IP_6 binds to bivalent cations such as Mg^{2+}, Zn^{2+}, Ca^{2+}, Fe^{2+}, and Mn^{2+} and forms phytases that cannot be broken down due to the lack of a predestined enzyme, contributing to the long term to deficiency of these minerals [10]. Newer studies indicated that approximately 50% of IP_6 can be degraded in the stomach and small intestine when the diet contains plant food phytases [11]. IP_6 is also digested by bacterial phytases and phosphatases [12]. On the other hand, IP_6 is a natural antioxidant. The thermal or mechanical treatment of the food such as cooking, soaking, baking and general processing significantly reduces the IP6 content [13]. It has been estimated that an average mixed Western diet can provide about 1 g of total inositol per day [14].

There are two types of transporters which are enabling MI cell uptake: sodium ion coupled (SMIT1/SMIT2) and proton coupled (HMIT1) [15–17]. HMIT1 expression is most significant in the brain [18].

MI can be also endogenously produced in the human kidney and liver from glucose-6-phosphate in just two reactions. The first one is catalyzed by MI-1-phosphate synthase (MIPS) and the second one by inositol monophosphatase-1 (IMPase) (Figure 1) [19–21]. To date, no dietary requirements regarding the amount of inositol daily intake have been established for humans. It is probably hampered due to the endogenous production of MI from glucose and differences in MI levels in individual organs and compartments [2].

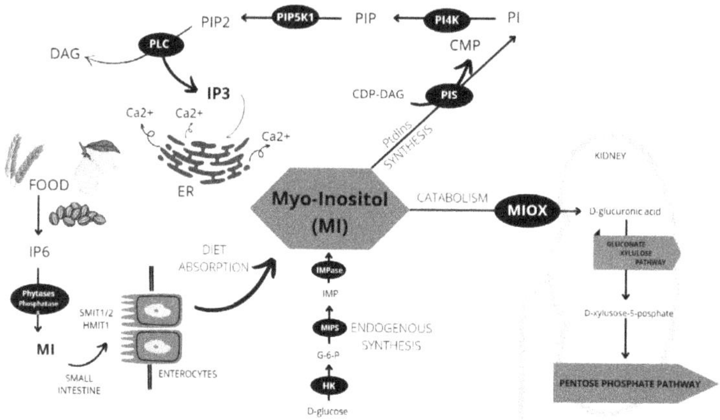

Figure 1. Metabolism of MI [IP6—phytic acid; HK—Hexokinase; G-6-P—Glucose-6-Phosphate; MIPS—Myo-inositol Phosphate Synthase; IMP—inositol Monophosphate; IMPase—Inositol Monophosphatase; MIOX—Myo-inositol Oxygenase; CDP-DAG—Cytidine Diphosphate Diacylglycerol; PIS—Phosphatidylinositol Synthase; CMP—Cytidine Monophosphate; PI—Phosphatidylinositol; PI4K—Phosphatidylinositol 4-Kinase; PIP—Phosphatidylinositol Phosphate; PIP5K1—Phosphatidylinositol Phosphate 5-Kinase 1; PIP2—Phosphatidylinositol Biphosphate; PLC—Phospholipase C; DAG—Diacyloglicerol; IP3—Inositol Triphosphate; ER—Endoplasmic Reticulum].

The kidney is the main organ of MI metabolism. Here, endogenous biosynthesis as well as catabolism takes place. MI is oxygenated to form D-glucuronic acid which can enter the gluconate xylulose pathway and be converted to D-xylulose-5-phosphate—one of the key components of the pentose phosphate pathway [8,22]. The pentose phosphate pathway is one of the most important processes in the human body. It allows the generation of energy and the maintenance of homeostasis, also being the principal source of nicotinamide adenine dinucleotide (NADPH), pentoses and ribose-5-phosphate—nucleotides synthesis precursor [23,24].

MI is a forerunner of many secondary messengers which play a key role in various intracellular processes. The most important derivatives are a family of phosphatidylinositols and inositol phosphates, especially inositol triphosphate (IP_3) [8].

5. Inositol Phosphates

Inositol phosphates (IP) are derivatives of MI. Among the IPs we can distinguish: IP, IP2, IP3, IP4, IP5 and IP6—also known as phytic acid. The level of IP6 is highest in nerve cells and is relatively constant regardless of the supply of IP6 in the diet [2]. IPs play a key role in the biochemistry and metabolism of cells. IP3 is an important secondary messenger, resulting from the breakdown of PIP2 by phospholipase C along with diacylglycerol (DAG). DAG remains bound to the cell intracellular membrane, while soluble IP3 is released into the cytoplasm and binds to the inositol 1,4,5-triphosphate receptor (IP3R). IP3R activation enables intracellular calcium (Ca^{2+}) signaling as it leads to the opening of Ca^{2+} ion channels located on the endoplasmic reticulum (ER) and the release of calcium ions into the cytoplasm.

There are three types of these receptors: IP3R 1, IP3R 2 and IP3R 3 [25]. IP3R 1 is the most common one expressed in neurons of all three types. Two receptors are responsible for the release of calcium form the ER: IP3R and the ryanodine receptor (RyR). RyR is the primary one in the striated muscle cells, while IP3Rs can be detected in all cell types. The function of these channels contributes to regulating various physiological functions such as muscle contraction, hormone secretion, reproduction, gene expression, cell life cycle, apoptosis, learning, memory and behavior [26].

Calcium release from the ER can be induced both by inositol (Inositol Induced Calcium Release; IICR) or calcium itself (Calcium Induced Calcium Release; CICR). While IP3Rs are solely responsible for IICR, CICR is responsible for the release of calcium from both IP3R and RyR, but with a significant advantage of RyR in this process [27]. Changes in the regulation of IP3Rs can lead to various abnormalities. Deregulation of these receptors disturbs intracellular homeostasis lowering the concentration of Ca^{2+} in the cytoplasm, changing the amplitude and frequency of calcium signaling and ultimately can even lead to cell death [25,28]. It was proven that improper function of these channels can lead to many neurological disorders including migraines, Alzheimer's disease (AD), Huntington's disease (HD) and spinocerebellar ataxias [25,26]. It is generally accepted that IP3Rs localize on the ER, but where else they may exist within the cell is under discussion. For the time being, it is known that these receptors may also appear on the inner nuclear membrane and within the plasma membrane. In neuronal cells presence of IP3R on the plasma membrane has so far been detected only in olfactory receptor neurons [29].

6. Inositol's Unproper Metabolism Impact on Neurodegenerative Process

In the brain, constant changes in inositol levels in extracellular and intracellular compartments regulate the activity of neuronal and glial cells [30]. MI and scyllo-inositol (SI) are the most common forms of inositol found in the brain. MI is found in large amounts in the glial cells and acts as an osmolyte. The concentrations of MI and SI are several times higher than the values found in the blood serum and are on average 100 times higher [31,32]. In the nervous system, the highest concentration of inositol is in the brain—6 mM. Then, MI occurs in cerebrospinal fluid (0,2 mM) and plasma of nervous cells (0.03 mM) [3,33,34]. SI is found in relatively high concentrations in the human brain than in other tissues, although it has a 12 times lower concentration than mI [35,36]. In nervous system diseases, we notice the occurrence of unproper MI's metabolism to phosphates and its secondary accumulation. MI has been found to be a marker of gliosis in demyelinating lesions. Elevated levels of MI have also been documented in glioblastomas. MI is also involved in the phosphatidylinositol secondary messenger system, which is associated with depression (91). Disorders in MI's metabolism and distribution have been found in many neurodegenerative diseases.

6.1. Alzheimer's Disease

Alzheimer's Disease (AD) is a chronic, progressive, neurodegenerative disease of the brain that causes nerve cell atrophy. AD is characterized by the occurrence of progressive dementia and at the same time is the most common cause of dementia among the elderly [37]. In the course of AD, we can distinguish symptoms such as memory loss and the progressive loss of cognitive functions [38]. Common neuropathological features of AD are neuronal loss, the aggregation of insoluble forms of β-amyloid (Aβ) forming plaques in extracellular spaces and microtubule τ protein hyperphosphorylation in the form of neurofibrillary tangles (NFTs) located in neuronal cells. Changes are usually located firstly in the cortex of frontal and temporal lobes and then slowly spread to the other parts of the brain tissue [39]. We can distinguish the sporadic form of AD (Sporadic Alzheimer's Disease—SAD) and the familial form (Familial Alzheimer's disease—FAD). FAD occurs much less frequently in about 5% of AD patients [40]. SAD tends to occur in the elderly and is the most common form of AD, while FAD will appear more frequently in middle age and is associated with mutations in the genes encoding the presenilin 1 and 2 proteins (PS 1,2) and the amyloid precursor protein (APP) [25,38,41–43]. APP is normally transformed through several reactions of proteolysis into two types of Aβ—Aβ40 and Aβ42. γ-secretase is one of the enzymes catalyzing these reactions and will be mentioned later in this paper, as a possible therapeutic target in AD treatment. The possible linkage between γ-secretase and inositol metabolism is the fact that PS1 is the main catalytic core of γ-secretase and PS1 is known to boost the activity of IP3R. These reactions and the cleavage of APP can be seen on Figure 2 [2,44,45].

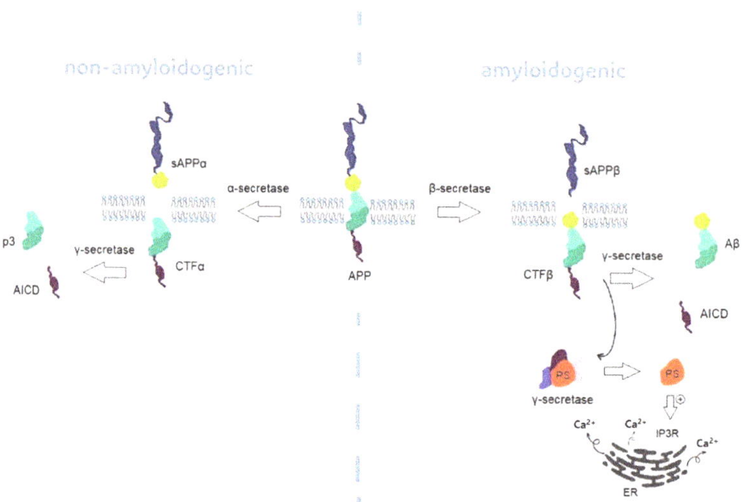

Figure 2. The amyloidogenic and non-amyloidogenic cleavage of amyloid precursor protein and the linkage between γ-secretase and IP3R [APP—amyloid precursor protein; AICD—APP intracellular fragment; CFT—APP C-terminal fragment].

In AD we can observe the unfavourable ratio of Aβ42 and Aβ40 levels, with a predominance of Aβ42—the more neurodegenerating one [46,47]. In AD patients according to the literature inositol metabolism is disturbed in several ways. It was proven that AD patients have higher concentrations of MI and SI in their brains compared to healthy people, despite of pathogenesis of the illness [48–50]. In Firbank et al. paper AD patients' MI levels seemed to be raised by about 15% but with no evidence for an increase in any particular brain region. Higher MI levels are also seen in adults with Down's syndrome and it has been shown that these patients will mostly develop AD in the future [51]. High MI levels are also detected in presymptomatic patients and those with mild cognitive impairment (MCI), which indicates the possibility of using MI as a marker of the early stages of AD [48,52–54]. The metabolism of inositol in AD patients can be impaired at every stage causing the deregulation of Ca^{2+} neuronal homeostasis which leads to neurodegenerative disorders. The intracellular calcium concentration must be constantly maintained at the appropriate level for all processes to take place properly. Disturbances in calcium levels can lead to serious malfunctions in its functioning. Calcium regulates the processes of growth, development and apoptosis, and its inadequate level can even lead to cell death [55–58]. In human cells, the level of calcium is regulated by several mechanisms. Calcium can enter cells from the extracellular space or it can be taken from the intracellular calcium store, which is the ER. Many studies indicate the enormous role of MI derivatives in regulating these processes. The role of IP3 in the elevation of intracellular calcium levels by releasing it from ER was described earlier in this work, but it is also worth mentioning that the activation of calcium influx from the extracellular space—the so-called Ca-influx also plays a significant role in the pathomechanism of AD and other neurodegenerative disorders [59,60]. There are reports indicating that Ca-influx can be as well stimulated by another MI derivative—Inositol 1,3,4,5-tetrakisphosphate (IP4) [61,62]. Many papers considering this topic focused on disruptions to the function of IP3R. Former literature report a decreased level of binding sites of IP3R in AD patients [63,64] and more recent studies highlight the over-activation of these channels. There is a strong correlation between the overactivity of IP3R and mutations in the presenilin genes [65–67]. In presenilin transgenic mice (PS1 FAD mutant mice) increased activity of IP3R was observed which subsequently enhances IICR and leads to increased intracellular calcium levels. Under conditions of increased Ca^{2+} levels, together with the additional oxidative stress characteristic of AD, a non-specific pore in the inner mitochondrial membrane is opened, known as the mitochondrial permeability transition pore (mPTP). The opening of mPTP allows the passage of molecules smaller than 1.5 kDa, and therefore, also protons. Consequently, this leads to the depletion of ATP stores and cell death [25,68–70]. It was proven that genetic modifications including the reduction of IP3R1 contributed to the equalization of Ca^{2+} levels [25,71]. Moreover, elevated levels of calcium activate calpain—a protein belonging to the family of calcium-dependent, non-lysosomal cystine proteases. Calpain has many isoforms, but to date, two of them have been most extensively studied—μ-calpain and m-calpain, otherwise known as calpain 1 and calpain 2, respectively. Both of them are activated by calcium ions and inhibited by a specific endogenous inhibitor—calpastatin (CAST). Calpain regulates many processes inside the cell, including the proper course of the cell cycle, cell proliferation, signal transduction, proper functioning of key protein kinases and phosphatases, apoptosis, memory, learning and in neurons—long term potentiation (LTP) which is a specific function for this type of cell [72,73]. With increasing age and in the course of neurodegenerative disorders such as AD, there is an excessive, uncontrolled activation of calpain, as a response to higher levels of intracellular Ca^{2+}. It was shown that CAST concentrations are additionally lowered in the prefrontal cortex in AD patients, thus, apart from the over-stimulation of calpain by calcium, its inhibition also does not work properly [74,75]. Overly elevated calpain promotes the aggregation of Aβ and NFTs, as well as induces the dephosphorylation (deactivation) of cAMP-response element-binding protein (CREB)—a key protein essential for converting a short-term memory to a long-term memory and other memory and learning processes [76]. Opinions about the role of calcium in the process of direct cell damage are divided, and the authors now tend to emphasize the subtle effects of calcium on the slow progression of neurodegenerative changes, rather than the rapid process leading to cell death [29,77]. Another interesting linkage between disturbances in MI metabolism and the presence of AD is MI's influence on catalase. Catalase allows the H_2O_2 to break down to harmless water and oxygen, and thus, together with other antioxidants such as glutathione peroxidase, reduces the formation of reactive oxygen species (ROS) and saves the cells from oxidative stress [78]. One of the most recent works on the influence of MI on the course of AD focuses on the inhibition of catalase function by MI, while other polyols such as mannitol, sorbitol and glycerol have been shown to have an activating effect on catalase. Researchers suggest that the inhibitory effect of MI may be due to MI binding to an active site of catalase or that MI causes conformational changes in the structure which can result in loss of activity. The loss of the antioxidant capacity of catalase may result in the occurrence of oxidative stress in cells, which was proven to be significantly increased in the course of AD and other neurodegenerative diseases [53,79]. On the other hand, previous reports suggest that MI supplementation results in an increase in the activity of antioxidant agents. Jiang et al. research has shown that antioxidative enzymes' activity such as catalase, glutathione peroxidase and glutathione reductase were improved along with the increasing MI levels in the diet of juvenile Jian carp (*Cyprinus carpio* var. *Jian*) [80]. Information on processes related to disturbances in the biochemistry of inositols that lead to neurodegeneration in the course of AD has been posted in Figure 3.

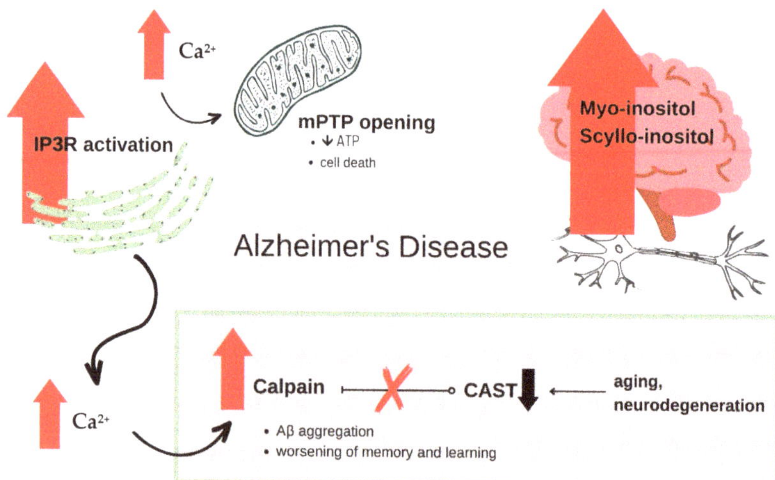

Figure 3. The summary of the mechanisms occurring in the course of AD in relation to inositol metabolism disorders. [ATP—adenosine triphosphate; mPTP—mitochondrial permeability transition pore; CAST—calpastatin; IP3R—inositol 1,4,5-triphosphate receptor].

6.2. Parkinson's Disease

Parkinson's Disease (PD) is the second most common neurodegenerative disease after AD, occurring in about 2–3% of people over the age of 65. In its course, there is a gradual loss of substantia nigra neurons leading to a decrease in dopamine levels in the striatal brain regions and the deposition of intracellular aggregates of α-synuclein. Many researchers also emphasize the important role of progressive dysfunction of mitochondrial function and the resulting increase in oxidative stress and increase in ROS. Clinical manifestations of PD include bradykinesia and at least one of the additional motor impairments: rigidity or rest tremor. Motor disorders usually occur asymmetrically [81].

Research on animals and cells has shown that IP6 has a protective effect on nerve cells in models of Parkinson's disease. Researchers have demonstrated significant protection against ROS and lipid peroxidation product malondialdehyde (MDA) in PD's model cells—6-OHDA (6-hydroxydopamine) previously exposed to IP6. IP6 was shown to inhibit the activation of key proteins involved in apoptosis. Therefore, IP6 due to its anti-apoptotic effect is proven to be neuroprotective against the loss of dopaminergic neurons in PD model cells [82,83].

Considering PD, the researchers also focused on examining the levels of receptors for IP3 and, as in older studies on AD, showed reduced levels of IP3 binding sites. A 50% reduced level of IP3 binding sites in the caudate nucleus, putamen and pallidum with no differences in the frontal cortex at the same time [84].

PD is still diagnosed based on the presence of characteristic clinical symptoms when the disease is already at a significant stage. Many authors have searched for potential diagnostic biomarkers of PD and other neurodegenerative diseases. Magnetic resonance spectroscopy (MRS) is a useful tool that allows for quantitative, non-invasive analysis of selected brain region biochemistry [85]. Of the substances present in the brain that have been studied, many researchers have focused on evaluating the concentration of MI. In Mazuel et al.'s research PD patients and healthy controls were examined with the use of hydrogen 1 proton magnetic resonance spectroscopy (^{1}H-MRS) for the assessment of the metabolic profile in the putamen. As a result, the MI was significantly lower in drug-off PD patients and the MI level did not change even when the therapy was reintroduced [86]. Gröger et al. also used ^{1}H-MRS to investigate the distribution of brain metabolites and focused on the ratios between different substations. It has been shown that the rostral substantia nigra regions of PD patients showed a trend towards decreased MI and total creatine (creatine + phosphocreatine, tCr) ratio compared with healthy controls whereas in the caudal substantia nigra regions the MI/Cr ratios were increased in PD patients compared with healthy controls [87,88].

Progressive Supranuclear Palsy (PSP) also known as Steele–Richardson–Olszewski syndrome is a chronic neurodegenerative disorder also involving the deposition of Tau protein aggregates, clinically resembling PD, and therefore, was often being misdiagnosed for this reason in the past. Typical symptoms of PSP include bradykinesia with disproportionate postural instability, upright posture with neck stiffness, frontal behavioral and cognitive changes, vertical gaze palsy and other brainstem deficits [89]. One of the areas of the brain affected by the disease is the Supplementary Motor Area (SMA). An Italian group of researchers focused on demonstrating PSP-specific neurobiochemical changes within the SMA using ^{1}H-MRS [36]. Research has shown reduced scyllo-inositol levels in the SMA portion of the brains of PSP patients. The researchers stress that there are reports stating the SI's neuroprotective ability against the deposition of protein aggregates in neurodegenerative diseases. In another paper, researchers administered 12 g of inositol daily to nine PD patients. They showed no significant positive MI effects but suggested possible beneficial effects of supplementation in patients with additional depressive symptoms and anxiety [90].

6.3. *Huntington's Disease*

Huntington's disease (HD) is a progressive, autosomal-dominant neurodegenerative disorder, manifested by chorea, dystonia, decreased motor coordination, cognitive decline and behavioral changes. Usually, the first symptoms of the disease appear in middle age but may occur at any stage of the patient's life [91,92]. The genetic basis of HD is an occurrence of expanded CAG repeat in exon 1 of the huntingtin gene (polyglutamine, polyQ expansion) causing the formation of mutant huntingtin (mHtt) protein. mHtt occurs is found in all types of cells, but it appears to be toxic only for neurons of specific brain regions: cortex, caudate nucleus and putamen [25]. Many reports confirm, that in HD deregulation of IP3R also takes place, this time due to the direct binding of mHtt protein to IP3R1 in its C-terminal region [29]. It was proven that mHtt sensitized activation of IP3R by IP3 in medium spiny striatal neurons (MSNs), while normal huntingtin protein showed no such ability. HD transgenic model mice used in research considering alterations in IP3R functions are yeast artificial chromosome (YAC) and mice with a targeted disruption of both Htt-associated protein-1A (HAP1) gene alleles. HAP1 was the first Htt-binding protein to be found. It was shown that HAP1 is present in MSNs and it intensifies the action of mHtt, resulting in increased IICR and elevated calcium levels [93]. Moreover, IP3R is an allosteric protein and its function can be disrupted by changes in its conformation. One of the enzymes that can disturb IP3R's allostery is transglutaminase type 2 (TG2) and its regulation is based on the covalent posttranslational modification of the Gln2746 residue which TG2 tethers to the communicating subunit [94]. Both Gln2746 changes and IP3R dysregulation were detected in HD models, confirming the involvement of IP3R dysregulation in disease pathogenesis [29,95]. TG2 ablation in model mice prolonged their lifespan and improved motor function [25]. Other researchers report that in the course of HD, there is an increase in the activity of inositol hexakisphosphate kinase type 2 (IP6K2), which, among other things, leads to a reduction in Akt phosphorylation, which may lead to cell death and promotes autophagy. Upon activation, IP6K2 is released from the nucleoplasm into the cytoplasm. It was shown that in HD lymphoblasts IP6K2 was present mainly in the cytoplasm of the cell, while in control cells it remained in the nucleus. IP6K2 catalyzes the reaction of transforming IP6 into inositol pyrophosphate diphosphoinositolpentakisphopshate (IP7; PPIP5). In HD lymphoblast cells, increased levels of IP7 were detected compared to control cells, and IP7 promotes cell death [96,97].

6.4. *Spinocerebellar Ataxias*

Another neurodegenerative disorder group that will be discussed in this paper is Spinocerebellar Ataxias (SCAs). SCAs are a group of hereditary autosomal dominant neurodegenerative disorders characterized by progressive ataxia. To date, there are more than 40 identified types of SCA [98]. Each of the SCA types are based on a mutation, deletion or polyglutamine (poly-Q) expansion at a different gene locus [99]. The characteristic symptoms in the course of SCA include loss of balance and coordination, dysarthria and nystagmus [100]. SCAs cause damage to the brain tissue and mostly affects the cerebellar Purkinje neurons, leading to cerebellar cortex atrophy, neuronal loss, and irreversible degeneration of spinocerebellar tracts, dentate nucleus and pontine[101]. There are many reports in the literature on the relationship between SCAs and dysregulation of IP3R function. Some papers indicate that reduced IP3R abundance is observed in SCAs, while others emphasize the phenomenon of hypersensitivity of IP3R for its ligand—IP3, and excessive IP3R activation [102].

SCA1, SCA2 and SCA3 are caused by intracellular poly-Q (CAG) expansions of cytosolic ataxin protein. It is already known that researchers are looking for potential diagnostic biomarkers for the effective detection of neurodegenerative diseases. In the Oz et al. paper, researchers focused on the analysis of levels of total NAA (*N*-acetylaspartate + *N*-acetylaspartylglutamate, tNAA), glutamate, glutamine, tCr and MI. The levels of tNAA and glutamate were decreased, while glutamine, tCR and MI levels were elevated. Along with increased neuronal loss and astrocytosis, elevated levels of MI were detected in the pons and cerebellar hemispheres of SCA 1 patients. Differences in MI levels in the study groups allowed for the complete separation of patient and healthy controls (104). In SCA2 there is the occurrence of Purkinje cells depletion and degeneration of the inferior olives, pontine nuclei, as well as pontocerebellar fibers. Ataxin protein-2 specifically binds the IP3R and increases IP3R sensitivity to its activation by IP3. Due to the IP3R overactivation supranormal calcium release from Purkinje cells' endoplasmic reticulum can be observed and as mentioned above in this paper, elevated levels of Ca^{2+} play a key role in the development of neurodegenerative pathologies. In the paper by Kasumu et al., the authors present a study on a SCA2-58Q transgenic mouse model. In SCA2-58Q mice the IP3R activation is chronically downregulated consequently lowering related calcium signaling. This downregulation is obtained through overexpression of the Inositol 1,4,5-phosphatase enzyme (5PP) in Purkinje cells of SCA2 transgenic mice. Their results supported the hypothesis that 5PP overexpression suppresses InsP3-induced Ca^{2+} release, and moreover, that Ca^{2+} release suppression prevents the progressive dysfunction of Purkinje cells in SCA2 mice [99]. SCA-3 is less severe than SCA-2 (25).

The deletion of the IP3R1 gene located on chromosome 3 leads to SCA type 15/16 with late/adult onset, SCA 29 with an early onset type, and also sporadic infantile-onset SCA [103–106]. Researchers suggest that deletion of the IP3R/ITPR1 gene leads to impaired IP3R function. A Western blot of lymphoblastoid cell line proteins confirmed reduced IP3R levels. In conclusion, gene mutations in the course of SCAs lead to reduced activity, as well as IP3R levels.

6.5. Other Neurodegenerative Disorders

The summary of other neurodegenerative disorders has been described in Table 2.

Table 2. The summary of other neurodegenerative disorders.

Disorder	Linkage to MI and It's Derivatives	References
Amyotrophic Lateral Sclerosis (ALS)	- increased MI in ALS patients brains - concentrations of MI were correlated with disease severity	[107]
	- inositol hexakisphosphate kinase 2 promotes cell death of anterior horn cells in the spinal cord	[108]
	- total *N*-acetylaspartate to myo-inositol ratio (tNAA/mIns) in motor cortex is significantly declined - motor cortex tNAA/mIns ratio shows promise as a potential ALS biomarker	[109,110]
Niemann-Pick Disease type C (NPC)	- genetic alterations in lysosomal cholesterol transporter NPC1 disrupt expression and distribution of IP3R1 in ER of neurons thus leading to elevated calcium levels in cells causing mitochondrial cytotoxicity and cell death	[111]
Epilepsy	- regions of brain, involved in seizures, have higher level of inositol - suggested that inositol can induce epilepsy	[112]
	- elevated levels of MI in hippocampus - suggested that MI can be used as early predicator of epilepsy	[113]

7. Possible Treatment Ideas

Changes in the level and metabolism of MI have long been attempted to relate to the occurrence of neurodegenerative diseases, and since these assumptions have been confirmed by many researchers, the next natural step has been to look for possible treatment ideas. From searching the research databases, much information on possible substances that affect the regulation of inositol metabolism can be found, some of them have already been tried, while others are only a vision of the future, knowing only the points of their grip in the cells, giving researchers the opportunity to discover them.

7.1. MI Itself

The first substance worth mentioning is the use of MI itself. MI is often administered in the form of D-pinitol (3-Omethyl-D-chiro-inositol), which is abundant in many plant families such as Pinaceae, Asteraceae, Caryophyllaceae, Zygophyllaceous, Cupressaceae, Aristolochiaceae and Sapindaceae [114]. In other diseases where MI levels are reduced, such as diabetes, PCOS, cancer and mental disorders: depression, panic disorder, obsessive-compulsive disorder and schizophrenia, inositol supplementation as a form of adjunctive therapy has already been better studied [21,115]. D-pinitol can be used in patients after stroke or epileptic seizures, where the loss of neuronal function and, at the same time, a decreased concentration of MI can be observed. In a study from 1996 in which inositol was administered to AD patients, there was a slight improvement in their condition, but these results were not statistically significant [116]. Other studies suggest that inositol may be a possible therapeutic agent of AD because of its positive effect on lowering the toxicity of Aβ oligomers due to the activation of insulin/IGF signaling components and at the same time regulation of γ-secretase activity. D-pinitol also has anti-inflammatory effects [115]. Currently, there are increasingly high hopes for the use of D-pinitol as an ameliorative agent in the treatment of AD. It is considered a selective γ-secretase modulator, and therefore, potentially it would not interfere with other enzymatic pathways, and could have a beneficial effect by inhibiting Aβ production. D-pinitol (NIC5-15) clinical trials are still unfinished, but this substance has a high potential for alleviating AD symptoms [114]. Insulin resistance contributes to the occurrence and worsening of symptoms of neurodegenerative diseases, so D-pinitol as an insulin sensitizer can play an important role in the inhibition of brain alterations. Medina-Vera et al. have shown that oral supplementation of D-pinitol lowered tau phosphorylation, by regulating cyclin-dependent kinase 5 (CDK-5) activity [117]. Scyllo-inositol, as mentioned above, is another naturally occurring stereoisomer of MI and it is also considered a potential remedy for neurodegenerative diseases. It was proven that SI is able to stabilize Aβ42, neutralize cell-derived Aβ trimers, promote low molecular weight Aβ in vivo and inhibit the aggregation of α-synuclein in Parkinson's disease [30,32,82]. SI treatment results in a higher level of MI in the brain and cerebrospinal fluid (CSF). Furthermore, it was shown that these elevated levels of SI have no effect on phosphatidylinositol lipid production and SI does not incorporate into brain PI lipids; therefore, it does not affect the proper functioning of the PI lipids dependent signal transduction pathways. What is more, SI can be supplemented in a convenient oral form, with a high ability to penetrate the blood-brain barrier [118]. There was scientific research on transgenic mice (TgCRND8 mouse model of AD) supplemented by SI for two months, starting at 5 months of age. Mice consumed about 25–30 mg of SI daily. The treatment resulted in a significant reduction in insoluble Aβ40 and Aβ42 levels in the brain, in comparison to the healthy controls. The SI supplementation also reduced the percentage of the brain area covered with plaques [119]. There were seven clinical trials for scyllo-inositol (drug name: ELND005). Four of them were completed, while two were terminated and one is currently under recruitment. One of the completed trials was a randomized, double-blind, placebo-controlled clinical trial of SI conducted on patients with Down Syndrome (DS). DS patients have a high risk of developing AD with an early onset, because of the constant overproduction of Aβ. In this clinical trial, 23 patients were dived into four groups: placebo and three ELND005 administered orally groups with different doses (250 mg, 1000 mg, 2000 mg). The last two groups with the highest SI doses were withdrawn, due to a higher risk of respiratory infections. Patients consuming 250 mg of SI were divided into two groups, considering the number of daily doses: BID—received 250 mg twice a day and QD—once a day. Both groups—250 mg and placebo were observed for 4 weeks. This study confirmed that the administration of SI was well tolerated by patients and no newly identified safety risks were observed. Another trial on 353 patients with the exact same doses, but 78 weeks observation time, also confirmed a higher risk of respiratory tract infections in the group consuming 1000 and 2000 mg of SI, which also lead to more frequent withdrawals in this group connected with adverse events [120,121]. Ways of producing SI through metabolic engineering are currently being sought. In one of the latest studies on this subject, researchers report the possibility of using the bacterium—Corynebacterium glutamicum as a promising host for the production of SI [122]. Another study also aimed at finding inexpensive ways of SI production on a larger scale has shown that different bacteria—Bacillus subtilis can also be used as a potential cell factory [123]. Another MI stereoisomer—epi-inositol—has the ability to stabilize small aggregates of Aβ42, which lowers the Aβ induced toxicity in Alzheimer's disease. It was proven that scyllo-insitol has the same effect on stabilizing Aβ [30,118].

7.2. Lithium and Valproic Acid

Lithium is currently the most widely used first-line mood stabilizer in the treatment of bipolar disorder. There are more and more reports about the possibility of using lithium also in neurodegenerative diseases. Lithium has many mechanisms of action, but the neuroprotective effects can be obtained due to its influence on inositol metabolism by inhibiting IMPase, causing the decrease in MI levels and consequently lowering the IP3 levels.

Lithium-induced autophagy leads to the clearance of neurodegenerative disease-related proteins such as mutant huntingtin fragments and mutant alfa-synuclein [124,125]. As lithium lowers MI levels, it has also been studied how the drug will act with an additional reduction in dietary MI during its use. The results of the research showed an increase in the effect of lithium when following a diet reduced in inositol. The administration of lithium alone reduced the concentration of brain MI by 4.7%, while combined with a low-MI diet by as much as 10.8% [125]. Other mechanisms of lithium action include the regulation of apoptosis and the down-regulation of calpain. The authors emphasize that further clinical studies are needed to determine, whether this drug can be used in the treatment of neurodegenerative diseases and that therapy based only on lithium should not be considered due to the inconsistent efficacy and the occurrence of potential side effects. Lithium should be considered as an adjuvant in the treatment of neurodegenerative diseases, administered along with other existing therapeutic methods [126]. Lithium may also be helpful in the treatment of spinocerebellar ataxias, thus it can alleviate the cerebellar symptoms in affected patients [127]. There are also clinical studies on specific IMPase inhibitor (L-690,330) that mimics the effects of lithium in reducing the MI levels which leads to inhibition of the phosphoinositide cycle, consequently inducing autophagy and clearance of mutant proteins occurring in HD, PD and other neurodegenerative disorders [128]. Another mood stabilizer also a candidate drug for the treatment of neurodegenerative diseases is valproic acid (VPA). Both VPA and other anticonvulsants, such as carbamazepine, also reduce the intracellular concentration of inositol in the brain, having the same effect as lithium and specific IMPase inhibitors. VPA, on the other hand, acts by inhibiting MIPS, which catalyzes the reaction preceding the formation of free MI conducted by IMPase, consequently leading to the same effect of promoting autophagy and mutant protein clearance [112,124]. Other authors also report that during pharmacotherapy with valproic acid and lithium, along with clinical improvement of the patient's health, there is a visible reduction in MI's biosynthesis and its concentration in brain regions such as the frontal and temporal lobes, basal ganglia and cingulate of the rim [3]. Many studies on mice models and rats have shown that lithium and VPA decrease the Aβ plaque formation, enhance Aβ degradation, reduce tau phosphorylation and generally improve neurodegenerative processes [128].

7.3. *γ-Secretase Inhibitors*

γ-secretase is one of three secretases participating in the cleavage of APP and it catalyzes the last reaction when the Aβ is formed. Under normal conditions, only small amounts of Aβ are produced in cells, but in cases of mutated PS 1,2 and APP, these proteins are more easily accessible for γ-secretase, which leads to uncontrolled overproduction of Aβ Attempts have been made to suppress the action of γ-secretase through its inhibitors and modulators. Modulator function was based on the increasing formation of soluble short-chain Aβ, creating a favorable ratio (Aβ37:Aβ40) and reducing the formation of Aβ42. Unfortunately, more than half of the clinical trials of γ-secretase inhibitors have not been finished, due to complications including limited effectiveness, large side effects and poor pharmacokinetics [129,130].

7.4. *Other Possibilities*

Additionally, some newly identified autoantibodies were described by Greek researchers and correlated with cerebellar disorders. In Purkinje neurons the antibody against receptor 1 for inositol was found. That autoantibody can be pivotal in seizures in mice with congenital defects for ataxy and epilepsy. That also gives a chance to develop immunotherapy in such disorders [131].

There are also reports about 2-aminoethoxy diphenyl borate—membrane-permeant IP3R blocker. The authors suggest its neuroprotective function through the inhibition of IP3R-related calcium release. The usage of 2-aminoethoxy diphenyl borate seems promising due to its therapeutic potential for the treatment of neurodegenerative disorders [25,132,

133]. The summary of possible therapeutic methods found in literature is presented in Table 3.

Table 3. The summary of possible therapeutic methods found in literature.

Substance (Drug Name)	Function	Results	Diseases	References
D-pinitol	Insulin-sensitizer; Inhibits γ-secretase; Lowers Tau phosphorylation	↓ Aβ production	AD, tauopathies	[114,117,134,135]
Scyllo-inositol (ELND005, AZD-103)	Stabilize Aβ42, neutralize cell derived Aβ trimers, promote low molecular weight Aβ in vivo; Inhibits the aggregation of α-synuclein in Parkinson's disease	Decreased neuronal toxicity, increased long-term potentiation (LTP) and ablation of cognitive deficits in multiple mouse models of AD	AD, PD	[30,120,122,123,136,137]
Epi-inositol	Stabilize Aβ42	Decreased aggregation of Aβ; Lowers anxiety	AD	[30,138]
Lithium; IMP-ase inhibitor (L-690,330)	Inhibits IMP-ase,	↓ MI ↓ IP3 ↑ clearance of autophagy substrates	HD, PD, SCAs	[112,124]
Valproic acid	Inhibits MIPS in human brain, lowers MI level, inhibits y-secretase	inhibits Aβ production	AD	[112]
γ-secretase inhibitors (Semagacestat (LY450139), MK 0752, E2012, GSI 136)	Inhibits γ-secretase and lowers β-amyloid in blood and spinal fluid in humans	Semagacestat did not slow disease progression, worsened cognitive functions in patients, study drug was stopped in all studies.	AD	[139,140]
Antibodies	Antibodies against IP3 receptor 1	This antibody may have a direct involvement in neurodegenerative process or can be a marker or cerebellar injury.	Cerebellar ataxia, epilepsy	[131]

8. Conclusions

In summary, the incidence of neurodegenerative diseases in society is still a significant problem, affecting mainly the elderly. The researchers are still looking for effective methods of detecting neurodegenerative diseases at their early stages, for which the level of MI can prove to be useful. Changes in MI metabolism at various stages can contribute to the development of diseases leading to atrophy of brain structures, either by promoting the deposition of mutant proteins or an enhancement of calcium release, which ultimately results in increased neuronal degeneration. The use of appropriate supplementation, which would significantly increase the quality of life in affected patients is highly desirable. Studies on the therapeutic efficacy of MI, D-pinitol, SI and other possible treatments should still be conducted. However, the use of MI appears to be beneficial, and supplementation with MI in appropriate doses may prove effective in patients with neurodegenerative diseases with associated symptoms of depression and anxiety.

Author Contributions: Conceptualization, J.W., M.D., P.M. and A.O.; formal analysis, J.W., M.D. and A.O.; writing—original draft preparation J.W., M.D., P.M. and A.O.; writing—review and editing J.W., M.D. and A.O. All authors have read and agreed to the published version of the manuscript.

Funding: This research received no external funding.

Institutional Review Board Statement: Not applicable.

Informed Consent Statement: Not applicable.

Data Availability Statement: Not applicable.

Conflicts of Interest: The authors declare no conflict of interest.

Abbreviations

^{1}H-MRS	Hydrogen 1 proton magnetic resonance spectroscopy
5PP	Inositol 1,4,5-phosphatase enzyme
6-OHDA	6-hydroxydopamine
AD	Alzheimer's disease
AICD	APP intracellular fragment
APP	Amyloid precursor protein
ATP	Adenosine triphosphate
Aβ	Amyloid β
CAST	Calpastatin
CDP-DAG	Cytidine diphosphate diacylglycerol
CFT	APP C-terminal fragment
CICR	Calcium induced calcium release
CMP	Cytidine Monophosphate
CSF	Cerebrospinal fluid
DAG	Diacylglycerol
ER	Endoplasmic reticulum
G-6-P	Glucose-6-Phosphate
GPI	Glycosyl-phosphatidyloinositol
GSIs	γ-secretase inhibitors
HAP1	Htt-associated protein-1A
HD	Huntington's disease
HK	Hexokinase
Htt	Huntingtin
IICR	Inositol induced Ca-release
IMPase	Inositol monophosphatase-1
IP	Inositol phosphate
IP3	Inositol 1,4,5-triphosphate
IP3R	Inositol 1,4,5-triphosphate receptor
IP6K2	Hexakisphosphate kinase type 2
IPG	Inositiol-phosphoglycan
LTP	Long term potentiation
MCI	Mild cognitive impairment
MDA	Malondialdehyde
mHtt	Mutant huntingtin
MI	Myo-inositol
MIOX	Myo-inositol Oxygenase
MIPS	MI-phosphate synthase
mPTP	Mitochondrial permeability transition pore
MRS	Magnetic resonance spectroscopy
MSNs	medium spiny striatal neurons
NADPH	Nicotinamide adenine dinucleotide
NFTs	Neurofibrillary tangles
PD	Parkinson's disease
PI/PtdIns	Phosphatidylinositol
PI4K	Phosphatidylinositol 4-kinase
PIP	Phosphatidyloinositide
PIP2	Phosphatidylinositol biphosphate
PIP5K1	Phosphatidylinositol phosphate 5-kinase 1
PIS	Phosphatidylinositol synthase
PLC	Phospholipase C
PPIP5	inositol pyrophosphate diphosphoinositolpentakisphopshate

PS 1,2	Presenilin 1,2
PSP	Progressive supranuclear palsy
ROS	Reactive oxygen species
RyR	Ryanodine receptor
SCA	Spinocerebellar ataxia
SMA	Supplementary Motor Area
tCr	Total creatine, creatine + phosphocreatine
TG2	Transglutaminase type 2
tNAA	Total NAA, *N*-acetylaspartate + *N*-acetylaspartylglutamate
VPA	Valproic acid
YAC	Yeast artificial chromosome

References

1. Antonowski, T.; Osowski, A.; Lahuta, L.; Górecki, R.; Rynkiewicz, A.; Wojtkiewicz, J. Health-Promoting Properties of Selected Cyclitols for Metabolic Syndrome and Diabetes. *Nutrients* **2019**, *11*, 2314. [CrossRef] [PubMed]
2. Bizzarri, M.; Fuso, A.; Dinicola, S.; Cucina, A.; Bevilacqua, A. Pharmacodynamics and Pharmacokinetics of Inositol(s) in Health and Disease. *Expert Opin. Drug Metab. Toxicol.* **2016**, *12*, 1181–1196. [CrossRef] [PubMed]
3. Owczarczyk-Saczonek, A.; Lahuta, L.B.; Ligor, M.; Placek, W.; Górecki, R.J.; Buszewski, B. The Healing-Promoting Properties of Selected Cyclitols—A Review. *Nutrients* **2018**, *10*, 1891. [CrossRef] [PubMed]
4. Wiśniewski, K.; Jozwik, M.; Wojtkiewicz, J. Cancer Prevention by Natural Products Introduced into the Diet—Selected Cyclitols. *Int. J. Mol. Sci.* **2020**, *21*, 8988. [CrossRef]
5. Murthy, P.P.N. *Biology of Inositols and Phosphoinositides: Subcellular Biochemistry*; Majumder, A.L., Biswas, B.B., Eds.; Subcellular Springer: New York, NY, USA, 2006; ISBN 9780387276007.
6. National Center for Biotechnology Information. PubChem Compound Summary for CID 892, Inositol. Available online: https://pubchem.ncbi.nlm.nih.gov/compound/Inositol (accessed on 18 April 2023).
7. Szkodziak, P.; Paszkowski, T. Wpływ Leczenia Mio-Inozytolem Na Insulinooporność u Pacjentek z Zespołem Policystycznych Jajników w Obserwacji 3-Miesięcznej. Available online: https://inofem.pl/wp-content/uploads/2022/03/Inofem-Badanie-kliniczne.pdf (accessed on 5 November 2016).
8. Croze, M.L.; Soulage, C.O. Potential Role and Therapeutic Interests of Myo-Inositol in Metabolic Diseases. *Biochimie* **2013**, *95*, 1811–1827. [CrossRef]
9. da Costa, L.L.; Adorian, T.J.; Goulart, F.R.; Leitemperger, J.; do Amaral, A.M.B.; Loro, V.L.; Robalo, S.S.; da Silva, L.P. Phytic Acid in Rhamdia Quelen Nutrition: Antioxidant or Antinutrient? *Anim. Feed Sci. Technol.* **2021**, *276*, 114915. [CrossRef]
10. Pramitha, J.L.; Rana, S.; Aggarwal, P.R.; Ravikesavan, R.; Joel, A.J.; Muthamilarasan, M. Diverse Role of Phytic Acid in Plants and Approaches to Develop Low-Phytate Grains to Enhance Bioavailability of Micronutrients. *Adv. Genet.* **2021**, *107*, 89–120.
11. Schlemmer, U.; Frølich, W.; Prieto, R.M.; Grases, F. Phytate in Foods and Significance for Humans: Food Sources, Intake, Processing, Bioavailability, Protective Role and Analysis. *Mol. Nutr. Food Res.* **2009**, *53*, S330–S375. [CrossRef]
12. Stentz, R.; Osborne, S.; Horn, N.; Li, A.W.H.; Hautefort, I.; Bongaerts, R.; Rouyer, M.; Bailey, P.; Shears, S.B.; Hemmings, A.M.; et al. A Bacterial Homolog of a Eukaryotic Inositol Phosphate Signaling Enzyme Mediates Cross-Kingdom Dialog in the Mammalian Gut. *Cell Rep.* **2014**, *6*, 646–656. [CrossRef]
13. Duhan, A.; Khetarpaul, N.; Bishnoi, S. Content of Phytic Acid and HCl-Extractability of Calcium, Phosphorus and Iron as Affected by Various Domestic Processing and Cooking Methods. *Food Chem.* **2002**, *78*, 9–14. [CrossRef]
14. Beemster, P.; Groenen, P.; Steegers-Theunissen, R. Involvement of Inositol in Reproduction. *Nutr. Rev.* **2002**, *60*, 80–87. [CrossRef] [PubMed]
15. Fu, H.; Li, B.; Hertz, L.; Peng, L. Contributions in Astrocytes of SMIT1/2 and HMIT to Myo-Inositol Uptake at Different Concentrations and PH. *Neurochem. Int.* **2012**, *61*, 187–194. [CrossRef] [PubMed]
16. Dai, G.; Yu, H.; Kruse, M.; Traynor-Kaplan, A.; Hille, B. Osmoregulatory Inositol Transporter SMIT1 Modulates Electrical Activity by Adjusting PI(4,5)P2 Levels. *Proc. Natl. Acad. Sci. USA* **2016**, *113*, E3290–E3299. [CrossRef] [PubMed]
17. Kiani, A.K.; Paolacci, S.; Calogero, A.E.; Cannarella, R.; Berardinis, E.D.E.; Giudice, F.D.E.L.; Stuppia, L.; Facchinetti, F. From Myo-Inositol to D-Chiro-Inositol Molecular Pathways. *Eur. Rev. Med. Pharmacol. Sci.* **2021**, *25*, 2390–2402.
18. Uldry, M.; Ibberson, M.; Horisberger, J.D.; Chatton, J.Y.; Riederer, B.M.; Thorens, B. Identification of a Mammalian H+-Myo-Inositol Symporter Expressed Predominantly in the Brain. *EMBO J.* **2001**, *20*, 4467–4477. [CrossRef]
19. Coldebella, D.; Buzzaccarini, G.; Ferrari, J.; Sleiman, Z.; D'Alterio, M.N.; Della Corte, L.; Cucinella, G.; Gullo, G. Inositols Administration: Further Insights on Their Biological Role. *Ital. J. Gynaecol. Obstet.* **2023**, *35*, 30–36. [CrossRef]
20. Loewus, M.W.; Loewus, F.A.; Brillinger, G.U.; Otsuka, H.; Floss, H.G. Stereochemistry of the Myo-Inositol-1-Phosphate Synthase Reaction. *J. Biol. Chem.* **1980**, *255*, 11710–11712. [CrossRef]
21. Wojciechowska, A.; Osowski, A.; Jóźwik, M.; Górecki, R.; Rynkiewicz, A.; Wojtkiewicz, J. Inositols' Importance in the Improvement of the Endocrine–Metabolic Profile in PCOS. *Int. J. Mol. Sci.* **2019**, *20*, 5787. [CrossRef]

22. Chang, H.H.; Chao, H.N.; Walker, C.S.; Choong, S.Y.; Phillips, A.; Loomes, K.M. Renal Depletion of *Myo*-Inositol Is Associated with Its Increased Degradation in Animal Models of Metabolic Disease. *Am. J. Physiol. Ren. Physiol.* **2015**, *309*, F755–F763. [CrossRef]
23. Kruger, N.J.; Von Schaewen, A. The Oxidative Pentose Phosphate Pathway: Structure and Organisation. *Curr. Opin. Plant Biol.* **2003**, *6*, 236–246. [CrossRef]
24. Alfarouk, K.O.; Ahmed, S.B.M.; Elliott, R.L.; Benoit, A.; Alqahtani, S.S.; Ibrahim, M.E.; Bashir, A.H.H.; Alhoufie, S.T.S.; Elhassan, G.O.; Wales, C.C.; et al. The Pentose Phosphate Pathway Dynamics in Cancer and Its Dependency on Intracellular PH. *Metabolites* **2020**, *10*, 285. [CrossRef] [PubMed]
25. Egorova, P.A.; Bezprozvanny, I.B. Inositol 1,4,5-Trisphosphate Receptors and Neurodegenerative Disorders. *FEBS J.* **2018**, *285*, 3547–3565. [CrossRef] [PubMed]
26. Serysheva, I.I. Toward a High-Resolution Structure of IP3R Channel. *Cell Calcium* **2014**, *56*, 125–132. [CrossRef] [PubMed]
27. Briggs, C.A.; Chakroborty, S.; Stutzmann, G.E. Emerging Pathways Driving Early Synaptic Pathology in Alzheimer's Disease. *Biochem. Biophys. Res. Commun.* **2017**, *483*, 988–997. [CrossRef]
28. Choe, C.; Ehrlich, B.E. (IP 3 R) and Its Regulators: Sometimes Good and sometimes bad teamwork. *Sci. STKE* **2006**, *363*, re15.
29. Takada, S.H.; Ikebara, J.M.; de Sousa, E.; Cardoso, D.S.; Resende, R.R.; Ulrich, H.; Rückl, M.; Rüdiger, S.; Kihara, A.H. Determining the Roles of Inositol Trisphosphate Receptors in Neurodegeneration: Interdisciplinary Perspectives on a Complex Topic. *Mol. Neurobiol.* **2017**, *54*, 6870–6884. [CrossRef]
30. López-Gambero, A.J.; Sanjuan, C.; Serrano-Castro, P.J.; Suárez, J.; De Fonseca, F.R. The Biomedical Uses of Inositols: A Nutraceutical Approach to Metabolic Dysfunction in Aging and Neurodegenerative Diseases. *Biomedicines* **2020**, *8*, 295. [CrossRef]
31. Haris, M.; Cai, K.; Singh, A.; Hariharan, H.; Reddy, R. In Vivo Mapping of Brain Myo-Inositol. *Neuroimage* **2011**, *54*, 2079–2085. [CrossRef]
32. Thomas, M.P.; Mills, S.J.; Potter, B.V.L. The "Other" Inositols and Their Phosphates: Synthesis, Biology, and Medicine (with Recent Advances in Myo-Inositol Chemistry). *Angew. Chem. Int. Ed.* **2016**, *55*, 1614–1650. [CrossRef]
33. Seaquist, E.R.; Gruetter, R. Identification of a High Concentration of Scyllo-Inositol in the Brain of a Healthy Human Subject Using 1H- and 13C-NMR. *Magn. Reson. Med.* **1998**, *39*, 313–316. [CrossRef]
34. Spector, R.; Lorenzo, A.V. Folate Transport in the Central Nervous System. *Am. J. Physiol.* **1975**, *229*, 777–782. [CrossRef] [PubMed]
35. Choi, J.-K.; Carreras, I.; Dedeoglu, A.; Jenkins, B.G. Detection of Increased Scyllo-Inositol in Brain with Magnetic Resonance Spectroscopy after Dietary Supplementation in Alzheimer's Disease Mouse Models. *Neuropharmacology* **2010**, *59*, 353–357. [CrossRef] [PubMed]
36. Barbagallo, G.; Morelli, M.; Quattrone, A.; Chiriaco, C.; Vaccaro, M.G.; Gullà, D.; Rocca, F.; Caracciolo, M.; Novellino, F.; Sarica, A.; et al. In Vivo Evidence for Decreased Scyllo-Inositol Levels in the Supplementary Motor Area of Patients with Progressive Supranuclear Palsy: A Proton MR Spectroscopy Study. *Park. Relat. Disord.* **2019**, *62*, 185–191. [CrossRef] [PubMed]
37. Cummings, J.L.; Cole, G. Alzheimer Disease. *Jama* **2002**, *287*, 2335–2338. [CrossRef]
38. Gaugler, J.; James, B.; Johnson, T.; Scholz, K.; Weuve, J. 2016 Alzheimer's Disease Facts and Figures. *Alzheimers Dement.* **2016**, *12*, 459–509. [CrossRef]
39. Masters, C.L.; Bateman, R.; Blennow, K.; Rowe, C.C.; Sperling, R.A.; Cummings, J.L. Alzheimer's Disease. *Nat. Rev. Dis. Prim.* **2015**, *1*, 15056. [CrossRef]
40. Harman, D. Alzheimer's Disease: Role of Aging in Pathogenesis. *Ann. N. Y. Acad. Sci.* **2002**, *959*, 384–395. [CrossRef]
41. Cruts, M.; Hendriks, L.; Van Broeckhoven, C. The Presenilin Genes: A New Gene Family Involved in Alzheimer Disease Pathology. *Hum. Mol. Genet.* **1996**, *5*, 1449–1455. [CrossRef]
42. Cruts, M.; Van Broeckhoven, C. Presenilin Mutations in Alzheimer's Disease. *Hum. Mutat.* **1998**, *11*, 183–190. [CrossRef]
43. Hutton, M.; Hardy, J. The Presenilins and Alzheimer's Disease. *Hum. Mol. Genet.* **1997**, *6*, 1639–1646. [CrossRef]
44. Gołaszewska, A.; Bik, W.; Motyl, T.; Orzechowski, A. Bridging the Gap between Alzheimer's Disease and Alzheimer's-like Diseases in Animals. *Int. J. Mol. Sci.* **2019**, *20*, 1664. [CrossRef] [PubMed]
45. Multhaup, G.; Huber, O.; Buée, L.; Galas, M.C. Amyloid Precursor Protein (APP) Metabolites APP Intracellular Fragment (AICD), Aβ42, and Tau in Nuclear Roles. *J. Biol. Chem.* **2015**, *290*, 23515–23522. [CrossRef] [PubMed]
46. Hansson, O.; Lehmann, S.; Otto, M.; Zetterberg, H.; Lewczuk, P. Advantages and Disadvantages of the Use of the CSF Amyloid β (Aβ) 42/40 Ratio in the Diagnosis of Alzheimer's Disease. *Alzheimers Res. Ther.* **2019**, *11*, 34. [CrossRef]
47. O'Neill, C.; Cowburn, R.F.; Bonkale, W.L.; Ohm, T.G.; Fastbom, J.; Carmody, M.; Kelliher, M. Dysfunctional Intracellular Calcium Homoeostasis: A Central Cause of Neurodegeneration in Alzheimer's Disease. *Biochem. Soc. Symp.* **2001**, *67*, 177–194. [CrossRef]
48. Huang, W.; Alexander, G.E.; Daly, E.M.; Shetty, H.U.; Krasuski, J.S.; Rapoport, S.I.; Schapiro, M.B. High Brain Myo-Inositol Levels in the Predementia Phase of Alzheimer's Disease in Adults with Down's Syndrome: A 1H MRS Study. *Am. J. Psychiatry* **1999**, *156*, 1879–1886. [CrossRef] [PubMed]
49. Chen, S.Q.; Wang, P.J.; Ten, G.J.; Zhan, W.; Li, M.H.; Zang, F.C. Role of Myo-Inositol by Magnetic Resonance Spectroscopy in Early Diagnosis of Alzheimer's Disease in APP/PS1 Transgenic Mice. *Dement. Geriatr. Cogn. Disord.* **2009**, *28*, 558–566. [CrossRef]
50. Griffith, H.R.; den Hollander, J.A.; Stewart, C.C.; Evanochko, W.T.; Buchthal, S.D.; Harrell, L.E.; Zamrini, E.Y.; Brockington, J.C.; Marson, D.C. Elevated Brain *Scyllo*-inositol Concentrations in Patients with Alzheimer's Disease. *NMR Biomed. Int. J. Devoted Dev. Appl. Magn. Reson. In Vivo* **2007**, *20*, 709–716.

51. Firbank, M.J.; Harrison, R.M.; O'Brien, J.T. A Comprehensive Review of Proton Magnetic Resonance Spectroscopy. *Dement. Geriatr. Cogn. Disord.* **2002**, *14*, 64–76. [CrossRef]
52. Jaworska, A.; Dzbek, J.; Styczynska, M.; Kuznicki, J. Analysis of Calcium Homeostasis in Fresh Lymphocytes from Patients with Sporadic Alzheimer's Disease or Mild Cognitive Impairment. *Biochim. Biophys. Acta Mol. Cell Res.* **2013**, *1833*, 1692–1699. [CrossRef]
53. Ali, F.; Manzoor, U.; Bhattacharya, R.; Bansal, A.K.; Chandrashekharaiah, K.S.; Singh, L.R.; Saraswati, S.M.; Uversky, V.; Dar, T.A. Brain Metabolite, Myo-Inositol, Inhibits Catalase Activity: A Mechanism of the Distortion of the Antioxidant Defense System in Alzheimer's Disease. *ACS Omega* **2022**, *7*, 12690–12700. [CrossRef]
54. Doraiswamy, P.M.; Charles, H.C.; Krishnan, K.R.R. Prediction of Cognitive Decline in Early Alzheimer's Disease. *Lancet* **1998**, *352*, 1678. [CrossRef]
55. Wang, X.; Zheng, W. Ca^{2+} Homeostasis Dysregulation in Alzheimer's Disease: A Focus on Plasma Membrane and Cell Organelles. *FASEB J.* **2019**, *33*, 6697–6712. [CrossRef] [PubMed]
56. Huang, H.M.; Toral-Barza, L.; Thaler, H.; Tofel-Grehl, B.; Gibson, G.E. Inositol Phosphates and Intracellular Calcium after Bradykinin Stimulation in Fibroblasts from Young, Normal Aged and Alzheimer Donors. *Neurobiol. Aging* **1991**, *12*, 469–473. [CrossRef] [PubMed]
57. Berridge, M.J. The Inositol Trisphosphate/Calcium Signaling Pathway in Health and Disease. *Physiol. Rev.* **2016**, *96*, 1261–1296. [CrossRef] [PubMed]
58. Seo, M.D.; Enomoto, M.; Ishiyama, N.; Stathopulos, P.B.; Ikura, M. Structural Insights into Endoplasmic Reticulum Stored Calcium Regulation by Inositol 1,4,5-Trisphosphate and Ryanodine Receptors. *Biochim. Biophys. Acta Mol. Cell Res.* **2014**, *1853*, 1980–1991. [CrossRef]
59. Hinterberger, M.; Fischer, P. Folate and Alzheimer: When Time Matters. *J. Neural Transm.* **2013**, *120*, 211–224. [CrossRef]
60. Blanchard, B.J.; Thomas, V.L.; Ingram, V.M. Mechanism of Membrane Depolarization Caused by the Alzheimer Aβ1-42 Peptide. *Biochem. Biophys. Res. Commun.* **2002**, *293*, 1197–1203. [CrossRef]
61. LÜckhoff, A.; Clapham, D.E. E. Inositol 1, 3, 4, 5-Tetrakisphosphate Activates an Endothelial Ca^{2+}-Permeable Channel. *Nature* **1992**, *355*, 356–358. [CrossRef]
62. Tsubokawa, H.; Oguro, K.; Robinson, H.P.C.; Masuzawa, T.; Rhee, T.S.G.; Takenawa, T.; Kawai, N. Inositol 1,3,4,5 Tetrakisphosphate as a Mediator of Neuronal Death in Ischemic Hippocampus. *Neuroscience* **1994**, *59*, 291–297. [CrossRef]
63. Haug, L.S.; Østvold, A.C.; Cowburn, R.F.; Winblad, B.; Bogdanovich, N.; Walaas, S.I. Decreased inositol (1, 4, 5)-trisphosphate receptor levels in Alzheimer's disease cerebral cortex: Selectivity of changes and possible correlation to pathological severity. *Neurodegeneration* **1996**, *5*, 169–176. [CrossRef]
64. Young, L.T.; Kish, S.J.; Li, P.P.; Warsh, J.J. Decreased Brain [3H]Inositol 1,4,5-Trisphosphate Binding in Alzheimer's Disease. *Neurosci. Lett.* **1988**, *94*, 198–202. [CrossRef]
65. Mak, D.O.D.; Cheung, K.H.; Toglia, P.; Foskett, J.K.; Ullah, G. Analyzing and Quantifying the Gain-of-Function Enhancement of IP3 Receptor Gating by Familial Alzheimer's Disease-Causing Mutants in Presenilins. *PLoS Comput. Biol.* **2015**, *11*, e1004529. [CrossRef] [PubMed]
66. Cheung, K.H.; Mei, L.; Mak, D.O.D.; Hayashi, I.; Iwatsubo, T.; Kang, D.E.; Foskett, J.K. Gain-of-Function Enhancement of IP3 Receptor Modal Gating by Familial Alzheimer's Disease-Linked Presenilin Mutants in Human Cells and Mouse Neurons. *Sci. Signal.* **2010**, *3*, ra22. [CrossRef] [PubMed]
67. Toglia, P.; Ullah, G. The Gain-of-Function Enhancement of IP3-Receptor Channel Gating by Familial Alzheimer's Disease-Linked Presenilin Mutants Increases the Open Probability of Mitochondrial Permeability Transition Pore. *Cell Calcium* **2016**, *60*, 13–24. [CrossRef]
68. Elder, G.A.; Sosa, M.A.G.; De Gasperi, R.; Dickstein, D.L.; Hof, P.R. Presenilin Transgenic Mice as Models of Alzheimer's Disease. *Brain Struct. Funct.* **2010**, *214*, 127–143. [CrossRef]
69. Halestrap, A.P. What Is the Mitochondrial Permeability Transition Pore? *J. Mol. Cell. Cardiol.* **2009**, *46*, 821–831. [CrossRef]
70. Baumgartner, H.K.; Gerasimenko, J.V.; Thorne, C.; Ferdek, P.; Pozzan, T.; Tepikin, A.V.; Petersen, O.H.; Sutton, R.; Watson, A.J.M.; Gerasimenko, O.V. Calcium Elevation in Mitochondria Is the Main Ca^{2+} Requirement for Mitochondrial Permeability Transition Pore (MPTP) Opening. *J. Biol. Chem.* **2009**, *284*, 20796–20803. [CrossRef] [PubMed]
71. Shilling, D.; Müller, M.; Takano, H.; Mak, D.O.D.; Abel, T.; Coulter, D.A.; Foskett, J.K. Suppression of InsP3 Receptor-Mediated Ca^{2+} Signaling Alleviates Mutant Presenilin-Linked Familial Alzheimer's Disease Pathogenesis. *J. Neurosci.* **2014**, *34*, 6910–6923. [CrossRef] [PubMed]
72. Nixon, R.A.; Saito, K.I.; Grynspan, F.; Griffin, W.R.; Katayama, S.; Honda, T.; Mohan, P.S.; Shea, T.B.; Beermann, M. Calcium-Activated Neutral Proteinase (Calpain) System in Aging and Alzheimer's Disease. *Ann. N. Y. Acad. Sci.* **1994**, *747*, 77–91. [CrossRef]
73. Sorimachi, H.; Hata, S.; Ono, Y. Calpain chronicle—An enzyme family under multidisciplinary characterization. 2011, 87, 287-327. *Proc. Jpn. Acad. Ser. B* **2011**, *87*, 287–327. [CrossRef]
74. Higuchi, M.; Tomioka, M.; Takano, J.; Shirotani, K.; Iwata, N.; Masumoto, H.; Maki, M.; Itohara, S.; Saido, T.C. Distinct Mechanistic Roles of Calpain and Caspase Activation in Neurodegeneration as Revealed in Mice Overexpressing Their Specific Inhibitors. *J. Biol. Chem.* **2005**, *280*, 15229–15237. [CrossRef] [PubMed]

75. Rao, M.V.; Mohan, P.S.; Peterhoff, C.M.; Yang, D.S.; Schmidt, S.D.; Stavrides, P.H.; Campbell, J.; Chen, Y.; Jiang, Y.; Paskevich, P.A.; et al. Marked Calpastatin (CAST) Depletion in Alzheimer's Disease Accelerates Cytoskeleton Disruption and Neurodegeneration: Neuroprotection by CAST Overexpression. *J. Neurosci.* **2008**, *28*, 12241–12254. [CrossRef] [PubMed]
76. Mahaman, Y.A.R.; Huang, F.; Afewerky, H.K.; Maibouge, T.M.S.; Ghose, B.; Wang, X. Involvement of Calpain in the Neuropathogenesis of Alzheimer's Disease. *Med. Res. Rev.* **2019**, *39*, 608–630. [CrossRef] [PubMed]
77. Frazier, H.N.; Maimaiti, S.; Anderson, K.L.; Brewer, L.D.; Gant, J.C.; Porter, N.M.; Thibault, O. Calcium's Role as Nuanced Modulator of Cellular Physiology in the Brain. *Biochem. Biophys. Res. Commun.* **2017**, *483*, 981–987. [CrossRef]
78. Sepasi Tehrani, H.; Moosavi-Movahedi, A.A. Catalase and Its Mysteries. *Prog. Biophys. Mol. Biol.* **2018**, *140*, 5–12. [CrossRef]
79. Nandi, A.; Yan, L.J.; Jana, C.K.; Das, N. Role of Catalase in Oxidative Stress-and Age-Associated Degenerative Diseases. *Oxid. Med. Cell. Longev.* **2019**, *2019*, 9613090. [CrossRef]
80. Jiang, W.D.; Feng, L.; Liu, Y.; Jiang, J.; Zhou, X.Q. *Myo*-Inositol Prevents Oxidative Damage, Inhibits Oxygen Radical Generation and Increases Antioxidant Enzyme Activities of Juvenile Jian Carp (*Cyprinus Carpio* Var. Jian). *Aquac. Res.* **2009**, *40*, 1770–1776. [CrossRef]
81. Poewe, W.; Seppi, K.; Tanner, C.M.; Halliday, G.M.; Brundin, P.; Volkmann, J.; Schrag, A.E.; Lang, A.E. Parkinson Disease. *Nat. Rev. Dis. Prim.* **2017**, *3*, 17013. [CrossRef]
82. Ibrahim, T.; McLaurin, J.A. α-Synuclein Aggregation, Seeding and Inhibition by Scyllo-Inositol. *Biochem. Biophys. Res. Commun.* **2016**, *469*, 529–534. [CrossRef]
83. Zhang, Z.; Hou, L.; Li, X.; Ju, C.; Zhang, J.; Li, X.; Wang, X.; Liu, C.; Lv, Y.; Wang, Y. Neuroprotection of Inositol Hexaphosphate and Changes of Mitochondrion Mediated Apoptotic Pathway and α-Synuclein Aggregation in 6-OHDA Induced Parkinson's Disease Cell Model. *Brain Res.* **2016**, *1633*, 87–95. [CrossRef]
84. Kitamura, N.; Hashimoto, T.; Nishino, N.; Tanaka, C. Inositol 1,4,5-Trisphosphate Binding Sites in the Brain: Regional Distribution, Characterization, and Alterations in Brains of Patients with Parkinson's Disease. *J. Mol. Neurosci.* **1989**, *1*, 181–187. [CrossRef] [PubMed]
85. Novotny, E.; Ashwal, S.; Shevell, M. Proton Magnetic Resonance Spectroscopy: An Emerging Technology in Pediatric Neurology Research. *Pediatr. Res.* **1998**, *44*, 1–10. [CrossRef] [PubMed]
86. Mazuel, L.; Chassain, C.; Jean, B.; Pereira, B.; Cladière, A.; Speziale, C.; Durif, F. Proton MR Spectroscopy for Diagnosis and Evaluation of Treatment Efficacy in Parkinson Disease. *Radiology* **2016**, *278*, 505–513. [CrossRef] [PubMed]
87. Ciurleo, R.; Di Lorenzo, G.; Bramanti, P.; Marino, S. Magnetic Resonance Spectroscopy: An in Vivo Molecular Imaging Biomarker for Parkinson's Disease? *Biomed Res. Int.* **2014**, *2014*, 519816. [CrossRef]
88. Gröger, A.; Chadzynski, G.; Godau, J.; Berg, D.; Klose, U. Three-Dimensional Magnetic Resonance Spectroscopic Imaging in the Substantia Nigra of Healthy Controls and Patients with Parkinson's Disease. *Eur. Radiol.* **2011**, *21*, 1962–1969. [CrossRef]
89. Morris, H.R. Progressive Supranuclear Palsy. *Blue Books Neurol.* **2010**, *34*, 361–374. [CrossRef]
90. Mishori, A.; Levine, J.; Kahana, E.; Belmaker, R.H. Inositol Is Not Therapeutic in Parkinson's Disease. *Hum. Psychopharmacol.* **1999**, *14*, 271–272. [CrossRef]
91. Walker, F.O. Huntington's Disease. *Lancet* **2007**, *369*, 218–228. [CrossRef]
92. Finkbeiner, S. Huntington ' s Disease. *Cold Spring Harb. Perspect. Biol.* **2011**, *3*, a007476. [CrossRef]
93. Tang, T.S.; Tu, H.; Orban, P.C.; Chan, E.Y.W.; Hayden, M.R.; Bezprozvanny, I. HAP1 Facilitates Effects of Mutant Huntingtin on Inositol 1,4,5-Trisphosphate-Induced Ca^{2+} Release in Primary Culture of Striatal Medium Spiny Neurons. *Eur. J. Neurosci.* **2004**, *20*, 1779–1787. [CrossRef]
94. Hamada, K.; Terauchi, A.; Nakamura, K.; Higo, T.; Nukina, N.; Matsumoto, N.; Hisatsune, C.; Nakamura, T.; Mikoshiba, K. Aberrant Calcium Signaling by Transglutaminase-Mediated Posttranslational Modification of Inositol 1,4,5-Trisphosphate Receptors. *Proc. Natl. Acad. Sci. USA* **2014**, *111*, E3966–E3975. [CrossRef] [PubMed]
95. Post, J.I.; Leergaard, T.B.; Ratz, V.; Walaas, S.I.; Von Hörsten, S.; Nissen-Meyer, L.S.H. Differential Levels and Phosphorylation of Type 1 Inositol 1,4,5-Trisphosphate Receptor in Four Different Murine Models of Huntington Disease. *J. Huntingtons Dis.* **2019**, *8*, 271–289. [CrossRef] [PubMed]
96. Nagata, E.; Nonaka, T.; Moriya, Y.; Fujii, N.; Okada, Y.; Tsukamoto, H.; Itoh, J.; Okada, C.; Satoh, T.; Arai, T.; et al. Inositol Hexakisphosphate Kinase 2 Promotes Cell Death in Cells with Cytoplasmic TDP-43 Aggregation. *Mol. Neurobiol.* **2016**, *53*, 5377–5383. [CrossRef] [PubMed]
97. Nagata, E.; Saiardi, A.; Tsukamoto, H.; Okada, Y.; Itoh, Y.; Satoh, T.; Itoh, J.; Margolis, R.L.; Takizawa, S.; Sawa, A.; et al. Inositol Hexakisphosphate Kinases Induce Cell Death in Huntington Disease. *J. Biol. Chem.* **2011**, *286*, 26680–26686. [CrossRef] [PubMed]
98. Sun, Y.M.; Lu, C.; Wu, Z.Y. Spinocerebellar Ataxia: Relationship between Phenotype and Genotype—A Review. *Clin. Genet.* **2016**, *90*, 305–314. [CrossRef] [PubMed]
99. Kasumu, A.W.; Liang, X.; Egorova, P.; Vorontsova, D.; Bezprozvanny, I. Chronic Suppression of Inositol 1,4,5-Triphosphate Receptor-Mediated Calcium Signaling in Cerebellar Purkinje Cells Alleviates Pathological Phenotype in Spinocerebellar Ataxia 2 Mice. *J. Neurosci.* **2012**, *32*, 12786–12796. [CrossRef]
100. Tipton, P.W.; Guthrie, K.; Strongosky, A.; Reimer, R.; Wszolek, Z.K. Spinocerebellar Ataxia 15: A Phenotypic Review and Expansion. *Neurol. Neurochir. Pol.* **2017**, *51*, 86–91. [CrossRef]
101. Klockgether, T.; Mariotti, C.; Paulson, H.L. Spinocerebellar Ataxia. *Nat. Rev. Dis. Prim.* **2019**, *5*, 24. [CrossRef]

102. Brown, S.A.; Loew, L.M. Integration of Modeling with Experimental and Clinical Findings Synthesizes and Refines the Central Role of Inositol 1,4,5-Trisphosphate Receptor 1 in Spinocerebellar Ataxia. *Front. Neurosci.* **2015**, *8*, 453. [CrossRef]
103. Novak, M.J.U.; Sweeney, M.G.; Li, A.; Treacy, C.; Chandrashekar, H.S.; Giunti, P.; Goold, R.G.; Davis, M.B.; Houlden, H.; Tabrizi, S.J. An ITPR1 Gene Deletion Causes Spinocerebellar Ataxia 15/16: A Genetic, Clinical and Radiological Description. *Mov. Disord.* **2010**, *25*, 2176–2182. [CrossRef]
104. Sasaki, M.; Ohba, C.; Iai, M.; Hirabayashi, S.; Osaka, H.; Hiraide, T.; Saitsu, H.; Matsumoto, N. Sporadic Infantile-Onset Spinocerebellar Ataxia Caused by Missense Mutations of the Inositol 1,4,5-Triphosphate Receptor Type 1 Gene. *J. Neurol.* **2015**, *262*, 1278–1284. [CrossRef] [PubMed]
105. Obayashi, M.; Ishikawa, K.; Izumi, Y.; Takahashi, M.; Niimi, Y.; Sato, N.; Onodera, O.; Kaji, R.; Nishizawa, M.; Mizusawa, H. Prevalence of Inositol 1, 4, 5-Triphosphate Receptor Type 1 Gene Deletion, the Mutation for Spinocerebellar Ataxia Type 15, in Japan Screened by Gene Dosage. *J. Hum. Genet.* **2012**, *57*, 202–206. [CrossRef] [PubMed]
106. van Dijk, T.; Barth, P.; Reneman, L.; Appelhof, B.; Baas, F.; Poll-The, B.T. A de Novo Missense Mutation in the Inositol 1,4,5-Triphosphate Receptor Type 1 Gene Causing Severe Pontine and Cerebellar Hypoplasia: Expanding the Phenotype of ITPR1-Related Spinocerebellar Ataxia's. *Am. J. Med. Genet. Part A* **2017**, *173*, 207–212. [CrossRef] [PubMed]
107. Weerasekera, A.; Peeters, R.; Sima, D.; Dresselaers, T.; Sunaert, S.; De Vocht, J.; Claeys, K.; Van Huffel, S.; Van Damme, P.; Himmelreich, U. Motor Cortex Metabolite Alterations in Amyotrophic Lateral Sclerosis Assessed in Vivo Using Edited and Non-Edited Magnetic Resonance Spectroscopy. *Brain Res.* **2019**, *1718*, 22–31. [CrossRef] [PubMed]
108. Nagata, E.; Fujii, N.; Kohara, S.; Okada, C.; Satoh, T.; Takekoshi, S.; Takao, M.; Mihara, B.; Takizawa, S. Inositol Hexakisphosphate Kinase 2 Promotes Cell Death of Anterior Horn Cells in the Spinal Cord of Patients with Amyotrophic Lateral Sclerosis. *Mol. Biol. Rep.* **2020**, *47*, 6479–6485. [CrossRef] [PubMed]
109. Cheong, I.; Deelchand, D.K.; Eberly, L.E.; Marjańska, M.; Manousakis, G.; Guliani, G.; Walk, D.; Öz, G. Neurochemical Correlates of Functional Decline in Amyotrophic Lateral Sclerosis. *J. Neurol. Neurosurg. Psychiatry* **2019**, *90*, 294–301. [CrossRef]
110. Srivastava, O.; Hanstock, C.; Chenji, S.; Mah, D.; Eurich, D.; Ta, D.; Seres, P.; Luk, C.; Zinman, L.; Abrahao, A.; et al. Cerebral Degeneration in Amyotrophic Lateral Sclerosis: A Prospective Multicenter Magnetic Resonance Spectroscopy Study. *Neurol. Clin. Pract.* **2019**, *9*, 400–407. [CrossRef]
111. Tiscione, S.A.; Casas, M.; Horvath, J.D.; Lam, V.; Hino, K.; Ory, D.S.; Fernando Santana, L.; Simó, S.; Dixon, R.E.; Dickson, E.J. IP3R-Driven Increases in Mitochondrial Ca^{2+} Promote Neuronal Death in NPC Disease. *Proc. Natl. Acad. Sci. USA* **2021**, *118*, e2110629118. [CrossRef]
112. Chhetri, D.R. Myo-Inositol and Its Derivatives: Their Emerging Role in the Treatment of Human Diseases. *Front. Pharmacol.* **2019**, *10*, 1172. [CrossRef]
113. Pascente, R.; Frigerio, F.; Rizzi, M.; Porcu, L.; Boido, M.; Davids, J.; Zaben, M.; Tolomeo, D.; Filibian, M.; Gray, W.P.; et al. Cognitive Deficits and Brain Myo-Inositol Are Early Biomarkers of Epileptogenesis in a Rat Model of Epilepsy. *Neurobiol. Dis.* **2016**, *93*, 146–155. [CrossRef]
114. Dubey, A.; Srivastava, K.; Tiwari, M.; Dubey, A. D-Pinitol-A Natural Phytomolecule and Its Pharmacological Effect. *Int. J. Pharm. Life Sci.* **2020**, *11*, 6609–6623.
115. Sánchez-Hidalgo, M.; León-González, A.J.; Gálvez-Peralta, M.; González-Mauraza, N.H.; Martin-Cordero, C. D-Pinitol: A Cyclitol with Versatile Biological and Pharmacological Activities. *Phytochem. Rev.* **2021**, *20*, 211–224. [CrossRef]
116. Barak, Y.; Levine, J.; Glasman, A.; Elizur, A.; Belmaker, R.H. Inositol Treatment of Alzheimer's Disease: A Double Blind, Cross-over Placebo Controlled Trial. *Prog. Neuro-Psychopharmacol. Biol. Psychiatry* **1996**, *20*, 729–735. [CrossRef] [PubMed]
117. Medina-Vera, D.; Navarro, J.A.; Rivera, P.; Rosell-Valle, C.; Gutiérrez-Adán, A.; Sanjuan, C.; López-Gambero, A.J.; Tovar, R.; Suárez, J.; Pavón, F.J.; et al. D-Pinitol Promotes Tau Dephosphorylation through a Cyclin-Dependent Kinase 5 Regulation Mechanism: A New Potential Approach for Tauopathies? *Br. J. Pharmacol.* **2022**, *179*, 4655–4672. [CrossRef]
118. McLaurin, J.A.; Golomb, R.; Jurewicz, A.; Antel, J.P.; Fraser, P.E. Inositol Stereoisomers Stabilize an Oligomeric Aggregate of Alzheimer Amyloid β Peptide and Inhibit Aβ-Induced Toxicity. *J. Biol. Chem.* **2000**, *275*, 18495–18502. [CrossRef]
119. Fenili, D.; Brown, M.; Rappaport, R.; McLaurin, J.A. Properties of Scyllo-Inositol as a Therapeutic Treatment of AD-like Pathology. *J. Mol. Med.* **2007**, *85*, 603–611. [CrossRef]
120. Rafii, M.S.; Skotko, B.G.; McDonough, M.E.; Pulsifer, M.; Evans, C.; Doran, E.; Muranevici, G.; Kesslak, P.; Abushakra, S.; Lott, I.T. A Randomized, Double-Blind, Placebo-Controlled, Phase II Study of Oral ELND005 (Scyllo-Inositol) in Young Adults with Down Syndrome without Dementia. *J. Alzheimers Dis.* **2017**, *58*, 401–411. [CrossRef]
121. Salloway, S.; Sperling, R.; Keren, R.; Porsteinsson, A.P.; Van Dyck, C.H.; Tariot, P.N.; Gilman, S.; Arnold, D.; Abushakra, S.; Hernandez, C.; et al. A Phase 2 Randomized Trial of ELND005, Scyllo-Inositol, in Mild to Moderate Alzheimer Disease. *Neurology* **2011**, *77*, 1253–1262. [CrossRef]
122. Ramp, P.; Lehnert, A.; Matamouros, S.; Wirtz, A.; Baumgart, M.; Bott, M. Metabolic Engineering of Corynebacterium Glutamicum for Production of Scyllo-Inositol, a Drug Candidate against Alzheimer's Disease. *Metab. Eng.* **2021**, *67*, 173–185. [CrossRef]
123. Michon, C.; Kang, C.M.; Karpenko, S.; Tanaka, K.; Ishikawa, S.; Yoshida, K. ichi A Bacterial Cell Factory Converting Glucose into Scyllo-Inositol, a Therapeutic Agent for Alzheimer's Disease. *Commun. Biol.* **2020**, *3*, 93. [CrossRef]
124. Sarkar, S.; Rubinsztein, D.C. Inositol and IP3 Levels Regulate Autophagy: Biology and Therapeutic Speculations. *Autophagy* **2006**, *2*, 132–134. [CrossRef] [PubMed]
125. Pietruczuk, K.; Witkowski, J.M. Lithium Salts-Mechanisms of Action | Mechanizmy Działania Soli Litu. *Psychiatria* **2008**, *5*, 51–57.

126. Lazzara, C.A.; Kim, Y.H. Potential Application of Lithium in Parkinson's and Other Neurodegenerative Diseases. *Front. Neurosci.* **2015**, *9*, 403. [CrossRef]
127. Morlet, É.; Hozer, F.; Costemale-Lacoste, J.F. Neuroprotective Effects of Lithium: What Are the Implications in Humans with Neurodegenerative Disorders? *Geriatr. Psychol. Neuropsychiatr. Vieil.* **2018**, *16*, 78–86. [CrossRef] [PubMed]
128. Schmukler, E.; Pinkas-Kramarski, R. Autophagy Induction in the Treatment of Alzheimer's Disease. *Drug Dev. Res.* **2020**, *81*, 184–193. [CrossRef] [PubMed]
129. Jia, H.; Wang, Z.; Zhang, J.; Feng, F. γ-Secretase Inhibitors for Breast Cancer and Hepatocellular Carcinoma: From Mechanism to Treatment. *Life Sci.* **2021**, *268*, 119007. [CrossRef]
130. Golde, T.E.; Koo, E.H.; Felsenstein, K.M.; Osborne, B.A.; Miele, L. γ-Secretase Inhibitors and Modulators. *Biochim. Biophys. Acta-Biomembr.* **2013**, *1828*, 2898–2907. [CrossRef]
131. Fouka, P.; Alexopoulos, H.; Chatzi, I.; Dedos, S.G.; Samiotaki, M.; Panayotou, G.; Politis, P.; Tzioufas, A.; Dalakas, M.C. Antibodies to Inositol 1,4,5-Triphosphate Receptor 1 in Patients with Cerebellar Disease. *Neurol. Neuroimmunol. NeuroInflamm.* **2017**, *4*, e306. [CrossRef]
132. Saleem, H.; Tovey, S.C.; Molinski, T.F.; Taylor, C.W. Interactions of Antagonists with Subtypes of Inositol 1, 4, 5-trisphosphate (IP 3) Receptor. *Br. J. Pharmacol.* **2014**, *171*, 3298–3312. [CrossRef]
133. Gambardella, J.; Morelli, M.B.; Wang, X.; Castellanos, V.; Mone, P.; Santulli, G. The Discovery and Development of IP3 Receptor Modulators: An Update. *Expert Opin. Drug Discov.* **2021**, *16*, 709–718. [CrossRef]
134. López-Sánchez, J.I.; Moreno, D.A.; García-Viguera, C. D-Pinitol, a Highly Valuable Product from Carob Pods: Health-Promoting Effects and Metabolic Pathways of This Natural Super-Food Ingredient and Its Derivatives. *AIMS Agric. Food* **2018**, *3*, 41–63. [CrossRef]
135. Azab, A. D-Pinitol—Active Natural Product from Carob with Notable Insulin Regulation. *Nutrients* **2022**, *14*, 1453. [CrossRef] [PubMed]
136. Ma, K.; Thomason, L.A.M.; McLaurin, J.A. *Scyllo-Inositol, Preclinical, and Clinical Data for Alzheimer's Disease*; Elsevier Inc.: Amsterdam, The Netherlands, 2012; Volume 64, ISBN 9780123948168.
137. Liang, C.; Savinov, S.N.; Fejzo, J.; Eyles, S.J.; Chen, J. Modulation of Amyloid-B42 Conformation by Small Molecules through Nonspecific Binding. *J. Chem. Theory Comput.* **2019**, *15*, 5169–5174. [CrossRef] [PubMed]
138. McLaurin, J.; Franklin, T.; Chakrabartty, A.; Fraser, P.E. Phosphatidylinositol and Inositol Involvement in Alzheimer Amyloid-β Fibril Growth and Arrest. *J. Mol. Biol.* **1998**, *278*, 183–194. [CrossRef] [PubMed]
139. Henriksen, K.; Byrjalsen, I.; Christiansen, C.; Karsdal, M.A. Relationship between Serum Levels of Tau Fragments and Clinical Progression of Alzheimer's Disease. *J. Alzheimers Dis.* **2014**, *43*, 1331–1341. [CrossRef]
140. Doody, R.S.; Raman, R.; Sperling, R.A.; Seimers, E.; Sethuraman, G.; Mohs, R.; Farlow, M.; Iwatsubo, T.; Vellas, B.; Sun, X.; et al. Peripheral and Central Effects of γ-Secretase Inhibition by Semagacestat in Alzheimer's Disease. *Alzheimers Res. Ther.* **2015**, *7*, 36. [CrossRef]

MDPI AG
Grosspeteranlage 5
4052 Basel
Switzerland
Tel.: +41 61 683 77 34

Nutrients Editorial Office
E-mail: nutrients@mdpi.com
www.mdpi.com/journal/nutrients

www.ingramcontent.com/pod-product-compliance
Lightning Source LLC
Chambersburg PA
CBHW062035220926
51850CB00010B/2554
9783725871384